Augmentative and Alternative Communication: New Directions in Research and Practice

Augmentative and Alternative Communication:

New Directions in Research and Practice

EDITED BY

FILIP T. LONCKE
JOHN CLIBBENS
HELEN H. ARVIDSON
LYLE L. LLOYD

W

WHURR PUBLISHERS
LONDON

British Library Cataloguing in Publication Data
A catalogue record for this book is available from the British Library.

ISBN 1 86156 143 1

Spelling
For this book, transatlantic English spelling has been used. This includes the American -ize spelling of words such as organize, realize, maximize, etc., but also has the British -our spelling of the words colour, behaviour, etc. Program/me is slightly peculiar in that the two spellings are used to differentiate computer programs from all other types of programmes. Transatlantic spelling is intended to appeal to readers from all over the world.

The choice for transatlantic spelling is partially made to reflect the international character of the International Society for Augmentative and Alternative Communication.

Printed and bound in the UK by Athenaeum Press Ltd, Gateshead, Tyne & Wear

Contents

SECTION IV: OUTCOMES MEASUREMENT IN AAC   205

Chapter 20   207

Outcomes Measurement in AAC
Mats Granlund and Sarah Blackstone

SECTION V: FAMILY ISSUES AND AAC   229

Chapter 21   231

Moving Forward with Families: Perspectives on AAC Research
and Practice
Lynn A. Sweeney

SECTION VI: CONSUMER ISSUES AND AAC   255

Chapter 22   257

An Introduction to Consumer Perspectives in AAC Research:
Approaches, Techniques and their Theoretical Underpinnings
Ralf W. Schlosser

Chapter 23   262

Challenging Oppression: Augmented Communicators'
Involvement in AAC Research
Susan Balandin and Pammi Raghavendra

Chapter 24   278

Nothing About Me Without Me: A Proposal for Participatory
Action Research in AAC
Hank Bersani Jr

Chapter 25   290

Examining the Perspectives of Families: Issues Related to
Conducting Cross-cultural Research
Mary Blake Huer and Howard P. Parette Jr

Contributors

Santiago Aguilera-Navarro
Laboratorio de Tecnologías de Rehabilitación
ETSI de Telecomunicación
Universidad Politécnica de Madrid
Madrid
Spain
aguilera@die.upm.es

Elisabeth Ahlsén
Department of Linguistics
Göteborg University
Box 200
SE 405 30 Göteborg
Sweden
eliza@ling.gu.se

Norman Alm
Applied Computing
University of Dundee
Dundee, DD1 4HN
United Kingdom
nalm@mic.dundee.ac.uk

Helen H. Arvidson
564 N. Old State Road 2
Westville, IN 46391
USA
arvidson@purdue.edu

Susan Balandin
Centre for Developmental Disability Studies
PO Box 6
Ryde, NSW 2112
Australia
susanb@med.usyd.edu.au

Hank Bersani Jr
Oregon Institute on Disability and Development
Assistive Technology Program
Oregon Health Sciences University
PO Box 574
Portland, OR 97207-574
USA
Bersanih@ohsu.edu

Sarah W. Blackstone
Augmentative Communication, Inc.
1 Surf Way, #237
Monterey, CA 93940
USA
sarahblack@aol.com

Alice Carlberger
Department of Speech, Music and Hearing
Royal Institute of Technology
Stockholm
Sweden
alice@speech.kth.se

John Clibbens
Centre for Thinking and Language
Department of Psychology
University of Plymouth
Drake Circus
Plymouth PL4 8AA
United Kingdom
J.Clibbens@plymouth.ac.uk

Ann Copestake
Center for the Study of Language and Information (CSLI)
Ventura Hall
Stanford University
Stanford, CA 94305-4115
USA
aac@csli.stanford.edu

Portia File
School of Computing
University of Abertay Dundee
Bell Street
Dundee DD1 1HG
United Kingdom
p.file@tay.ac.uk

Dan Flickinger
Center for the Study of Language and Information (CSLI)
Ventura Hall
Stanford University
Stanford, CA 94305-4115
USA
danf@csli.stanford.edu

Juan I. Godino-Llorente
Laboratorio de Tecnologías de Rehabilitación
ETSI de Telecomunicación
Universidad Politécnica de Madrid
Madrid
Spain
godino@die.upm.es

Mats Granlund
ALA Research Foundation
Sibyllegatan 7 1 tr.
114 51 Stockholm
Sweden
mats.granlund@ala.fub.se

Nicola Grove
Centre of Clinical Communication Studies
City University
Northampton Square
London EC10 0HB
United Kingdom
N.C.Grove@city.ac.uk

Dave Hershberger
Prentke Romich Company
1022 Heyl Road
Wooster, OH 44691
USA
dhh@prentrom.com

Marianne Hickey
(formerly:)
Applied Computing
University of Dundee
Dundee, DD1 4HN
(now at:)
Hewlett-Packard Laboratories,
Filton Road
Bristol, BS12 6QZ
United Kingdom
mh@hplb.hpl.hp.com

Erland Hjelmquist
Department of Psychology
Gothenburg University
Haraldsgatan 1
S-413 14 Göteborg
Sweden
psyhjelm@pew.psy.gu.se

Mary Blake Huer
Department of Speech Communication
Program in Communicative Disorders
California State University, Fullerton
PO Box 6868
Fullerton, California 92834-6868
USA
mbhuer@fullerton.edu

Sheri Hunnicutt
Department of Speech, Music and Hearing
KTH
SE-100 44 Stockholm
Sweden
sheri@speech.kth.se

Stefan Langer
CIS, Munich University
Oettingenstr. 67
D-80538 München
Germany
stef@cis.uni-muenchen.de

Lyle L. Lloyd
Special Education and
Audiology & Speech Sciences
Purdue University
West Lafayette, IN 47907-1446
USA
lloydaac@purdue.edu

Filip T. Loncke
International Project Coordination Fracaritatis
43 Jozef Guislainstraat
9000 Gent
Belgium
ftl4n@virginia.edu

José L. Martin-Sánchez
Laboratorio de Tecnologías de Rehabilitación
ETSI de Telecomunicación
Universidad Politécnica de Madrid
Madrid
Spain
jlmartin@depeca.alcala.es

Kathleen F. McCoy
CIS Department
103 Smith Hall
University of Delaware
Newark, DE 19716
USA
mccoy@cis.udel.edu

Shirley H. McNaughton
Department of Speech-Language Pathology
Faculty of Medicine
University of Toronto
Tanz Neuroscience Building
6 Queen's Park Crescent West
Toronto, Ontario
Canada M5S 3H2
smcn@freespace.net

Gillian M. Nelms
The ACE Centre
92 Windmill Road
Headington
Oxford , OX3 7DR
United Kingdom
info@ace-centre.org.uk

Judith D. Oxley
Department of Communication Disorders
Louisiana State University Medical Center
1900 Gravier Street
New Orleans, LA 70112-2262
USA
oxley@lsumc.edu

Sira E. Palazuelos-Cagigas
Laboratorio de Tecnologías de Rehabilitación
ETSI de Telecomunicación
Universidad Politécnica de Madrid
Madrid
Spain
sira@die.upm.es

Howard P. Parette Jr
Department of Elementary, Early, and Special Education
Southeast Missouri State University
One University Plaza
Cape Girardeau, MO 63701
USA
pparette@semovm.semo.edu

Pammi Raghavendra
Communication Therapy Services
Crippled Children's Association of South Australia
PO Box 2438
Regency Park, SA 5942
Australia
mwhitela@biochem.adelaide.edu.au

José L. Rodrigo-Mateos
Universidad Complutense de Madrid
Madrid
Spain
rodrigo@die.upm.es

Ralf W. Schlosser
Department of Speech-Language Pathology and Audiology
Northeastern University
360 Huntington Avenue
151B Forsyth Building
Boston, MA 02115
USA
r.schlosser@nunet.neu.edu

Martine Smith
School of Clinical Speech & Language Studies
184 Pearse Street
Trinity College
Dublin 2
Ireland
mmsmith@mail.tcd.ie

Gloria Soto
Department of Special Education and Communication Disorders
San Francisco State University
San Francisco , CA 94132
USA
gsoto@sfsu.edu

Sven Strömqvist
Department of Linguistics
Göteborg University
Box 200
SE 405 30 Göteborg
Sweden
msven@ling.gu.se

Ann Sutton
Mackay Center
3500, Boulevard Decarie
Montreal, PQ H4A 3J5
Canada
asutton@mackayctr.org

Lynn A. Sweeney
Sweeney Communication and Consultation Services
Mt Pleasant, Michigan
USA
and
Psychology Department
Central Michigan University
Mt Pleasant, Michigan
USA
Sween1l@mail.cmich.edu

John Todman
Department of Psychology
University of Dundee
Nethergate
Dundee, DD1 4HN
United Kingdom
j.todman@dundee.ac.uk

Hans van Balkom
Institute for the Deaf (IvD)
Department of Research, Development & Support (RDS)
42 Theerestraat
5271 GD Sint-Michielsgestel
The Netherlands
h.vanbalkom@rdt.ivd.nl

Stephen von Tetzchner
Department of Psychology
University of Oslo
PO Box 1094 Blindern
N-0317 Oslo
Norway
s.v.tetzchner@psykologi.uio.no

Foreword

PRUE FULLER
ISAAC PRESIDENT

The mission of the International Society for Augmentative and Alternative Communication (ISAAC) is to improve communication and, therefore, the quality of life for individuals with severe communication disabilities throughout the world. By providing appropriate and viable communication channels, augmentative and alternative communication (AAC) makes this goal possible. In terms of research, AAC is still a young field, but one that is currently expanding rapidly throughout the international community. In the 15 years since ISAAC was founded, the study of AAC has evolved into a solid and diverse body of research which informs and guides practice in the field.

It is central to ISAAC's mission that ISAAC play a key role in providing both a forum for discussion on AAC issues and a mechanism for sharing ideas amongst researchers, clinicians, educators, AAC users, and all individuals in the community of users. One major vehicle for discussion, debate and sharing has been *Augmentative and Alternative Communication*, ISAAC's peer-reviewed journal which has influenced and furthered the field since it was first published in 1985. A CD-ROM version of all back issues provides an invaluable research tool. The high standards of the journal have guaranteed the recording of top quality research, and a fruitful forum has resulted in discussion that has been held in high esteem both inside and outside the community of individuals who have an interest in AAC. The unique work in language acquisition from the viewpoint of AAC, for example, has been of great interest to individuals involved in other disciplines.

Another important activity of ISAAC is the biennial research symposium, the only international symposium devoted to research into the psychological, social and technical mechanisms of communication and the ways in which AAC can contribute to a better quality of life for individuals with severe communication disabilities. At the 1998 research symposium in Dublin, researchers, clinicians, educators, and AAC users with special interests in research development met to discuss a variety of themes. The ISAAC research symposia are unique in that, in addition to the introduction of new AAC research themes, selected established themes are carried over from symposium to symposium creating focus and continuity for the biennial meetings. Presentations and discussions are in the form of seminars and workshops with pre- and post-symposium papers which provide a view of the state of the art in critical AAC research areas. Brainstorming between participants, prior to, during and after each symposium facilitates the identification of important issues for future research. In all papers, authors seek to analyse how specific issues fit within the larger context of understanding the nature of AAC, as well as within the broader theoretical concepts related to communication, information processing, and service delivery. Thus the outcomes of the symposia are of interest to individuals from a number of related disciplines.

For these reasons, it seems only logical that the Dublin Research Symposium and its outcomes be oriented toward a publication that will be widely accessible. This book is the result of a collaborative endeavour by participants, authors and editors to produce individually readable chapters with a collective intent that will meet the goals jointly set by ISAAC and the editors. The intent is to demonstrate the importance of critical AAC research and theory building, interest and enlighten individuals involved in related disciplines, and ultimately play a role in improving the lives of AAC users.

We at ISAAC would like to thank the European Commission TIDE office for its support for the 1998 Dublin Research Symposium. We would also like to thank everyone who contributed to making the 1998 Research Symposium such a fruitful, stimulating and productive meeting. In particular, we thank the members of the research committee, Peter Lindsay, Filip Loncke and John Clibbens; and all the section editors, Stephen von Tetzchner, Sheri Hunnicutt, Lyle Lloyd, Lynn Sweeney, Sarah Blackstone and Ralf Schlosser. We are greatly indebted to the editors of this volume, Filip Loncke, John Clibbens, Helen Arvidson and Lyle Lloyd, whose untiring energies have so greatly enriched the field of AAC research.

Prue Fuller
ISAAC President

Introduction

FILIP T. LONCKE, JOHN CLIBBENS,
HELEN H. ARVIDSON AND LYLE L. LLOYD

As a field, the study and applications of augmentative and alternative communication (AAC) lie at a crosspoint of multidisciplinary discussion. The very existence of AAC is the result of multiple developments in several domains in educational sciences, clinical psychology, speech-language pathology, engineering, speech synthesis, sociology, and psycholinguistics. One of the interesting aspects of AAC research is that it is not 'owned' by any one single discipline. *Augmentative and Alternative Communication*, the scholarly journal reporting research and developments in the field, for example, contains articles from a wide variety of professional disciplines and orientations. In addition, the biennial research symposia, exceptionally fruitful events organized by the International Society for Augmentative and Alternative Communication (ISAAC), update and balance several state of the art critical research areas within the field of AAC. It is exciting that scholars who have been developing several specific research areas have succeeded in maintaining and strengthening a common interest in AAC.

This book is based on the presentations and discussions held at the 1998 ISAAC Research Symposium in Dublin, Ireland, August 28–29. The previous research meeting, held in Vancouver, Canada in August 1996, led to the publication of *Communication...Naturally: Theoretical and Methodological Issues in Augmentative and Alternative Communication*, a book of proceedings edited by Björk-Åkesson and Lindsay (1998), acclaimed to be extremely useful in guiding the course of research as well as in orienting clinical and educational aspects of AAC. It was felt during the early planning stages of the Dublin Research Symposium that the momentum of the meeting could be a major springboard into a process leading to a new high-quality roundup of the status of research within

AAC. Publishing a book with a research perspective could be an effective means to keep symposium presenters and participants focused on defining the essentials in current AAC research and examining ways that might contribute to a better general understanding of processes related to AAC use and implementation. Most of the presenters and several of the participants are the authors and co-authors of this book. All authors have been encouraged to include discussion matters and ideas that were raised during the sessions. In fact, many unnamed participants have been directly or indirectly providing ideas and guidelines for the chapters.

This book is organized around six sections, reflecting the themes that were discussed in parallel during the research symposium. For each theme, a theme leader, presenter(s), and participants worked out their own method of discussion and exchange of ideas. This is reflected in the way the book is structured. Each section (Language Development, Natural Language Processing, Graphic Symbol Use, Outcomes Measurement in AAC, Family Issues and AAC, and Consumer Issues and AAC) corresponds with a theme discussed during the symposium. The organizers of the symposium and the editors of this book do not want to suggest that these themes are the main categories of AAC research. Without pretending to be exhaustive, other major themes critical to AAC research are literacy development, theory building, ageing, unaided communication (including the use of gestures and manual signs) and telecommunications. The reader will notice that while these themes are not presented as whole sections, they are indeed discussed, sometimes in more than one section. Gestural and manual communication, for example, are important elements in both the Language Development and Graphic Symbol Use sections. Section editors and authors have been encouraged to cross-reference to increase the internal consistency of the book.

A main consideration in the field of AAC should be to preserve communication between subareas of research within a broad context. The balance between analytically investigating specific, essential subareas and keeping sight of the big picture has proven to be extremely useful. It is a priority that AAC research continues to delve into specific areas of interest while maintaining connections with broader fields of discipline such as communication research, psycholinguistics and service delivery. It is hoped that the present book responds to this challenge.

Section I
Language Development

Chapter 1
Introduction to Language Development

STEPHEN VON TETZCHNER

The present section is concerned with alternative communication systems within a developmental framework. Its main foci are descriptions of developmental paths of spoken language and non-vocal communication systems, the processes underlying these paths, the untangling of influences of spoken language and various other factors, and explanations of why alternative communication systems may be acquired when speech fails to develop. The chapters specifically address how representations of alternative forms of communication are formed; how different modes and modalities are applied; the construction of grammar; and the implications new theoretical models and empirical evidence may have for intervention practice. The last chapter in the section discusses a number of issues that were brought up by the participants during the symposium presentations. This introduction clarifies some issues related to terminology and constitutes a prologue to the developmental issues discussed in the section.

Terminology

Descriptions of development within a particular domain depend on availability of appropriate terms. As augmentative and alternative communication develops as a theoretical and empirical field, traditional and new conceptual distinctions become more pertinent, and with them a need for a more refined terminology. However, it is not evident how language acquisition involving alternative communication systems is best described. The differences related to the various modes may mainly be related to form, while the symbolic function that constitutes language is essentially independent of the mode(s) applied. On the other hand, form may influence pragmatic and grammatical function and hence create a need for new terminology in these areas.

One terminology issue concerns the use of 'sign' and 'symbol'. In the literature on augmentative and alternative communication, it has been usual to call manual signs 'signs' and graphic representations 'symbols' (and vocal and orthographically written utterances 'words'), in spite of the fact that they are both used symbolically for communicative purposes. In the present section, in order to distinguish the various forms of expression and avoid attributing symbolic function to only one of them, 'sign' is used as a generic term for all modes of communication, with mode added, such as manual signs, graphic signs and tangible signs. (Spoken words are vocal signs.)

It is important to distinguish between mode and sensory modality. With the exception of tangible signs and manual signs used in a deaf–blind mode (where the sender leads the receiver's hands through the signs), most alternative communication systems are based on vision. There are thus several, quite different systems whose signs are perceived visually and thus belong to this modality. However, productively they differ in the use of movement: manual signs require complex hand movements, while graphic signs require pointing or another form of indicating with or without the help of switches and other technical aids.

Both normally speaking children and children who use alternative communication systems usually employ several modes of communication. Normally developing children typically use pointing and other deictic gestures before they start to speak, and gestures continue to fulfil various communicative functions throughout life. It is debatable whether gestures should be considered part of the linguistic system, but in any case, it is necessary to distinguish between the development of language (vocal and non-vocal) and diverse non-verbal forms of communication. This is also true for hearing intellectually impaired children who develop manual signs (which are verbal but not vocal), and where this distinction may appear blurred. Similarly, pointing (with the hand, eye, etc.) and other ways of indicating are essential for productive language with graphic signs. In descriptions of aided language, it is often said that children point to a particular graphic sign on the communication aid, implying that the indication is not part of the linguistic production. However, like articulation of speech and sign, the indicating 'gesture' uses part of the cognitive resources in graphic production. Moreover, the use of pointing as part of graphic sign production should be distinguished from the traditional pointing gesture that may be used in isolation or to accompany verbal language forms, in the same way as pointing is distinguished from the formal use of the pointing movement in the execution of a manual sign.

Finally, the expression augmentative and alternative communication, or rather the acronym AAC, is often used in unreflective ways (usually referring to aided communication). Children do not develop augmentative and alternative communication, but learn to comprehend and use alternative (i.e. non-speech) communication systems to substitute or augment spoken language. A particular child may develop one or several manual, graphic and/or tangible modes of communication, and their functions may differ as the child grows older. For the individual, some systems may be used more in early phases of development, others at more advanced stages. Some children eventually acquire a good mastery of spoken language and stop using the alternative system that augmented speech in the early phases of their development. In descriptions of language acquisition involving the use of alternative communication systems, it is important that the actual modes of communication applied are specified, including comprehension and use of spoken language. In order to be specific and clear, one should restrict the use of global terms.

Developmental processes and intervention

The acquisition of alternative language systems implies the learning of one or several modes of communication that replace or supplement the comprehension and use of spoken language. The systems may function as a linguistic system to a greater or lesser degree, and as in the normal acquisition of spoken language, there is a gradual change in complexity and function, from a mainly non-verbal mode (vocalizations, gestures and pointing at, for example, objects and pictures) to a mainly verbal mode (manual, graphic and tangible signs and speech). This implies that the linguistic, communicative and cognitive processes underlying the development of alternative language forms may both differ and share qualities with typical language development.

The emergent characteristics of children who need an alternative language system are therefore likely to differ in important ways from those of children who learn to speak normally, although both groups show significant within-group variation. The communication mode itself implies the use of different motor and cognitive strategies, as well as linguistic and communicative skills and strategies. Different constraints and possibilities may apply. For example, the cognitive resources needed for using a communication aid to construct an intended message may differ from those needed for speaking and signing. Also the life-worlds of normal speakers and aided speakers differ in the sense that their experiences and possibilities and abilities to direct other people's attention and be directed by other people differ.

There is one particular characteristic that distinguishes the development of alternative language systems from spoken language development. For children growing up with manual, graphic or tangible signs as their main form of communication, development is a planned rather than a 'natural' course, where the scaffolding properties of the language environment depend on communicative acts and the explicit beliefs and strategic acts of professionals and other people in the environment. Discussion on

augmentative and alternative communication is dominated by intervention issues, and within this field, studies based on a language development
framework may actually be regarded as basic research. The chapters in the
present section attempt to raise questions that are critical for understanding the developmental process. They address issues related to
descriptions of developmental courses of spoken language and different
non-speech communication systems, the processes underlying these
courses, the untangling of the influence of various factors, and explanations of why alternative communication systems may be acquired when
speech development is not.

An important issue is the until now limited empirical material about
typical and atypical developmental paths of language development
involving alternative language systems. It is not possible with any degree
of certainty to predict the acquisition of alternative language forms on the
basis of existing knowledge. The history and language background of non-
speaking adults, including the intervention provided to them at different
periods, is rarely known. There is a dearth of descriptions of developments that extend over a year or two. The transactional processes underlying intervention and development are simply not known: on the one
hand, it is a planned course; on the other, a fuzzy process characterized by
ad hoc strategies and a lack of clearly defined milestones. Moreover, the
forms provided to children acquiring graphic language competence tend
to remain static and leave little room for the child to change them or vary
the expression in a creative manner. Even the end point, competent and
mature adult functioning, is obscure.

The fact the chapters in this section are concerned with the developmental processes underlying the acquisition of alternative communication
modes does not mean that intervention is not included in the discussion.
On the contrary, it is the implicit and explicit assumptions of professionals
about language and the language acquisition process that are the bases of
innovation and determine their choice of intervention strategies. There
may in fact be constraints on intervention – and thereby acquisition –
caused by prejudices and inappropriate conceptual and theoretical understanding of development. Nevertheless, the basic premise of all language
intervention is that it is possible to influence the acquisition of language
and communication skills through environmental adaptations. The
essence of language intervention is a systematic restructuring of the
environment in such a manner that the way it interacts with the
individual's developmental realization (the result of earlier interactions
between organism and environment) is changed. This applies to all
language intervention and should not be confounded with 'milieu
teaching'. Intervention represents an induced change in the language
environment, whether it takes the form of isolated training or consists of
introducing more global changes of the natural environment. It follows
that all forms of intervention with children can only be understood from a

truly developmental perspective, where all influences are taken into account. The chapters in this section thus have a double objective: to increase knowledge about the acquisition process and to use this knowledge to change the process through intervention measures when this seems to be needed.

Chapter 2
The Bimodal Situation of Children Learning Language Using Manual and Graphic Signs

MARTINE SMITH AND NICOLA GROVE

The bimodal situation of children learning language using alternative communication systems has been described as unique in many respects, not least of which is the frequently asymmetrical organization of modes of communication across input and output, with speech the dominant input mode, and manual or graphic signs the dominant output required (Grove and Smith, 1997). Whilst typical communication involves harnessing several modes of expression, early communication development is characterized by changes in intra- and intermodal organization, usually with one mode taking on the burden of linguistic communication. Children apparently manage to separate out communicative gestures from multilayered linguistic organization with remarkable consistency, even when both occur within the same mode (Petitto, 1993).

Clearly, not all communication needs evidence linguistic, or more specifically, morphosyntactic organization. Locke (1995) distinguishes between a specialization in social cognition, which allows children to achieve a working vocabulary without an elaborated linguistic system, and a grammatical analysis module, an analytical, computational system, dealing in rules and representations. In a somewhat similar vein, many authors have made reference to distinctions between two cooperative processes at work in language acquisition – a strategy of reproducing what are variously termed 'rote', 'frozen' or 'unanalysed' forms and a subsequent process of analysis and revision of such forms, whether in spoken (e.g. Bates, Bretherton and Snyder, 1988; Karmiloff-Smith, 1992; Lieven, Pine and Baldwin, 1997; Pine and Lieven, 1993) or signed language acquisition (Reilly, McIntire and Bellugi, 1990). A strict dichotomy between 'gestalt' and 'analytic' strategies is somewhat simplistic, in that the extraction of a single phrase from a conversational context requires analysis in itself and it is not at all clear that the distinction reflects two autonomous strategies. However, the principle of a dual orientation towards wholes and parts seems to fit well with much of the data on early child language. It is the latter focus on analysis of component elements which is frequently regarded as pivotal to linguistic development, reflecting the engagement of, in Locke's (1995) terms, a grammatical analysis module, or the operation of Petitto's (1993) structure-seeking mechanism, typically referred to as the 'language acquisition device'.

Both Locke's grammatical analysis module and Petitto's structure-seeking mechanism are regarded as being 'blind to modality' (Petitto, 1993) in the sense that they are not constrained in their operation to a single modality. Children acquiring language using alternative modes of communication therefore potentially have available to them two complementary strategies which can be applied across multiple modes. What seems likely is that at least one of the modes must have available to it data which have the potential for segmentation and recombination, given that such combinatorial potential of structure is a universal feature of natural languages. Alternative modes of communication offered to people with communication disorders differ in their potential for such linguistic organization (Grove and Smith, 1997; Smith and Grove, 1996).

Thus, individuals learning language using alternative modes must juggle not only the asymmetries inherent in the intermodal relationships across input and output situations, but must also deal with the challenge of combining modes of communication which may differ fundamentally from each other. The focus in this chapter is on the juggling act itself and possible changes in juggling skill over time. The interrelationship between speech and manual or graphic signs is discussed with reference to three different groups: two children with cerebral palsy, who use Picture Communication Symbols (PCS)-based communication boards; six children with moderate intellectual impairments, using manual signs in conjunction with speech; and four typically-developing pre-school children using PCS. The initial focus is on the interpretation of graphic signs provided as input; we then look at the use of manual and graphic modes for output.

Bimodal situations

A bimodal situation means the harnessing of more than one modality for the purposes of communication. However, relationships across modes can be very complex. Loncke, Vander Beken and Lloyd (1998) distinguish between two types of multimodality. 'Parallel multimodality' refers to the typical speech + gesture situation, where speech is accompanied by multiple modes of communication in the expression of a message. 'Recoded multimodality' refers to the reformulation of a message from one mode into another. Such recoding may typically be interpreted as a recoding from speech to an alternative mode, although where manual or graphic sign use is in advance of spoken language skills, presumably recoding may also occur in the other direction (von Tetzchner et al., 1998). A third possibility also exists, that is the formulation of a message within the non-speech alternative mode without any recoding. All three types of multimodality may be available to, and used by, individuals using manual and graphic signs. Identifying the network of complex relationships for each individual may be extraordinarily difficult.

Most children learning language using alternative means, as referred to in this chapter, are exposed to speech as their dominant input, but must encode their expressive output in a different mode. Thus the term 'bimodal situation' may refer to a uniquely asymmetrical language learning context for many such children. As a further complication, it must be noted that the mere presence of more than one mode of input or output does not guarantee that individuals will necessarily avail themselves of the opportunity to use them.

For example, von Tetzchner and Martinsen's (1992) alternative language group may not be able to make effective use of spoken input, even if it is, from the point of view of the interaction partner, the primary input mode. Finally, it is important to note in discussing all these issues that a further gap in our knowledge is the role of input itself, and the relationship between input, the problem space created by the child, and the processing mechanisms brought to bear on that problem space to determine uptake (Harris, 1992; Snow, 1995).

Identifying a bimodal situation

One can artificially create the need to use manual or graphic signs, or their use may be necessitated by factors intrinsic to the individual – specific disabilities which preclude the use of speech. However, is the mere presence of a non-speech mode within a communication interaction sufficient to justify terming the communication context bimodal, or is there a sense in which the term refers to a set of relationships, a complex system, rather than to a single feature such as a communication board or a manual sign? Is the concept of a homogeneous bimodal situation useful? Should one more appropriately be exploring whether each individual using manual and graphic signs develops his or her own bimodal context, reflecting the developments in intermodal relationships occurring within that individual's communication system (Heim and Baker-Mills, 1996; Smith, 1996a)?

In other words, as a child develops particular skills within a mode, does this affect the overall organization of communication across modes? In exploring some of the above questions, we look first at the ability of children to process messages presented in either speech or PCS; we then look at the messages produced by children using PCS, manual signs and speech, and how the structuring of those messages across modes changed over time and across contexts.

One of the tools used in gathering some of the data reported here is a picture task, devised for the purposes of contrasting comprehension of messages presented in speech and in PCS and for contrasting comprehension of PCS-encoded messages and the construction of PCS messages expressively. The picture test presents a series of plates of either three or four pictures. The subjects (a group of four typically-developing pre-school children and a second group of two children with cerebral palsy) were required to identify a stimulus picture on the basis of either a spoken or a PCS description (see Tables 2.1 and 2.2 for subject descriptions). The typically-developing pre-school children were introduced to PCS during weekly sessions over a 10-week period. The focus of intervention was on introducing the concept of using PCS to communicate with a bird puppet who could not hear, establishing PCS-referent links, encouraging communication board use and gradually increasing utterance length (see Smith, 1996b for a more complete description).

Table 2.1. Age and language scores of typically-developing pre-school children

Subject	Chronological age	Information score: age equivalent	Grammar score: age equivalent
Oisin	3 years 7 months	3;6–3;11	4;6–4;11
Natalie	4 years 2 months	8;0–8;5	8;0–8;5
Olwen	4 years 3 months	5;6–5;11	5;6–5;11
James	4 years 7 months	6;0–6;5	6;0–6;5

Speech was by far the most familiar mode of communication for all subjects, at least in input. Therefore one might predict higher accuracy on test items where the picture description was spoken, rather than presented in PCS, and further that those individuals who were highly familiar with PCS (i.e. Laura and Yvonne) would find the processing of messages presented in PCS easier than their speaking pre-school peers, who had only limited exposure to PCS. The first prediction was fulfilled in that on the whole, the children were most likely to identify pictures correctly when the description was spoken for them. However, in processing PCS input, two patterns emerged (see Figure 2.1). Three of the four pre-schoolers had comparable scores regardless of whether the picture description was spoken or presented in PCS. By contrast, Natalie and the two PCS users did very poorly on the latter task.

In exploring possible explanations for the discrepancy in performance across the contexts, it was noted that, when presented with a message encoded in PCS, James, Olwen and Oisin typically verbalized the description, effectively recoding it into speech. By contrast, Natalie rarely vocalized during this task. Instead, she seemed to concentrate on using PCS. It seems likely that the task of decoding a message presented in PCS may be accomplished via at least two different processing routes, one involving recoding into speech, the other essentially unimodal (Figure 2.2).

Table 2.2. Summary of information on PCS users

Name	Yvonne	Laura
Chronological age (CA) through study	5;0–7;0	4;6–6;8
Psychological assessment	Average (Leiter, sections of WISC-R)	Average (Leiter, sections of WISC-R)
Communication board	PCS, 200+ at start of study	PCS, 200+ at start of study
Physical accessing of board	Direct finger pointing, though often unclear	Direct finger pointing; rarely ambiguous
Receptive language	Within normal limits (SLT report)	Within normal limits (SLT report)
Speech production ability	Primarily reflexive vocalization; no functional speech	Generally intelligible to mother; unintelligible to others without considerable contextual support
Educational placement	Local mainstream school, no special supports	Local mainstream school, no special supports
Speech and language therapy input	Monthly therapy with local therapist; consultation with specialist centre; focus on developing sentence structure	Regular (monthly) therapy with local therapist; consultation with specialist centre; focus on increasing use of PCS
Test of Reception of Grammar (Bishop, 1982)	CA 5;1: LA 4;06: %ile 25 CA 6;11: LA 8;00: %ile 50–75	CA 4;7: LA 5;3: %ile 50–75 CA 6;7: LA 8;0: %ile 50–75

WISC-R, Wechsler Intelligence Scale for Children - Revised; SLT, speech and language therapist; LA, language age.

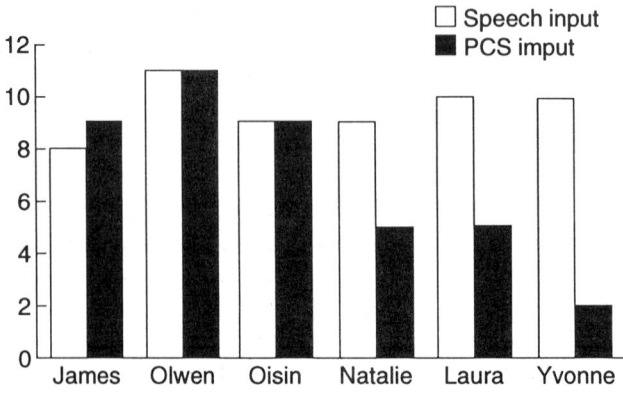

Figure 2.1. Performance on tasks using spoken description and PCS description.

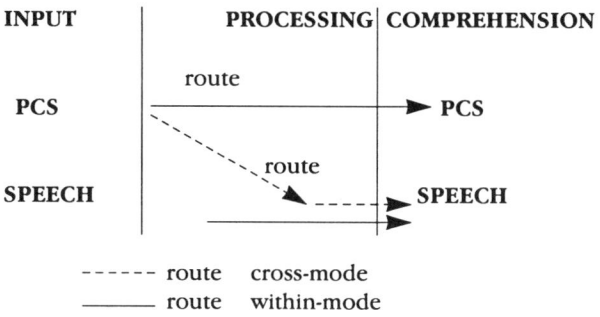

Figure 2.2. Possible processing routes.

The first strategy is that presumed to be used by most of the speaking children – unit-by-unit translation to speech, with the spoken utterance then processed as a whole to identify the target picture – analogous to Romski and Sevcik's (1996) cross-modal processing. This route may be supported by overt verbal rehearsal.

The second strategy might be viewed as essentially unimodal or intramodal – the message presented is processed as PCS, without direct reference to a spoken language model. Indicators suggesting operation of the latter strategy might include a lack of overt vocalization during PCS tasks, or a contrast in performance across spoken-PCS conditions – the features of Natalie's performance. There may of course be other explanations of the profiles of performance. For example, although Laura frequently audibly rehearsed/translated the PCS to speech, she nonetheless did just as poorly as Yvonne and Natalie in identifying a picture based on a PCS description. What might account for her performance?

One possibility is that Laura may be more vulnerable to the loading of the additional step of 'translation', due to a number of factors such as physical effort, or articulatory demands. Her strategy may be similar to that of the speaking children, in that she translates the PCS to speech, with the subsequent utterance processed as a spoken, rather than a PCS utterance. However, the pre-school children, by virtue of their learning experiences with PCS, may have had considerably more experience in working directly with tasks involving speech-PCS recoding. In many instances during intervention, they produced spoken messages and were then supported in recoding the messages into PCS so that the 'bird' could understand. For Laura, the extra effort of translation and retaining in memory either the unfamiliar visual sequence of PCS, or the recoded utterance may militate against accurate performance. A second possibility is that her familiarity with PCS is in fact working against her, in that it is biasing her away from a clear selection of either strategy (intramodal or cross-modal) so that there is, in a sense, 'interference' across the strategies.

A third factor which may affect a preference for within-mode or cross-modal processing may relate to individual preferences (Barnes, personal communication, 1998). Natalie, for instance, may view the task as one of working either with PCS or with speech. It is possible that, unlike speech or manual signs, graphic signs such as PCS cannot be visually 'rehearsed', adding to both memory demands and task complexity, if one opts to pursue the within-mode processing route (von Tetzchner, personal communication, 1998).

In all of the above explanations, in essence the point is that what looks on the surface like the same task may well be tackled in very different ways. The nature of the bimodal context is influenced not only by the modes introduced, but also by the experience and expertise of the individuals involved in that context. Individuals who have experience with 'recoding', or those for whom this has been a focus in intervention may learn to a certain extent to resolve the input–output asymmetry by referring always to a single code and effectively restoring symmetry through recoding non-speech input into speech. Other individuals may not use this strategy either regularly or effectively. The question of intermodal relationships is perhaps even more critical in considering output tasks. Observations of individuals who use manual signs as an alternative to speech, or to augment speech, offer another source of evidence when considering variation in processing style. Smith and Grove (1996) provide examples which illustrate a remarkable similarity in patterns of output between users of graphic and manual signs. These similarities include a slow transition to multi-sign utterances, and word order differing from that of the spoken input. In the next section we explore graphic and manual sign use separately initially, and then consider similarities across both contexts.

Graphic output: PCS within a multimodal context

Laura and Yvonne, the two PCS users, were similar in many respects, one important difference being their speech production abilities. Yvonne's vocalizations were extremely limited; Laura could produce speech which was intelligible to her mother for much of the time, and which could be understood by unfamiliars given considerable contextual support. Both were exposed to speech as input, and had similar experience with using PCS for expressive communication. However, over the period of observation considerable differences in their use of PCS emerged.

From the initial contact with Laura at 4;6 years, she was a 'reluctant' PCS user and tended to rely on speech. Initially, her PCS messages were predominantly single-sign selections. Yvonne had very little speech and her PCS output was initially similar to Laura's. In the first visit, she produced 28 PCS messages with her mother as her primary communication partner. Only one utterance contained more than a single PCS (PUT WET), yielding a mean length of utterance (MLU) of 1.03. From these initially similar profiles, the developments for both users over the subsequent two years were in many respects apparently quite different.

Yvonne's PCS output very gradually increased in quantity and complexity. During her final visit, she produced 34 PCS utterances, of which 26 (76%) were single signs. She produced 6 two-sign utterances, and 1 three- and 1 four-sign utterance. Such utterances included: SPOON CUP (glossed as put the spoon in the cup); DRINK DOLL (describing a picture of a doll drinking); I LOOK I VIDEO (relating that she had seen a clip of herself from an earlier video).

Laura's development over the two years reflects not so much changes in PCS, but rather in the intermodal organization of speech and PCS. She produced remarkably few PCS utterances in the early visits, and these tended to be produced without speech. On later visits, not only were more PCS utterances produced, but they were far more likely to be produced in addition to speech, and were likely to be longer than the early unimodal PCS utterances, with one 7-sign utterance recorded, and an overall PCS MLU of 2.0.

Table 2.3. Laura: comparison of proportion of utterances based on PCS alone or in combination with speech, and length of utterances produced using PCS alone and in combination with speech

	No. of PCS utterances	No. of PCS + speech utterances	Length of utterance	No. in PCS utterances	No. in PCS + speech utterances
Visit 1	2	0	1-PCS	14	9 (33.3%)
Visit 3	2	1	2-PCS	1	7 (26%)
Visit 4	6	7	3-PCS		6 (22.2%)
Visit 5	1	6	5-PCS		4 (14.8%)
Visit 6	4	13	7-PCS		1 (3.7%)

In Laura's multimodal output, the relationship of the selected PCS to a spoken message varied. Utterances which were produced using only PCS tended to consist primarily of 'substantive' PCS, such as: BOAT DRINK (referring to a play activity with a boat which squirted water); GUN; HOUSE; TRAIN; SHEEP; STOP; CAR; THREE. In fact, of the 15 utterances she produced using PCS alone, 14 consisted of items selected from the people/object and action sections of her chart, and the other item (THE) almost certainly represents a false start on a succeeding utterance which combined speech with PCS, and which was initiated using {THE: the}.

In other utterances, PCS were used in combination with speech. These utterances were categorized into three groups based on information distribution across modes. Utterances where the complete message was produced in one modality (whether sign or speech), and elements were produced in another modality were categorized as supplementary use of speech or sign. Where an exact match occurred between speech and sign, utterances were categorized as redundant. (Due to Laura's poor speech intelligibility when speaking to unfamiliar listeners, it is difficult to classify any of her PCS output as redundant.) Finally, where information was shared across modes, so that the full message could only be understood by reference to both modes, utterances were categorized as evidencing complementary use of speech and sign. These patterns have also been found in the communication of hearing and deaf children using sign and speech (de Villiers, Bibeau, Ramos and Gatty, 1993; Mills, van den Bogaerde and Coerts, 1994) and thus appear to be highly robust features of multimodal communication.

Supplementary PCS messages

Some of Laura's utterances (11 in total) were classified as 'telegraphic', in that the PCS represented the substantive words within the spoken utterance, resembling Radford's (1990; p. 3) description of telegraphic speech with 'non-essential constituents' omitted. Examples include:

1. {I: I} went on a {BUS: bus}
2. I {I} will {WILL} {GO: go} {TO: to } my MINISTER MOTHER FATHER
3. the {MAN: man} {IS: is} standing ON {THE: the} {HORSE: horse}
4. the {TEDDY} holding the {DOLL: dolly}
5. the {MOTHER} holding the teddy TEDDY
6. mammy /unintelligible / IN the THE /unint./ SIOPA.

The group of utterances above contrasts with instances where the PCS component of a message was reduced relative to the spoken message, but where the elements selected in PCS were not substantives, and could not be interpreted as adding necessary information. Examples include the following:

7. THE {CAR: car} {IS: is } {IN: in} {THE: the} box
8. the car {IS: is} {ON: on} {THE: the} road
9. {I: I } {BREAK: break} {THE: the} door
10. the car {ON: on} {THE: the} road
11. sleeping SLEEP {ON: on} {THE: the} bed.

In some instances, failure to select a PCS for a particular lexical item might reflect constraints of the communication board (e.g., BOX was not available in 7 above).

However, in other instances (CAR in 8, 10; DOOR in 9; BED in 11) the relevant PCS were available and had been used previously in other utterances. Laura's motivation in selecting PCS for relatively unimportant elements of the message and omitting symbols for other more semantically important items is unclear. Given that she was able to access her PCS directly, considerations of physical effort are insufficient. Constraints on

PCS utterance length also fail to explain a selection of ON and THE and not BED, when other utterances included as many as seven PCS.

Redundancy

In a further group of utterances, the information communicated in speech matched almost exactly that produced in PCS. These utterances included some examples where it is hard to avoid the impression that Laura is very consciously 'translating' her spoken message into PCS, as she searches for PCS during the message formulation.

12. {HAPPY: happy}
13. THE – where girl – GIRL {ON: on} A {THE: no, the} {CHAIR: chair}
14. THE {GIRL: girl} where sit – sit down – SIT {UNDER: down} {DOWN: down} ON {THE: the} {TABLE: table}

In utterances 13 and 14 above, Laura pays particular attention to formulating an utterance in PCS which matches the correct syntactic form for a spoken utterance, searching for items on her chart, correcting the selection of the determiner A in favour of the more appropriate THE, and behaving much as any speaking adult might if asked to communicate using PCS.

Complementarity

A final small group of three utterances consisted of complementary information shared across both modalities.

15. {HOUSE: a black} retelling a story of a black house
16. {CAR: the man} describing a picture of a man in a car
17. {GO: go} {TO: to} {BED: there}

The last example is not entirely congruent with the definition of complementary as given above, but nonetheless suggests that information in both modalities needs attention if the message is to be interpreted correctly.

In summary, Laura's PCS utterances are reduced relative to her spoken output, with shorter utterances which are structurally less complex. In some instances they are produced without any speech, typically in single-sign utterances with a heavy reliance on common nouns, suggestive of a lexical-conceptual dominance. When PCS are used in combination with speech, there is evidence to suggest grammatically-based organization. PCS may augment the spoken message in varying ways, highlighting key semantic elements of a message (resulting in 'telegraphic' PCS utterances), or partially augmenting a message, with relatively less important items selected in PCS. In yet other utterances, Laura seems to be attempting to recode a spoken utterance into PCS, in much the same way as any speaking adult might, faced with a similar task. Finally, in a small number of utterances, complementary information is communicated in speech and PCS, both modes contributing substantively to the message.

A comparison of output from Yvonne and Laura

The bimodal situation for Yvonne and Laura appears similar in many respects. Nonetheless, at first glance their use of PCS looks very different. Laura produced many different types of PCS utterances, even within a very small corpus, with an MLU of 2.0 and an upper boundary of seven signs, suggesting an integration of lexical and grammatical systems, or the coming on stream of Locke's (1995) grammatical analysis module. Yvonne's PCS MLU was only 1.23, with an upper boundary of four signs, more suggestive of lexical system dominance. There is evidence of lexical and functional categories in Laura's PCS output, whilst only lexical categories can be attested in Yvonne's data, allowing for the possibility that her output is dominated by Locke's specialized social cognition system. And yet a small subset of Laura's PCS utterances were similar to Yvonne's. They were produced without speech.

Fourteen of these 15 messages (93%) were single-sign utterances, and referred almost exclusively to objects or people within her environment. Yvonne's PCS utterances were produced without speech and 177 of 206 (85%) were single-sign utterances, but were distributed across all the lexical categories available on her chart. Laura's single-mode use of PCS decreased over the course of observation, so that by the final visit PCS were three times as likely to be produced in combination with speech as they were to be produced unimodally, so that the pattern of combining modes changed over time. The next section concerns multimodal relationships with manual signs and speech.

Bimodality and manual signs

In exploring the use of manual signs by individuals with learning difficulties, Grove studied 10 hearing children with moderate intellectual impairments, six of whom had some intelligible speech, but all of whom appeared to rely on manual signs as their main means of communication (Grove, 1995; Grove, Dockrell and Woll, 1996). Data were collected from three contexts: picture description (a set of pictures depicting transitive verbs, attributes and locative relationships), a five minute conversation with a teacher, and up to two minutes of recall of a story from a silent video narrative of actions depicting contrasts in the size and shape of objects, facial expressions and locative relationships. The input to all the children by teachers and parents was predominantly spoken, with a relatively low sign density (typically one sign per clausal unit, if signs were used at all). Thus it would be predicted that, since the children could hear and understand spoken language, word order would follow the pattern of the spoken input, and that since the children had received no input from native signers, they would be unlikely to use any of the visuospatial features characteristic of sign languages.

Mode dominance: sign and speech

A measure of sign dependence was determined for each participant, by calculating the proportion of intelligible utterances which were expressed in the manual mode (total of intelligible signs/total intelligible signs + intelligible spoken words). Subjects with a score of 0.6 or over may be regarded as sign dependent, since only 40% of their output is intelligible in speech. Table 2.4 shows that four of the children had virtually no functional speech. Three others were sign dependent, and another two used signs and words in about equal proportions. Using the groupings suggested by von Tetzchner and Martinsen (1992), this measure suggests that seven children could be regarded as expressive users of sign, and three as augmentative users. However, mode dependence varied considerably among the subjects, confirming the need to be cautious in treating disparate individuals as groups.

Table 2.4. Sign dependence in the output of hearing children with intellectual impairments

	Total signs	Total words	Sign dependence
Adam	108	1	0.99
Michael	36	1	0.97
Jonathan	74	3	0.96
Louise	61	9	0.87
Ana	54	25	0.68
Mark	43	26	0.62
Amita	123	79	0.61
Jayesh	138	113	0.55
Bina	54	50	0.52
Pardeep	69	99	0.41

This functional measure of intelligibility conflates speaker and listener variables, and may be misleading when it comes to determining the underlying strategies used for processing. This is because the number of unintelligible vocalizations produced by the children greatly exceeded the number of intelligible spoken words. To make inferences about processing, one probably needs to transcribe and analyse data in far more detail than has been common practice to date in the field of augmentative and alternative communication.

When the relationship between sign and speech production was explored in more detail, identical patterns were found to those produced by the PCS users: one modality alone (sign or speech); supplementary use of sign or speech; redundant messages; and complementary messages (information shared across modes).

Bimodality and context: Pardeep

Of the ten individuals discussed above, Pardeep showed the lowest dependence on sign, and it was clear that although she still used sign to a considerable extent, she was developing beyond MLU Stage I (Brown, 1973) in spoken language. Pardeep was a 15-year-old girl of Punjabi origin, with a mental age of 4;6 obtained on the *Snijders–Oomen Scale of Nonverbal Intelligence* (Snijders and Snijders-Oomen, 1976). Although English was not her first language, she spoke it consistently at school, paired with sign, and there was no evidence of interference from Punjabi. On the *Derbyshire Language Scales* (Knowles and Masidlover, 1982), her understanding of receptive language was assessed by her speech and language therapist as 'five or more information-carrying words'. Her data show evidence of phrase structure (e.g. *my little baby, bite it, at home*) and word level morphology (e.g. *pulling, pulled*). However, her sign dependence score of 0.41 masks critical differences between contexts. In fact, when mode dependence was calculated separately by task, it was found to be 0.31 in conversation, and 0.56 in story recall. Other measures, shown in Tables 2.5–2.8, confirm that signs are used more extensively in the story task.

Table 2.5 shows the extent of lexical overlap by context: the number of word or sign types produced in each mode alone, and in both modes. In conversation, the majority of lexical types are produced in speech alone, or sign and speech. This pattern is reversed in the story recall. Two measures of utterance length are shown in Tables 2.6 and 2.7. For the purpose of this study, an utterance was equated with a conversation turn.

Table 2.5. Lexical overlap for Pardeep in two contexts: proportion of types represented in each modality (raw frequencies)

Context	Speech only	Sign + speech	Sign only
Conversation	0.58 (23)	0.38 (15)	0.05 (2)
Story recall	0.14 (3)	0.52 (11)	0.33 (7)

Table 2.6. Length of utterance (manual signs or words) for Pardeep in two contexts

	No. of words per utterance				No. of signs per utterance			
Context	1	2	3	4+	1	2	3	4+
Conversation	22	10	2	4	23	2	1	1
Story recall	6	6	2	3	2	2	0	7

Table 2.7. Mean length utterance (morphemes) for Pardeep in two contexts

Context	MLU-Words	MLU-Signs
Conversation	2.03	1.32
Story recall	2.22	4.60

The number of signs and words per utterance is a conservative measure. Table 2.5 indicates that Pardeep's utterance length in speech did not change much between contexts: she produced multi-word utterances in both. However, her use of sign differed dramatically. In conversation she was mainly using single signs, whereas in the story recall, 9 of her 11 signed utterances were multi-term. A richer interpretation of Pardeep's communication was used to calculate MLU. Her spoken utterances were sometimes hard to decipher exactly, but the syllable structure often indicated an inflection on the verb. In the story recall, she changed the handshape of GIVE from a flat hand (the citation form) to a bunched hand, indicating that something small (a sweet) was given, GIVE-SMALL. She also produced RUN with intensity, indicating a meaning of 'run-fast'. In sign language, these would be examples of verb morphology and would be counted towards utterance length. Table 2.6 shows Pardeep's MLU score in sign and speech by context. Again, MLU for speech remains fairly consistent, but MLU for sign increases in the story recall context.

Finally, Table 2.8 shows the different patterns of distribution of meaning across modality by context. In conversation, Pardeep seems to be recoding key content words into sign. She never uses sign without speech, produces several utterances in speech alone, and her supplementary utterances are always more complete in the spoken than in the sign modality. Signs are produced singly, and the prosodic carrier in the output is vocal. By contrast, in story recall Pardeep is clearly drawing on both modes simultaneously to communicate more complex meanings. Her longest utterances are strings of signs accompanied by speech. A high proportion of utterances show complementary distribution and it is only in this context that she shows some use of specific gestural morphology. Speech output is characterized by single words and short phrases, with very little elaboration of clausal and phrasal structure. Although she consistently ordered information so that subjects preceded verbs, there was one example of an object preceding the verb, rather than following it (*cake eat*).

Table 2.8. Distribution of semantic content for Pardeep in two contexts

	One modality		Supplementary		Redundant	Complementary
	Speech	Sign	Speech > sign	Sign > speech		
Conversation	0.37	0.12	0.33	0	0.19	0
	(16)	(5)	(14)		(8)	
Story recall	0	0	0.18	0.27	0	0.55
			(2)	(3)		(6)

There are at least two explanations for her different patterns of communication. First, the story recall task specifically targeted visuospatial contrasts, which may have predisposed her to produce more signs and gestures (McNeill, 1992). Alternatively, the story recall task could be considered more cognitively demanding than the conversation task. In order to produce a coherent narrative, the child must recall events in sequence and relate them to a naive listener. There is less co-construction in the dialogue evident here than in the conversation, placing more responsibility on the narrator. Possibly Pardeep's skills in spoken language were unequal to the task, and she was driven to introduce precision through the recruitment of an alternative mode (Rimé and Schiatura, 1991). Thus, when required to communicate information which is both visual and complex, Pardeep seems to shift the problem space of linguistic organization from speech to a shared vocal–manual base.

The above data on both PCS and manual sign processing show that one should be wary of assuming that bimodality is a fixed characteristic of manual and graphic signs (see also Mills, van den Bogaerde and Coerts, 1994). It may well be the case that not only does the situation vary according to each individual's abilities and experiences, so that there are as many bimodal situations as there are users of alternative communication systems, but that each communicative situation impinges on the organization of modes. For some individuals, or for certain contexts, speech may serve as the reference point for input and output purposes, so that symmetry is restored. In other cases, asymmetry may be the hallmark. Careful recording of prosody and temporal relationships between output in different modes may yield critical information about the processing and organization of language.

Representational redescription in two modes - the problem of word order

Research to date suggests that two contrasting patterns of word order development may be observed in groups of individuals using manual or graphic signs. Some individuals seem to develop strategies for sequencing their output to match the word order available in the input (e.g. Bruno, 1998, personal communication; Kraat and Brune, 1998), whereas others appear to disregard the word order of the input, and fail to match it in their output (Smith and Grove, 1996). We have suggested that part of the reason may lie in the nature of the task, which involves internalizing the rules governing word order in speech, and recoding them into manual or graphic signs when constructing the output. Our evidence suggests that some individuals may not adopt this strategy, or may adopt different strategies in different contexts. The essential questions are what processes generate the different surface representations that we find in the data, and what influences the adoption of different processing styles?

Our starting point is the nature of the shift from pre-linguistic to linguistic development, which has been characterized by Karmiloff-Smith (1992) as a process of 'representational redescription'. A set of existing representations is reorganized under pressure to accommodate new problems. In the development of communication, for example, the increasing need to provide complex and elaborate information which extends beyond the immediate context seems to be important in creating a problem space for the child, and motivating the shift towards grammatical analysis. For the users of alternative communication systems faced with communicating information about an event, the problem is whether to develop a system for expressing relationships between constituents, and how to do it. Existing data show that individuals sometimes string constituents together in no particular order (Smith and Grove, 1996), sometimes develop consistent ordering patterns which differ from the input (Goldin-Meadow, 1995), and sometimes follow the pattern provided in the input (Kraat and Brune, 1998). Thus in a verb–object phrase, one may see:

biscuit eat

or

eat biscuit

We suggest that both patterns could be generated by different underlying processes, reflecting different stages of language development (see Atkinson, 1992). It has been argued that the earliest stage of word combinations, corresponding to Brown's (1973) MLU Stage 1, is essentially pre-syntactic, governed by lexical, thematic and pragmatic, rather than syntactic constraints (Atkinson, 1992; Locke, 1997; Radford, 1990). At this stage, the individual simply lists the constituents involved in an action, without paying attention to ordering cues in the spoken input, or patterns of relationships between constituents. One would expect, therefore, in samples collected over time and across different contexts, to see random variation in the positioning of objects in relation to verbs.

In typical development, there is a swift transition from these pre-syntactic sequences to the rule-governed, analytic behaviour. The second stage of word combinations is accompanied by the development of functional categories, and morphological inflections (McDonald, 1997; Radford, 1990), perhaps as a consequence of the application of a computational, analytic strategy (Locke, 1997). If the user's production of a verb–object sequence is linguistically governed, then one might expect to see the consistent use across time and space of either object–verb, or verb–object patterning, resulting from two alternative types of redescription: recoding or reformation.

The recoding route

In the process of recoding, the assumption is that the individual becomes sensitized to the rules governing word order in the spoken input, which then regulates the development of inner speech. Output is generated from this base, with the individual recoding from speech to manual or graphic sign, resulting in the order 'eat biscuit'. The problem space which motivates representational redescription is intermodal.

The reformation route

In the process of reformation, the assumption is that the individual becomes sensitized to the need for a rule-based system to express relationships between constituents. In this case, the spoken input may be disregarded in favour of other sources of structure.

For example, Goldin-Meadow's subjects showed a semantic bias in favour of the constituent affected by an action, placing patients before actions or recipients, and treating intransitive actors as patients (ergative structures) (Goldin-Meadow, 1995).

Consistent pragmatic priorities might lead to a topic–comment organization as suggested by Livingstone (1983) and Mohay (1990). Such priorities could generate the order 'biscuit eat' or 'eat biscuit' depending on whether the topic is the act of eating, or what is eaten. The individual's own output then acts as input, and the problem space is intramodal, leading in some cases to the development of gestural morphology as well as patterns of constituent order.

If the model or recoding or reformation is correct, development may not necessarily follow an intermodal route. The question arises therefore whether the assumption of bimodal processing is a useful one when deciding what input may best support language acquisition in children using manual or graphic signs.

Is bimodal better?

The use of augmented input seems a logical way to support 'symmetry' across input and output modes and is therefore potentially a useful intervention approach (e.g. Calculator, 1988; Romski and Sevcik, 1996). The provision of multimodal input is not entirely without controversy. Iacono, Mirenda and Beukelman (1993) and Iacono and Duncum (1995) report a comprehension advantage in bimodal communication situations for the children with learning disabilities they studied. By contrast, Remington and Clark (1993a,b), working with cognitively impaired individuals, suggest that multimodal input can be either facilitative or inhibiting, in that individuals may attend to only one mode of stimulus presentation, although there may have been other task-related factors contributing to the patterns of performance observed in their subjects.

Two other sources of evidence suggest that bimodal processing may be problematic for linguistic development. Research on bilingualism in both signed and spoken language suggests that for children to become proficient in both signed and spoken language, the two languages need to be separated by the child learner. Providing such separation in input by adopting a one person–one language approach is commonly reported as facilitative of language learning (Baker, 1995). Language mixing by the child, with elements from two languages coexisting in one utterance does occur, but usually one language is dominant, and the 'guest language' element is a single free morpheme, typically a noun (de Houwer, 1995) (a pattern remarkably like that demonstrated by Pardeep in the conversation context).

A second source suggesting a need for caution in introducing bimodal processing in input is research by McNeill and his colleagues on the shift towards language-like organization in the manual–gestural mode. Their work (McNeill, 1992; Singleton, Goldwin-Meadow and McNeill, 1995) suggests that this shift is only likely to happen when speech is suppressed and the individual is relying on visuospatial processing (i.e. on one mode). In other words, for individuals who have extremely limited speech skills, an alternative mode may offer the best opportunity for the development of linguistic potential. It remains an open question, however, whether such potential is best developed by exploiting the specific characteristics of a mode – graphic or visuospatial – or by attempting to represent the structure of the spoken language completely in the alternative modality. The failure of manually signed speech with deaf populations should caution us that the latter strategy is fraught with logical problems, even for individuals who can hear and understand some speech.

Clearly, it cannot be assumed that simply simultaneously indicating key words of a spoken message on a communication board will provide the necessary input for manual or graphic sign-users to abstract the relevant information about cross-modal equivalences, and subsequently generate their own messages (Romski, Sevcik and Adamson, 1997b). Whilst there are many apparently strong arguments supporting the provision of bimodal and multimodal input, substantial empirical evidence to support these arguments is still lacking. It may be that certain kinds of messages can be relatively easily and usefully presented bimodally, but that in other instances the simultaneous presentation of non-equivalent information may actually increase the processing difficulties. Pairing speech with PCS when referring to objects which can be easily depicted may support the building of equivalence links across modes. However, when communicating a message where the match between the PCS and the referent is somewhat less optimal, any uncertainty on the part of the user may be exacerbated by the potential ambiguity of the graphic sign. The apparent iconicity of PCS reflects the experience of the perceiver as well as the characteristics of the sign. As many (e.g. Stephenson and Linfoot, 1996) have pointed out, iconicity is in the eye of the beholder. Furthermore, the effects of iconicity on language processing may be highly context-dependent and may differ across concrete or abstract language use (Paivio, 1986). Well matched imagery across PCS and speech, for example, may support processing of concrete linguistic information more than it does abstract linguistic information, but equally, poorly matched visual images may disrupt processing of concrete linguistic messages to a greater extent than abstract linguistic messages. It may be that the potential value of the apparent iconicity of PCS is highly dependent on the content of any given communication message, even for children adopting a predominantly recoding approach, bimodality may at times distract the juggler.

There are therefore many questions to which there are as yet no satisfactory answers. Is bimodal input always better and should it therefore be a key strategy in therapeutic intervention? Are there developmental trends which interact in significant ways in determining the usefulness or otherwise of simultaneous presentation of information in more than one modality? Are certain kinds of messages more suited to bimodal representation than others? Are there benefits other than supporting linguistic organization which derive from presentation of information across modes? Inferences regarding the processing of language across manual and graphic modes can only be speculative at this stage. However, a model which allows for either intramodal or intermodal problem-solving, through processes of either recoding or reformation does account for the different patterns of expressive communication seen cross-modally in users of manual and graphic signs. The question which follows is, what factors influence the development of one type of process rather than the other? What processes and properties can emerge, given particular interactions between biological bases and environmental influences? For children with severe speech impairments, one crucial environmental influence is the type of non-speech mode of communication offered to them.

Producibility as an essential requirement for linguistic organization

Regardless of the mode within which a language system is constructed, it seems plausible that the grammatical analysis module suggested by Locke (1995) must have available to it data which are perceivable, producible and segmentable (Petitto, 1993), in order to construct a rule-governed, hierarchically structured system. There has been some recent discussion as to the extent to which non-speech systems which are provided to people with communication disorders match the feature of segmentability (e.g. Light, 1997; Smith and Grove, 1996). Less frequently discussed is the question of 'producibility'. If the development of a syntactically organized system requires not only units which can be segmented and recombined, but also segments which can be produced, then production itself may be presumed to have a role in the process.

In returning, if somewhat clumsily, to the juggling analogy, even if one can provide materials which have the potential for reorganization and combination, is it also necessary to be able to provide direct experience of juggling itself in order for the full potential of the system to develop? Is such experience essential for the hierarchical potential of segmentable units to become evident?

The role of production in spoken language acquisition remains somewhat unresolved. Elbers (1995) and Platt and MacWhinney (1983) argue that children acquiring language use data from all available sources in their experimentation in analysis of structure, thus creating their own unique error forms, which over time are subjected to further analysis. In fact, Elbers (1995) argues that children's own productions are a privileged source of data for analysis, the 'output as input hypothesis'. Production may also be central to two common features of early communication and language behaviour: repetition and non-social uses of language.

In discussing repetition, Scollon (1979) and Veneziano, Sinclair and Berthoud (1990) propose that in the transition to multi-word speech, children initially create a structural form with two components simply by repeating one element of a message and only subsequently progress to adding new information within a multi-term structure. In a similar vein, when using 'non-social language' (Elbers, 1995; Elbers and Wijnen, 1992; Ervin-Tripp, 1979; Weir, 1962), children may be playing with both the structural and conceptual aspects of language productions, without the need to divide an attentional focus across own-productions and other-productions. Thus, the ability to actually produce language may facilitate many aspects of the analytical process underlying language acquisition.

For children for whom the language problem space is intramodal, that is, those children constructing a system for relating constituents within a single mode, production may play a particularly crucial role. With very restricted access to input from others in the manual or graphic mode (and possibly also reduced access to spoken input), children's own 'output as input' may become an atypically important source of data for analysis, facilitating the reformation of a within-mode system for relating constituents, which differs from that provided in the spoken input – for example the kinds of morphological creativity reported by Grove, Dockrell and Woll (1996).

As pointed out by von Tetzchner and Martinsen (1992), unlike manual signs, graphic signs such as PCS are selected, not produced; even if they have segmental potential, they cannot be directly manipulated. The effort involved in selecting each PCS is likely to militate against the use of repetition. Indeed, as PCS can only be used with a communication partner, it is quite possible that if a child repeats a selection, the communication partner assumes that an error is being corrected or that the repetition is caused by a motor problem. Thus repetition is unlikely to be a frequently used strategy. Equally, it is hard to imagine non-interactive monologues for children using PCS. These additional constraints on individuals using PCS may make the task of constructing a hierarchically structured system more difficult, limiting the extent of within-mode reformation which is either possible or demonstrable. PCS productions may remain structurally very simple and reduced relative to spoken language models, (i.e. governed by lexical, thematic or pragmatic constraints) either because of the limited 'reformation' potential of the graphic signs, or because our definitions of complexity derive from a spoken language perspective and are not appropriate to the graphic mode (Soto, 1998).

Conclusion

It seems clear that a unitary view of 'the bimodal situation' is overly simplistic, and that the focus needs to be on a complex system of relationships between modes. The model proposed in this chapter suggests two possible routes to the development of complexity. One route (recoding) hinges on the insight that a spoken message may be recoded into manual or graphic form – hence implicating intermodal development. As a spoken language base expands, parallel developments are seen in the non-speech mode, within the constraints intrinsic to the non-speech system and the communicative context. An alternative route involves a focus on intramodal development. Increases in complexity derive from the reformation or development of a system of relationships between constituents within the manual or graphic mode, without direct reference to a spoken language system.

The factors which motivate the selection of one or other processing strategy may be many and varied. Individual preferences or biases may interact in complex ways with experience (both in the sense of experience of spoken language and direct teaching or intervention experience), task demands, skill level across modes and the communicative context. The input provided may alert a child to the possible relationships which may exist across modes, but only if the child can access both modes simultaneously, share attention cross-modally, infer the partner's communicative intent and then draw conclusions regarding the structuring of information across modes. The ability to produce some speech may predispose towards a recoding strategy, although the performance of Natalie, the typically-developing pre-schooler, suggests caution is warranted in making this assumption. Access to a system which is not only perceivable and segmentable, but also producible (Petitto, 1993) may strongly influence the extent of within-mode reformation or development which can be achieved or demonstrated.

The 'sleeping partner' to be considered in attempting to introduce more than one mode of communication, whether relating to strategies of recoding or reformation, is the influence of the mode of communication itself. Systems for structuring complexity translate poorly across modes, so that for example the linear sequencing characteristic of spoken language is inefficient within the visuospatial mode, where simultaneous multi-layering of information is possible. Within-mode developments are likely to require a mode-specific system of description and analysis. Likewise, addressing the question of intermodal relationships will necessitate detailed task description, as well as the transcription of information regarding prosody and temporal relationships within and across modes, in a level of detail as yet not widely included in research on augmentative and alternative communication.

Finally, the implications for intervention with children with severe speech impairments learning language using manual or graphic signs are far from clear. The mere provision of input in more than one mode may be insufficient in demonstrating recoding strategies, without an additional focus on the task of recoding itself. If a strategy of within-mode development is that being pursued by the child, then the information presented in one of the modes may well be redundant, if not distracting.

It seems clear that researchers are only starting to unravel the complexities which are at the heart of the language learning experience of children using manual and graphic signs. The juggling act which faces each individual is influenced by many factors, in ways which we are only beginning to explore. The apparent shifts in mode-dominance and cross-modal organization over time for Laura, or across contexts for Pardeep, raise questions about the nature of the underlying organizational structures or problem processing space for the individuals involved. Capturing information which allows objective exploration of such phenomena raises a methodological problem: how to best capture cross-modal communication within a transcript so that such relationships can be further explored. The challenge is to not only describe the product of juggling, but to explore the process by which individuals can become expert jugglers and how the tools and experiences which we offer them facilitate or hinder their progress.

Chapter 3
Form and Meaning in Alternative Language Development

ERLAND HJELMQUIST

The questions discussed in this chapter are whether there are restrictions on the form in which meanings can be expressed, whether certain meanings are more amenable to certain forms than others, and whether meaning actually changes when the form of communication is changed (see also Hjelmquist, 1997). There are no direct answers to these questions, of course, but they are fundamental for understanding alternative language development.

The approach chosen here implies that language acquisition is viewed from the perspective of input–output relations. The focus is essentially the same as in Hjelmquist (1997), that is, in what ways and to what extent linguistic communication can be achieved in an alternative language mode. Motor-impaired children without speech belonging to the *expressive group* (Martinsen and von Tetzchner, 1996) are the focus of this chapter, and for this group, the divide between input and output is located in the speech mode. The communicative environment of these children comprises speech, text, graphic signs, pictures, facial and body expressions, and for some, manual signs. The children's output is restricted to writing and other forms of graphic communication, facial and body expressions, and possibly manual signs. Synthetic speech always presupposes some kind of proxy medium, such as indicating or touching graphic signs.

I have claimed elsewhere that the use of artefacts for communication among disabled children forces them to take a metaperspective on communication in ways that are different from those of naturally speaking children (Hjelmquist, 1991; 1997; Hjelmquist, Dahlgren Sandberg and Hedelin, 1994). Acquisition of an understanding of the layers of communicative discourse, such as messages, words and subword structures is a prerequisite for learning to use communicative tools. In fact, these are two sides of the same coin: coming to understand that communicative tools can be used to represent something is a crucial first step for starting to manipulate them for communicative purposes. This is true for all communicative modes, and has been a major theme in studies of the acquisition of orthographic reading and writing skills. The systematic relationship between speech sounds and graphic signs in the form of letters has to be discovered and mastered to enable reading and writing, demanding an analysis of speech. Such an analysis seems to require a certain developmental level, and in literate societies, naturally speaking children usually start to learn to read when they are around 5-6 years of age. The same principle, that is, that children have to understand a representational relationship, seems to hold also for iconic graphic representations. DeLoache, Pierroutsakos, Uttal, Rosengren and Gottlieb (1998) found that 9-month-old infants tried to grasp a pictured object and concluded that the children actually understood the difference between a real object and a picture of it, in the sense that they discriminated between them, but did not understand that pictures are not tangible (DeLoache, Uttal and Pierroutsakos, 1998).

Basic insights such as the ones presented by DeLoache, Uttal and Pierroutsakos (1998) are relevant for the understanding of alternative language development. Understanding the environment in its broadest sense requires learning to interpret experiences. When it comes to communication, children in literate societies, beside the face-to-face interaction with adults, early on meet pictures, movies, television and books. All these cultural artefacts must be understood as representations of something.

To sum up: the perceptual input to children takes many forms: speech, pictures, text and facial and bodily expressions. Naturally speaking children eventually also produce the same forms. Non-speaking children cannot produce natural speech, and facial and bodily expressions and manual signs are in general very restricted due to motor problems. The situation is summarized in Figure 3.1.

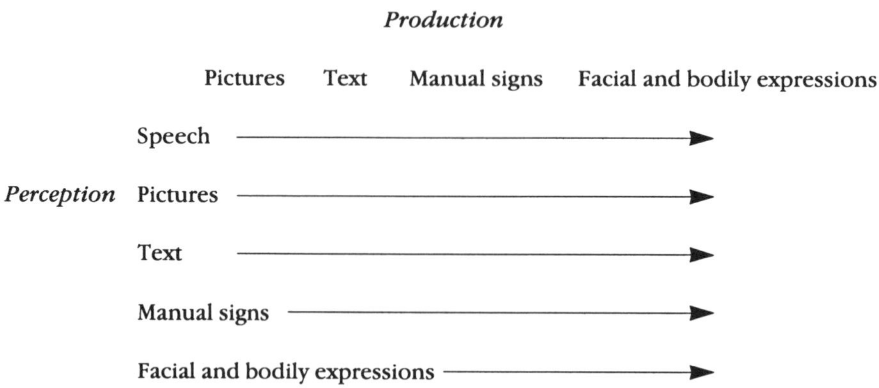

Figure 3.1. Input–output relations in the communication of non-speaking children belonging to the expressive language group.

The illustration in Figure 3.1 is simplified in the sense that pictures and text could be specified and classified in various ways. For the present purpose this is not necessary though. The main point is that speech as output has to be substituted with graphic signs of one or the other kind, facial and bodily expressions, and possibly manual signs. In the following, only speech and graphic communication modes will be discussed.

As already pointed out, the obvious expressive communication for non-speaking children is written language (Hjelmquist, 1997). However, this meets with problems as evidenced in several studies (Dahlgren Sandberg and Hjelmquist, 1996,a,b; 1997). Non-speaking children have great difficulties with an orthographic written language. These difficulties are in contrast to their ability to analyse spoken language. Speech perception seems to function 'normally' even though the developmental process might be delayed. Perception and analysis of the three standard aspects of spoken language, phonology, grammar and semantics, are within the repertoire of non-speaking children (Hjelmquist, Dahlgren Sandberg and Hedelin, 1994; Dahlgren Sandberg and Hjelmquist, 1996,a,b; 1997). Consequently, there is no doubt that non-speaking children can develop representations of all three levels of language, though they cannot produce them in speech. Given these facts, the main issues are whether, in what way, and to what extent, mental representations of the three aspects of language are different among non-speaking children compared with naturally speaking children.

Phonology

Studies of non-speaking children's and adults' perceptual phonological skills show that they vary from normal to below normal compared with normally speaking individuals (Dahlgren Sandberg and Hjelmquist, 1996a,b; 1997). These skills refer to analysis of the phonemic level, and the fact that such skills exist is in itself a noteworthy finding. By definition, these persons cannot produce any spoken language, but nevertheless develop the ability to analyse speech sounds in a similar manner as other people in the same language environment. However, because speech production is lacking, assessment procedures have to be changed and adapted compared to assessment of normally speaking persons, implying that participants have to respond by pointing to, nodding, or by using any other means to indicate a choice among the items that are available.

Given these circumstances, it is possible that the representation of speech is affected by the lack of motor and acoustic feedback, hearing what one says and subvocal articulation. In view of the often crucial importance attributed to subvocal articulation, the results are striking. Fine-grained analysis of spoken language can be attained despite lack of such articulation. This is in line with the findings of Bishop and Robson (1989a) who showed that short-term memory involving verbal components can function within a normal range despite dysarthria. Altogether, there is by now compelling evidence that non-speaking children develop phonological skills similar to those of speaking children. In most cases though, the results of non-speaking children are somewhat below those of speaking children, though statistically not significant. There are thus indications that non-speaking children may be quantitatively but not qualitatively different from normally speaking children. However, quantitative differences may give rise to qualitative differences in other aspects. There is an empirically well established positive relationship between phonological skills and literacy among naturally speaking children (Goswami and Bryant, 1990; Lundberg, Frost and Petersen, 1988). Difficulties in acquiring literary skills may be the result of not reaching a 'critical level', in quantitative terms, of phonological skills.

It is not only the skill level that might be important, but also other aspects related to representation. Since linguistic units, such as the phoneme, are very abstract, it presupposes a representation mode that is abstract enough to handle the infinite variation in the way specific phonemes might be realized, due to internal characteristics of speech, such as coarticulation and speaker characteristics like dialect, age and sex. Such a representation may be more or less developed and established. Elbro (1994, 1996) used the concept 'distinctiveness' to refer to how well representations of phonemes are available to the individual. Among speaking and otherwise non-disabled individuals Elbro found that those with dyslexic problems tended to have less distinctive representations of phonemes. Ideas about the nature of representation of speech sounds may have a bearing on the way non-speaking persons develop such representations. It is possible that a lack of articulatory skills leads to less clear representation of what one hears.

Closely related to the ability to sound out is the ability to repeat verbal information one has heard, more or less silently to oneself, and the ability to pronounce words and utterances before they are definitely delivered. The latter is evident in the normal acquisition of foreign languages. In view of the lack of possibilities for non-speaking children to engage in activities such as the ones mentioned above, it is even more remarkable that these children develop phonological representations to the extent actually found in empirical studies. This shows that development can take other routes than the typical ones and that compensatory mechanisms can be very effective. Non-speaking children develop basic skills in segmenting and combining speech; the fundamentals of any linguistic system. However, these skills must be used productively in other modes than speech.

The relatively well developed phonological skills among non-speaking children can be compared with those of deaf children. Aaron and associates (1998) found that deaf children with little or no phonological ability were also poor spellers. These results make sense; without a phonology, spelling of an orthographic language will pose problems. Non-speaking children present another picture: they have well-developed phonological skills but still have poor spelling and reading skills.

The resilience of receptive phonological skills to severe motor impairments must be understood in an evolutionary perspective. Linguistic communication and speech are a characteristic of *Homo sapiens*, a species which is at least 100 000 years old. The origins of spoken linguistic communication must probably be sought long before that, implying that the biological basis for this particular type of communication is the result of an evolution which has turned out to be exceedingly successful. However, this long evolutionary history has created a tool of communication which may be difficult to replace with another. The effectiveness of orthographic reading and writing systems is due to the systematic relationship between spoken language and graphic signs. The way spoken language 'sounds' is 'depicted' in graphic forms. This is a crucial component of the technology of writing. In a deep sense, there is a natural relationship between the orthographic system and spoken language, while at the same time, writing is not natural at all, but a cultural product. The mental representation of a spoken language in the form of knowledge of the orthographic graphic mode is thus extremely flexible since it can take care of any linguistic form, irrespective of meaning, as long as it conforms to the phonological structure of the specific language. Non-orthographic graphic modes of communication, on the other hand, seem to build on the basic conception that iconicity, more or less salient in different systems, is an essential ingredient of such communication. Iconicity in this case refers to a similarity between the sign and its meaning, a similarity within the semantic domain. This is in contrast to the relationship between speech and an orthographic system, where abstract forms are related to each other.

Grammar

A crucial question is to what extent and in what ways non-speaking children develop a structural analysis, a grammar, of the spoken input and their alternative output mode (Soto, 1997, this volume; Sutton, 1997). One major methodological problem is that non-speaking motor-impaired children constitute a heterogeneous group. Their impairments vary in respect of such characteristics as aetiology, degree of severity and presence of other impairments.

The fact that grammar is often raised as a crucial issue is partly due to the fact that there is very little productive language data. There is no doubt, though, that non-speaking children develop substantial insights into the grammar of the language that is spoken around them and that they have structural and combinatorial abilities (Hjelmquist, Dahlgren Sandberg and Hedelin, 1994). These abilities may also be applied to alternative modes of communication (Soto, 1997).

In a study reported by Hjelmquist, Dahlgren Sandberg and Hedelin (1994), non-speaking individuals were told a message orally by one person and instructed to repeat this message to another person using Blissymbols. The spoken messages were compared with Blissymbol productions and the children's judgement of what they had expressed in Blissymbols. The evidence for a structural analysis of the spoken message was indirect, since there was no systematic variation of grammatical structure in the test questions. Nevertheless, the children showed that they could remember a spoken sentence and its constituent components very well, and compare the memorized sentence with another spoken sentence.

Discussion about the formal aspects of non-orthographic graphic communication often takes the structure of spoken language as point of reference (Soto, 1997, this volume). This implies that there is a generative, creative capacity, not only a fixed set of signs, or vocabulary. This is a reasonable expectation in view of the enormous variation between natural languages and the fact that new languages are created in the interplay between different languages when speakers are motivated to communicate though they do not understand each other's languages. Pidgin languages are products of such intercultural encounters where adults find ways of creating systems which are effective for certain communicative purposes. However, if a pidgin language is creolized, children who acquire that language change what they hear by introducing linguistic devices such as inflections and functional word order. This is perhaps the best example of how children's potential for developing language can evolve a language in a short time. One may ask whether similar developments may be happening when children learn to communicate with a graphic communication system. The evidence summarized by Soto (1997, this volume) seems to support such a possibility, though empirical evidence is much too scarce to allow any firm conclusions.

There are several reasons, though, to doubt that graphic systems will work in this way. One fundamental problem is the lack of a natural cultural habitat for the development and use of such systems. The graphic systems are not generated by children on the basis of spontaneous input from users of the same mode of communication. There is no language community, where a non-vocal communication form is used as the primary mode of communication (except sign language in communities with deaf people). The most frequent spontaneous input to a non-speaking child is speech, not messages produced with graphic system(s). Furthermore, the 'lexical' units of most present graphic communication systems are fixed and petrified and allow very little innovative and creative use, a ubiquitous feature of the way a speaking child treats spoken language. There are also other characteristics of the output of graphic communication modes, to be discussed below, which cast further doubt on the analogy to a creolization process.

Semantics

Human communication is about conveying meaning. This is done symbolically, using semantic representations also available to non-speaking persons. In this context, symbolic functioning is defined as the level of cognitive function which is usually attained at around 12 months of age and is manifest in the first words used for communicative purposes. This excludes profoundly intellectually disabled persons.

Human communication starts with intentions and meaning which have to find a manifest form. It has been shown that non-speaking children analyse spoken linguistic communication at a semantic level (Hjelmquist, Dahlgren Sandberg and Hedelin, 1994). From a very early age, non-speaking children, similarly to speaking children, are made aware of the systematic connection between objects, events, qualities, etc., and lexical items such as nouns, verbs and adjectives. Young children, whether speaking or not, usually have developed the ability to extract meaning from speech when approaching 12 months of age. For non-speaking children, however, there is no further development of articulated speech. The question is then how these analytic abilities can be used for productive communication in alternative communication modes, in particular in graphic ones.

Soto (1997) suggests that the use of alternative communication systems might give rise to specific productive rules that are different from the ones in the spoken input to the child, implying a generative structure. Such a structure must have as one of its origins the representational system used for speaking. This system is capable of handling any natural spoken language, but it is not certain that it is powerful enough, or is offered enough substance by graphic systems, to develop a semantic system suitable to non-speaking persons.

A crucial factor is that graphic systems are artefacts, in a similar manner as orthographic writing systems. However, in contrast to orthographic systems, it is not clear what non-orthographic graphic systems model. An absolutely crucial feature of orthographic writing systems is that they are models of natural spoken languages. This feature makes it possible, for example, to decipher scripts of languages no longer spoken, as in the case of Linear B (there are other necessary conditions for such a reconstruction, including a large enough sample of writing). The main point is that it is known what is sought for in terms of some general structural features. It is unclear, though, what graphic communication systems used for non-speaking people are models of. Therefore it is unclear what the structural features of an alternative system would be.

Conclusions

A hypothetical model of input–output conditions for non-speaking children who belong to the expressive language group (Martinsen and von Tetzchner, 1996) is presented in Figure 3.2.

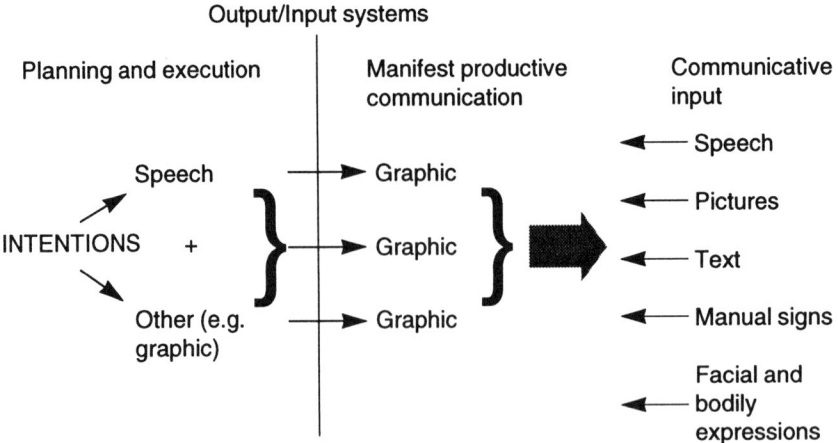

Figure 3.2. A model of multimodal communication of non-speaking children belonging to the expressive language group.

One question is what role phonology plays in the production of messages up to the actual execution, and what role the alternative communication modes play. One may refer to this as the planning stage in the communication process. In spoken communication the distinction between the planning stage and the production of an utterance has been criticized (Linell, 1982). It is problematic because spoken communication is interactive and dialogical. In spoken communication it is difficult to make a clear distinction between the planning of an utterance and the actual saying of an utterance. Immediate feedback from what the speaker hears of his or her own utterance and feedback from the listener has direct effects on what is said. In spoken communication there is a continuous adjustment of the form and content of the message according to demands from the 'audience' and the speaker. According to Hjelmquist and Dahlgren Sandberg (1996), this is in sharp contrast to the communication situation for a non-speaking child where the distinction between planning and execution is clear. Children using graphic communication systems often seem as if they follow a plan when they slowly construct an utterance. It is likely that the characteristics of the communication device used by the child influence the planning process. This indicates that the cognitive processes and strategies applied in spontaneous communication are different for non-speaking children and speaking children.

One obvious feature is that the speed of communication is very slow, implying among other things, that the memory processes must be different, especially in certain processes related to working memory functions such as 'rehearsal'. It seems very unlikely, though, that speech-related processes are not activated in the production of alternative communication among children who understand spoken language. As indicated in Figure 3.2, one reasonable hypothesis is that subvocal speech and the characteristics of the graphic system used jointly constitute the planning stage, possibly together with other 'imageless thoughts'. The presence of two pre-execution modes of planning raises the question of what mode has priority, if any. From a nativist perspective on language acquisition, the default mode should be speech (Pinker, 1995). The orientation towards analysis of spoken language input is powerful enough to compensate for peripheral problems, such as limited articulatory capacity. Because the 'language instinct' is specialized, it is not expected to be particularly useful for analysing and synthesizing other modes of communication. Instead, the general perceptual and cognitive functions should be expected to do the work. Very simplified, this amounts to a kind of problem-solving activity at a high level of awareness. Such processes are characterized by being relatively slow and taxing, for example on memory processes.

It is implied in the claims above that an analogy between learning to use an alternative communication system and developing a creole language is improper. What goes on when an individual uses an alternative system is probably a combination, or mixture, of highly specific and rapid 'language instinct' processes and general and slow 'problem-solving'. A child's development of a creole language implies a creative use of the 'language instinct' and this is not applicable to alternative communication systems (except to sign languages which are a language proper). In this sense there is a definite divide between language perception and language production among non-speaking children.

Chapter 4
Understanding the Impact of Graphic Sign Use on the Message Structure

GLORIA SOTO

Language production of individuals who use graphic signs as their primary means of expression has been shown to differ from that of normally speaking individuals (e.g. Collins, 1996; Smith, 1996b; Soto and Toro-Zambrana, 1995; Sutton and Morford, 1998; van Balkom and Welle Donker-Gimbrère, 1996; von Tetzchner and Martinsen, 1996). In addition, research appears to indicate that the structure of messages constructed by individuals using graphic signs is remarkably similar across subjects, regardless of age and disability (Soto, 1997a).

Two explanations are frequently presented in the literature as to why the structure of graphic sign messages differs so much from that of spoken utterances. First, the 'process' or 'compensation' hypothesis suggests that the message structure of graphic sign communication reflects compensatory strategies utilized by graphic sign users and their partners to circumvent the cognitive, physical and linguistic constraints involved in aided communication (e.g. van Balkom, 1998; van Balkom and Welle Donker-Gimbrère, 1996). Second, the modality-specific hypothesis relates the structural characteristics of graphic sign communication to constraints specific to the visual graphic mode (e.g. Smith, 1996b; Soto, 1997a; Sutton and Morford, 1998). The purpose of this chapter is to speculate about the modality-specific variables that may affect the structure of messages constructed with graphic signs. The chapter will close by outlining barriers to proving or disproving this hypothesis due to existing difficulties in graphic sign research.

Structural regularities in graphic sign communication

In 1997, Soto synthesized the findings from a number of published studies aimed at analysing the language production of individuals who used different graphic sign systems to communicate. Soto found that, despite subject and language elicitation task variability, all existing studies reported remarkably similar results. First, single-sign turns appear to dominate both in spontaneous and elicited conditions for users of pictorial signs, resulting in a prevalence of simple clauses, with very few examples of questions, commands, negatives and auxiliary verbs. Second, the structure of graphic messages does not seem to parallel the constituent order of the user's spoken language background regardless of the graphic system being used. Third, graphic sign users tend to omit morphosyntactic structures that appear frequently in the user's spoken language background, such as verbs and articles, even when those structures are available in the participants' communication boards. Fourth, graphic sign users utilize multimodal combinations (e.g. gestures + sign, facial expressions + sign, vocalizations + sign, alphabet + sign, and pointing + sign) while constructing their messages. Fifth, users of graphic systems apply an abundance of metalinguistic strategies to compensate for the lack of appropriate graphic signs and the inability to generate new signs as needed. These strategies could be summarized as (a) semantic bypasses – using another sign with similar assigned meaning, (e.g. *LET ME FINISH* instead of *Don't interrupt me*; *COOKIE* instead of *pie*); (b) phonological similarity – using another sign whose spoken label sounds like the intended one (e.g. *BEE* instead of *be*; *EYE* instead of *I*); and (c) word modification markers afforded by some graphic systems (e.g. Blissymbolics *THE OPPOSITE OF*; *COMBINATION*; *OBJECT OF*; *SIMILAR TO*). Lastly, most published studies described the atypical role assumed by the speaking communicative partner, both in terms of interaction 'dominance' and meaning 'co-construction' (for examples see Collins, 1996; von Tetzchner and Martinsen, 1996). Speaking communicative partners often enhanced and interpreted the message using strategies such as word order adjustments, syntactic corrections and semantic clarifications.

Investigating the modality hypothesis

As described above, the literature reports remarkable similarities in the structure of graphic sign messages. Because the existing studies have used participants that varied in age and ability level and varied tasks for language elicitation, the reported similarities in message structure cannot be attributed solely to user or context variables. Rather, observed structural regularities in the graphic messages have been speculated to be associated with constraints specific to the graphic modality (Smith, 1996b, 1997; Soto, 1997a; Sutton and Morford, 1998).

The human linguistic capacity has been described as a structure-seeking mechanism whereby the individual must be able to perceive, produce and combine a restricted and consistent set of meaningful segments (Petitto, 1993). The way an individual perceives, produces and combines those meaningful segments depends on the constraints imposed by the execution mode (e.g. gestural or spoken) and perception modality (e.g. visual or auditory). The influence of mode and modality on language structure has been observed through differences in phonological, morphological, syntactic and semantic structures between something that is said and something that is signed (e.g. Petitto, 1987).

While the impact of the gestural and visual mode on language structure is well documented, modality factors associated with graphic communication have received little attention (Sutton and Morford, 1998). In order to describe the influence of the graphic modality on the structural characteristics of graphic sign messages, structural regularities in messages produced using graphic sign systems must be identified and described under highly controlled conditions. Finding structural regularities will help researchers in the field of augmentative and alternative communication address an important theoretical question: is graphic output linguistic in nature (i.e. constructed according to an intrinsic and consistent system of organization) or is it a mere 'translation' or 'adaptation' of the user's spoken language? If, in fact, graphic sign communication is linguistic in nature (i.e. language-based), there must be an intrinsic 'graphic' system of organization yet to be understood and described. The description of the modality effects of graphic communication should encompass both a cross-sectional and developmental perspective.

Empirical evidence suggests developmental patterns in the way children use graphic signs to communicate. In one study that addresses the role of the visual graphic mode in constituent order patterns, Sutton and Morford (1998) asked 32 normally developing children (ages 5:9–12:7) to retell a series of transitive actions displayed on videotape. The retelling task was presented in two conditions. In the pointing condition, the children watched a video clip and then were asked to describe what they had seen by pointing to pictures available on a board. After the pointing condition, the same clip was shown and the children were asked to retell the story using their speech. Both oral and graphic responses were videotaped, transcribed and coded according to the number and order of constituents used. The data analysis revealed a significant effect of modality and a significant effect of age on the use of English constituent order, which was used more consistently by older children. In the pointing condition, use of English order increased with age, but was still not at ceiling even among the oldest children. These findings indicate that the children did not automatically transfer their knowledge of English grammar to their use of a picture board. Sutton and Morford (1998) noted that the English syntax was used more regularly as the children got older. In addition, the use of non-English constituent order pattern was not random, OV (object–verb) pointing sequences being significantly more frequent than non-OV responses across all age groups. They propose that the prevalence of OV order pattern may be related to changes in modalities of language expression.

Developmental patterns were also identified with the use of multi-unit graphic utterances. The youngest children produced single-sign utterances more often, and it was the action information (verb-label) they attempted to encode with their single points. Older children tended to produce more multi-unit sequences, transitioning onto English-constituent order. Sutton and Morford (1998) suggest that OV order pattern may serve as a transitional step between single constituent responses and full SVO (subject–verb–object) English constituent order in aided communication.

Developmental influences within the graphic modality may explain the findings by Smith (1996b). In her study, Smith (1996b) taught five normally developing pre-schoolers to use picture boards. She found that the children used mostly single-sign points in a picture description task. These results were interpreted as support for the modality hypothesis since all five children had intact linguistic competence and physical abilities.

In order to apply the above findings to aided communication, similar studies need to be conducted with children with severe speech impairments who use graphic signs as their primary means of expression and are at different developmental stages with regard to the use of graphic communication. However, there are a number of variables unique to graphic-based interactions that need to be addressed when describing the structural consistency of graphic sign communication. Among them, I will refer to (a) the multimodal nature of graphic sign communication; (b) the input–output asymmetry; (c) the existing heterogeneity frequently found among aided communication users and graphic sign systems; and (d) the sociocultural and linguistic contexts in the acquisition of graphic communication competence.

The multimodal nature of graphic communication

Researchers have repeatedly described graphic communication as a multimodal process in which various aided and unaided modes are used in combination to convey meaning (e.g. Heim and Baker-Mills, 1996). The choice of modes seems to depend on the individual's physical, cognitive and linguistic capacities as well as on the communicative situations (e.g. communicative functions and discourse roles). Because the individual's abilities change over time, the study of the effects of multimodality on the structure of aided communication would necessarily entail a description of the developmental processes within modes and across modes; that is, it would describe the possible dominance of one mode at a particular point in time, but also the changes in mode dominance in the course of the child's development (Heim and Baker-Mills, 1996).

Smith (1997) raised a number of issues that need to be addressed in the study of multimodality. First, she described the process of developing language through alternative modes as restricted by the range of available modes and by the users' motor limitations. Second, the development and coexistence of multiple modes of communication raises the issue of the supplementary and complementary relationships that emerge across modes. In complementary relationships, at least two communication modes provide different propositional information in a single turn. In supplementary relationships, most of the propositional information is conveyed through one mode while other modes add information that is not regarded as strictly necessary. The study of intermodal organization would involve the description of mode dominance both developmentally and cross-sectionally (Smith, 1997).

Third, in the course of the child's development, one of the available modes of communication acquires linguistic status (Petitto, 1993). In typically developing children, the choice of linguistic mode naturally depends on their linguistic input. In their search for structure, children developing language utilize the consistency afforded by their linguistic input to learn new signs and novel sign combinations (Slobin, 1985). However, for many children with severe physical impairments, the choice of 'linguistic' mode becomes a decision made by someone else, usually a professional or a caregiver, and it is usually based on graphic signs. As Smith (1997) notes the 'extraordinary' nature of the language learning environment of most children using graphic signs is characterized by the asymmetry between the modality of their linguistic input and their linguistic output.

The input–output asymmetry

Individuals who use graphic signs as their primary means of expression are for the most part hearing and live immersed in spoken language environments where they constantly receive speech input. In fact, they hardly ever see graphic systems being used in their environment, and thus, are very frequently deprived of expressive language models outside structured teaching situations (von Tetzchner and Jensen, 1996). Thus, graphic sign users are faced with a distinct asymmetry between the primary channel of language input and their primary channel of language output because they continue to receive auditory input in the spoken language of their environment while they are expected to express themselves through a graphic sign system that differs from that spoken language (Smith and Grove, 1996).

The input–output asymmetry is further complicated by the fact that the user's graphic sign selection is often 'translated' and extended into spoken language by the listener or a previously programmed voice output communication aid. Even when users of graphic systems communicate to each other, they may be unable to do so directly and may depend on a speaking person to translate and formulate their message (von Tetzchner and Martinsen, 1996). Thus, in graphic communication, meaning is 'co-constructed' by the communicative partner, usually an adult, through 'translation' of the user's graphic output. In communicative interactions augmented through graphic means, the communicative partner frequently uses contextual knowledge about the user, the task, and the graphic system to infer meaning through a process where sign interpretations are highly based on extra-linguistic information (see Collins, 1996, for an example).

The extraordinary implications of the input–output asymmetry continue to puzzle researchers who raise multiple questions with regard to modality dominance, intermodality organization and the effect of spoken language comprehension on the structure of graphic messages (see Smith and Grove, Chapter 2, this volume).

Heterogeneity in graphic sign communication

The issue of the influence of modality on the structure of graphic messages is further confounded by the heterogeneity of graphic sign users. Graphic sign users may vary in chronological age, ability level, level of spoken language proficiency, and experience with graphic communication among other factors. Additionally, available graphic sign systems may vary according to their physical characteristics. Some graphic systems primarily include signs designed for their iconic or conceptual relationship with their referent (e.g. pictures, photographs). Other sign systems may utilize a combination of iconic signs along with graphic classifiers and other morphological markers to establish sign meaning (e.g. Blissymbolics, combination of pictures and alphabet boards). Therefore, in order to understand the impact of modality on the structure of graphic messages, the relationship between regularities observed in graphic sign communication and type of graphic sign system must be further explored. This will require cross-system comparisons of graphic sign messages constructed with different graphic sign systems from users of the same linguistic background.

With regard to user variability, an unresolved issue in graphic sign communication is the role of spoken language comprehension on the structure of graphic-based messages. Despite the critical role of spoken language comprehension in the overall communicative competence of people who use alternative communication systems as well as in the acquisition of grammatical knowledge and graphic sign learning (Nelson, 1992; Romski and Sevcik, 1991, 1992, 1996; Sutton and Morford, 1998), the role of the spoken language in graphic message formulation is yet to be systematically analysed. There is no empirical evidence as to whether graphic sign users formulate their messages by directly translating from their spoken language (e.g. paralleling spoken language as in the case of Morse code or Braille), according to the graphic modality's own intrinsic constraints, or combine both depending on the language task or the method of instruction. If graphic sign users follow the graphic modality's intrinsic system of organization, then graphic sign users from different language backgrounds and differing levels of spoken language comprehension would tend to construct messages with similar structures and word order and would also understand the graphic output of other users.

In order to investigate spoken language effects, it is necessary to obtain cross-linguistic data from graphic sign users with varying levels of spoken language comprehension who belong to different spoken language backgrounds where there are very different rules for word order, tense marking and other grammatical artefacts. Yet, in reality, graphic sign users with poor spoken language comprehension skills might exhibit concomitant difficulties in other areas related to language and cognition. This would make cross-group comparisons rather difficult.

In an effort to explore the use by individuals of non-English-speaking cultures of graphic-based communication aids developed in English-speaking countries, Nakamura and his colleagues (1998) asked 80 Japanese and 43 English speakers to compose picture-based sentences using a computer-based system with a dynamic screen. The screen displayed a subject button, a verb button and an object button that were linked to a list of appropriate words. The three buttons were presented in SVO order and in SOV order respectively. In one of the conditions, the Japanese subjects were offered the possibility of using Japanese morphological markers to be combined with the pictures. The results of their investigation show that in all conditions both the Japanese and the English subjects omitted words when using graphic signs as compared with using speech. Additionally, the results show that whenever morphological markers were available, the Japanese subjects tried to compose sentences that more closely matched their verbal response and respected the Japanese word order (e.g. SOV, OSV). By contrast, all English-speaking subjects used English word order (SVO) while composing the sentences.

These results provide preliminary data regarding the influence of the graphic modality on the structural characteristics of graphic sign messages. The findings of Nakamura and his colleagues are consistent with earlier studies that show a predominance of single-sign utterances and simple clauses in messages constructed using pictographic signs. Additionally, these findings suggest that whenever vocal and graphic modalities appear together, the structure of the dominant modality will prevail, which supports the idea of modality dominance previously raised. It would be very informative to conduct the same kind of cross-cultural study with individuals for whom the graphic modality is more dominant than the vocal one (e.g. individuals with low levels of spoken language comprehension or individuals who have been using graphic signs for many years).

When interpreting the results of Nakamura's study, certain limitations should be kept in mind. First, the fact that most subjects transferred the word order of their spoken language into the sentence building task is not surprising since the available sign options were already categorized according to their function in the sentence. Additionally, all subjects were fluent speakers of their home language and had not used graphic signs for expressive purposes before. The graphic sentences were elicited as a response to a written paragraph with reading comprehension questions. Therefore, it is quite likely that subjects transferred the written language word order onto their graphic messages. Further research addressing the impact of modality on the message structure of graphic sign messages is therefore needed.

Challenges in graphic sign research

Perhaps one of the biggest challenges in addressing the impact of modality on graphic communication is the development of a theoretical model that could support the study of the many factors that might potentially influence language acquisition augmented through graphic means (Loncke, Vander Beken and Lloyd, 1997; von Tetzchner et al., 1996). According to von Tetzchner and his colleagues, the model should be compatible with existing general models of communication but at the same time, provide a framework to investigate the specific characteristics of alternative forms of communication, such as the use of multimodal communication, the use of derived forms of language, the dynamic relationship between linguistic and non-linguistic information and the physical, cognitive, interactional and sociocultural aspects that may be specific for the community of users of alternative communication systems. As described by a number of researchers (e.g. Calculator, 1997; Collins, 1996; Light, 1997; Romski, Sevcik and Adamson, 1997; von Tetzchner and Martinsen, 1992, 1996), the sociocultural and linguistic aspects of aided language acquisition include, among others: (a) restricted access to the physical environment due to the child's disabilities (Light, 1997); (b) restricted access to social and play routines due to the fact that children with aided communication needs usually spend more time in care routines (Light, 1997; von Tetzchner and Martinsen, 1992); (c) restricted access to pre-symbolic forms of communication such as vocalizations, babbling and gestures (Paul, 1997); (d) restricted access to spoken language input due to a lower rate in adult initiations (Calculator, 1997); (e) restricted access to expressing intentions due to others' anticipation of the user's needs (Calculator, 1997; Collins, 1996; von Tetzchner and Martinsen, 1996); (f) restricted access to their existing systems (von Tetzchner and Martinsen, 1992); (g) restricted access to proficient graphic sign use models (Light, 1997; Romski, Sevcik and Adamson, 1997); and (h) restricted access to an aided system with full linguistic potential (Soto, 1998).

All the above conditions may result in an impoverished experiential base for conceptual, lexical, social and linguistic development, which in turn, may explain differences found in the communicative behaviour of children using graphic sign systems. An added difficulty in the development of a comprehensive model of augmented language development is the already mentioned heterogeneity of individuals who need an alternative communication system in terms of age, disability, spoken language proficiency, cultural and linguistic background, system, vocabulary content, means of representation and method of instruction.

Additionally, there is a number of methodological issues that deserve special consideration in addressing the impact of modality on message structure of graphic communication. First, is the delineation and transcription of what constitutes an 'utterance' or unit for structural analysis (Bedrosian, 1997; Smith, 1996b, 1997). This issue poses a special challenge to researchers due to (1) the multimodal nature of most graphic messages – which often incorporate graphic and non-graphic productions, (2) the proliferation of speech output devices – which incorporate whole messages under a single key stroke, and (3) the unusual role that the communicative partner assumes in co-constructing the final message (Collins, 1996; von Tetzchner and Martinsen, 1996).

Other methodological considerations relate to sample size and sample characteristics. For example, finding a group of graphic sign users with similar ability levels and the same level of spoken language comprehension and graphic communication proficiency from the same spoken language background could be extremely difficult. In addition, assessing spoken language comprehension of individuals with severe speech impairments has proven to be very difficult (Nelson, 1992), due to the fact that one can never be sure whether test results are a true reflection of the individual's abilities or his or her inability to respond to the task demands. Without homogeneous groups, conclusions made from group comparisons can be misleading.

The message elicitation task can also be an issue to consider in graphic sign research. For instance, using verbal stimuli or even verbal directions could be problematic due to the fact that they could trigger a modality dominance effect for individuals with a good level of spoken language comprehension and they could be difficult to understand for individuals with a lower one.

Thus, additional work remains to be done in order to determine how modality influences the structure of graphic sign messages. Variables such as spoken language comprehension, spoken language background, ability to understand the graphic output of other users and graphic system characteristics must be further explored.

Acknowledgement

The author thanks Stephen von Tetzchner for his comments on earlier drafts of this paper.

Chapter 5
Linking Language Learning Experiences and Grammatical Acquisition

ANN SUTTON

Children may require graphic communication systems for a variety of reasons (Martinsen and von Tetzchner, 1996). Children with motor impairment with good comprehension of spoken language may use graphic communication systems for expressive communication or to support its development, rather than for comprehension in addition to production. Language learning environments and experiences for these children differ in important ways from those of typically developing children (see Goldbart, 1998). It may be problematic for them to acquire grammatical knowledge, that is, the implicit understanding of syntax and morphology that supports comprehension of the spoken language of the environment and that provides the foundation for structures used in graphic sign utterances. Comparison of this atypical language learning situation with strong versions of language acquisition theories focusing on comprehension (e.g. Chomsky, 1986; Crain, 1987; Crain and Fodor, 1993) or production (e.g. Clark, Hutcheson and van Buren, 1974; Ninio and Snow, 1988) suggests that neither of these positions can be fully adopted as explanations of grammatical knowledge acquisition in children with motor impairment who use graphic systems (Sutton, 1997). Available research suggests that their grammars are not exactly like those of speaking individuals (e.g. Blockberger, 1998; Soto and Toro-Zambrana, 1995; Sutton and Gallagher, 1993), in contrast to what would be implied by comprehension-based theories. Nor are they completely different (e.g. Berninger and Gans, 1986; Hjelmquist, Chapter 3, this volume; Smith 1992; Sutton and Dench, 1998; Sutton and Gallagher, 1995) in contrast to what would be implied by production-based theories.

Three current models of grammatical development present more moderate positions and suggest that acquisition of grammatical knowledge might be problematic but not necessarily unachievable for children with motor impairment who need graphic systems. They all emphasize the developmental process and involve the notion of a threshold of processed input, termed uptake by Harris (1992), needed to initiate further progress. In the representational redescription model (Karmiloff-Smith, 1992), knowledge within content domains (e.g. mathematics and language) is repeatedly redescribed at a higher level of abstraction. At each level, a certain quantity of representations activates the process of redescription. Knowledge (representations) already stored, not only the external environment, can be exploited in learning more about grammar. Thus development may be internally as well as externally motivated.

The second proposal is that infants store unanalysed utterances in memory (Locke, 1997). When this store reaches a critical mass, analytic and computational mechanisms are pressed to operate due to storage limitations. Analysis identifies common patterns within and across utterances. Analytic mechanisms require a threshold of perceived input (Locke, 1997) and will not fully activate if there is not enough work for them to do (Locke, 1998). New input is thus organized by previous analyses, which facilitates further learning.

The third proposal is that grammatical acquisition is lexically based (Clark, 1995). Children learn the syntactic characteristics of individual words along with their meanings. As more words are learned, the frequency of words that have similar syntactic properties also increases. Once a sufficient number of individual words have been acquired, regularities across items can be analysed to form grammatical categories and syntactic patterns. Children progress in lexical and grammatical acquisition by attempting to reconcile representations they construct based on their comprehension with those they construct for production (Clark, 1995).

There are several potential obstacles to attaining the threshold of input suggested by these models to be needed to drive progress in acquisition of grammatical knowledge for children with motor impairment who need graphic systems. For example, these children may face a more difficult language learning task than is the typical process of acquisition of language comprehension and production through the auditory–oral (or visual–manual) modalities from native speakers. In addition, early social–cognitive experiences may provide weak preparation for attending to the structural features of the language of the environment. Further, it may be challenging to acquire sufficient vocabulary to prompt the onset of grammatical processes in comprehension and in production. Each of these characteristics of the language learning experiences of children with motor impairment who need graphic systems could impede progress in acquisition of grammatical knowledge. Although the specific impact of these potential obstacles is not fully understood, a brief review permits speculation about the types of influence that might be predicted and suggests implications for intervention.

The language learning task

Children typically learn their language from hearing and interacting with native speakers within a cultural context. The modality and mode of communication they learn to use to produce language are the same as those used by the native speaker models. Comprehension and production (of words and grammar) are usually coordinated but not fully synchronized. Comprehension typically precedes consistent productive use (Clark and Hecht, 1983), but production may also support learning by providing practice and by eliciting responses and feedback from listeners (Bloom and Lahey, 1978).

The transition from non-linguistic (illocutionary) to linguistic (locutionary) communication in typically developing children seems to be facilitated by their use of speech (Paul, 1998). The automaticity of speech production acquired through prior motor experience (babbling) may support use of the vocal mode for linguistic communication, although direct causal relationships are difficult to establish. Children typically demonstrate considerable facility (although far from complete mastery) in vocal production before beginning to produce words. However, children prevented from babbling by temporary tracheotomies seem to experience short-term delays but no obvious long-term deficits in spoken language production following decannulation (e.g. Bleile, 1998). It has also been suggested that early communication intents expressed by single words tend to overlap with intents expressed non-verbally (Paul, 1997) and that children begin using speech for intents that they already successfully communicate non-linguistically. They may make the transition to spoken words because speech is a more conventional form of communication and is a closer match to the spoken language input.

In contrast to the typical developmental situation, children with motor impairment who use graphic signs acquire language comprehension and production in different modalities (auditory versus visual). Knowledge of the grammar of the spoken environmental language is acquired primarily through comprehension and there is an atypical mismatch between the modes of communication that are comprehended (speech) and produced (graphic signs) (e.g. Smith, 1997; Smith and Grove, Chapter 2, this volume). As a consequence of these differences, the relationship between structures comprehended in spoken language and those used in production is not straightforward for children with motor impairment who use graphic systems. Modality-specific and pragmatic variables in production may influence the need to include grammatical features and the kinds of grammatical structures and markers used (Smith, 1996b; Sutton and Morford, 1998). Whether pictographic signs used in many graphic systems are even perceived as linguistic symbols by the children using them has been questioned (Hjelmquist, 1997; Hunt-Berg and Schick, 1995).

Children who are acquiring language production using graphic signs do not have the benefit of native speaker models for production. Adults who do provide models of communication using the graphic system are typically speaking adults, not 'native speakers' of graphic signs. Opportunities for acquiring graphic sign production are therefore reduced relative to spoken language production opportunities for typically developing children and relative to spoken language comprehension opportunities for children who need graphic systems.

The transition from illocutionary to locutionary communication for children needing graphic systems may be difficult. Their non-linguistic experience with the graphic sign mode may not support its use for linguistic communication, and opportunities to attempt to match the limited graphic input they receive may be infrequent. Attempts to match spoken language input would also have limited success when motor speech production is impaired. Further, the drive to approximate input more closely, assumed to underlie the transition to use of single words in speaking children, may be weak in children with motor impairment given their previous reduced experience in vocal production.

Difficulty in attaining a level of automaticity that would support the transition to linguistic communication using graphic systems may be compounded by the additional motor effort required to communicate when the vocal mode is unreliable or not available. Attentional and cognitive resources for observing and perceiving the physical, social and linguistic environment may be reduced as a consequence (Blockberger, 1995) and it may be difficult to attend to ongoing activities while trying to produce a message for children who are learning to communicate with graphic systems.

In intervention, an adequate solution has not yet been discovered for reconciling the asymmetry between comprehension and production modes that is inherent in using graphic systems. The use of voice output communication devices for young children may serve to reduce the gap between comprehension and production because of the auditory feedback which may enhance the link between the child's own production and the spoken language of the environment. However use of voice output is still mediated by a visual-graphic display even when based on traditional orthography. Thus the modality asymmetry remains an issue.

One implication of the primacy of spoken language comprehension over production for typically developing children would be an early focus on comprehension in intervention involving alternative communication systems. Establishing spoken language comprehension is important in order to ensure progress in that mode while exploring other means of production. Comprehension of graphic signs is also critical; in order to lay the foundation for their later use as a production mode. If graphic signs are not perceived as linguistic symbols, as suggested by Hunt-Berg and Schick (1995), highlighting a possible correspondence with spoken language may help children make this transition. However, if research shows that the likelihood of coming to interpret graphic signs as linguistic is very small, then intervention strategies would be needed to develop the metalinguistic skills required to permit use of non-linguistic symbols for linguistic communication.

Establishing automaticity in graphic sign production that would support the transition to linguistic communication may require specific attention. Automaticity could be addressed through practice opportunities in which fully linguistic communication is not required (Harris and Vanderheiden, 1980). Some early intervention strategies may provide such opportunities by presenting only those response options (or a single response option) that are acceptable in the context so that the child's behaviour results in appropriate communication (e.g. Goossens, 1998). Whether opportunities could be provided this way that would be sufficiently frequent to develop the automaticity required to make the transition to linguistic communication remains an open question. For example, practice using motor activity for a communicative purpose is possible very early with the help of technology such as the *Baby Babble Blanket* (Ferrier et al., 1996). Five-month-old infants used body movement to activate their mother's voice. Whether sustained and expanded motor experience for communication would provide sufficient practice to attain automaticity requires study (Calculator, 1997).

Social–cognitive preparation for acquiring grammar

Infants seem predisposed to attend to communicative behaviours in which linguistic input is incorporated. For example, very young infants prefer faces to other visual stimuli (Johnson, Dziurawiec, Ellis and Morton, 1991; Slater and Butterworth, 1997). They respond differentially to speech versus other auditory stimuli (Columbo and Bundy, 1981) and to the language of the environment versus other languages (Moon, Cooper and Fifer, 1993). Whether these sensitivities are innate, are learned easily by a general learning mechanism, or are the result of variations in pre-natal exposure to environmental auditory stimuli is a matter of debate (Locke, 1997). Nonetheless, these social–cognitive biases may serve to guide infants toward the linguistic input in their environments (Locke, 1997, 1998).

While refining their ability to focus on linguistically relevant features of communication, infants also progress through stages in which their own non-verbal communication behaviour becomes more precise. Although there is not complete agreement in the literature regarding the nature of the stages and their transitions, early communication assessment formats are frequently based on descriptions of these stages (e.g. Wetherby and Prizant, 1993). Very young infants communicate by engaging in social interaction with adults through eye contact, affective behaviour, and gesture. Then they begin to communicate to regulate the behaviour of their conversation partners (i.e. to direct their attention, to request objects and actions). These skills develop into joint attention, in which infants seem to attempt to share communication about an object or activity with communication partners (Mundy and Gomes, 1997).

Infants with motor impairments may start out with similar social–cognitive biases that would facilitate progress towards language but they may experience non-optimal interactive environments (Paul, 1998) in which interaction from their caregivers may be reduced and more directive (Hanzlik, 1990). That the language learning experiences for children who may need graphic systems are restricted when compared with those of typically developing children is acknowledged in the literature (e.g. Calculator, 1997; Goldbart, 1998; Light, 1997; Light, Collier and Parnes, 1985a; Paul, 1997, 1998), experiences characterized by sparse communication, misinterpretation and reduced experience with the physical environment (Paul, 1998). These early experiences for children with motor impairments therefore may not be sufficiently rich and varied socially and cognitively to facilitate filtering through communication input in order to attend to linguistic structure. The guiding benefit of early social–cognitive experience towards linguistic analysis may be weakened.

Development of pre-linguistic communication skills may also be problematic for children with motor impairments. They may have developed limited awareness of the fact that their own behaviour can be used to influence others due to lack of motor control (Dunst, Cushing and Vance, 1985). Atypical gestures and affective behaviours may be difficult to decipher and therefore may be misinterpreted by communication partners (Calculator, 1997). The benefit to development believed to be provided by adult response to infants' own communication skills may be reduced as a consequence of caregivers' difficulties in interpreting diminished and atypical communication behaviours.

These potential difficulties in early social–cognitive experiences and pre-linguistic communication skills highlight the importance of early intervention for children with motor impairment who may need graphic systems. The risk of communication difficulties is known from the time of diagnosis of cerebral palsy (Billeaud, 1993), the medical condition of most children with severe physical and speech impairments who use graphic systems (Mirenda and Mathy-Laikko, 1988). Communication intervention could in principle begin at that time, and it is believed that appropriate intervention could serve to prevent or minimize the risk of severe communication disorders (Blackstone, 1990) by avoiding the development of unfavourable communication and interaction behaviours in both caregivers and infants. Social interaction, exploration and verbal input are typically stressed in early intervention with alternative communication systems for their value in social, affective, cognitive and general language development. However, the potential impact of these early experiences on later grammatical development should also be highlighted. The sooner children sort out the physical and social aspects of their world, the speech they hear, and the link between the two, the sooner they can start to focus in on grammar.

Intervention strategies designed to encourage communication partners to assign interpretations of infant communication behaviours and to shape them into more conventional forms (e.g. Cress, 1998) should also be helpful in preparing children for linguistic analysis. Increasing communication partners' frequency and contingency of interaction could also serve to bypass some of the potential adverse influence of atypical interaction patterns among users of alternative communication systems and may facilitate development of pre-linguistic communication skills believed to support linguistic development. The impact of early intervention on grammatical knowledge specifically requires further study, especially for children who need graphic communication systems. For young speaking children with language impairment, it seems that parent training alone may increase interaction for both parents and children but may not have a direct influence on children's language (Tannock, Girolometto and Seigel, 1992). Whether altering interaction patterns of caregivers would have a wider influence on language development for children needing graphic communication systems, who are more dependent on caregiver assistance in experiencing the world, than for children with normal motor and speech development is an important question for research.

Lexical preparation for acquiring grammar

Even though infants seem pre-disposed to attend to communication behaviours, they are still faced with the task of figuring out which aspects of the environment correspond to which aspects of the speech that they hear. Infants' sensitivities to relevant aspects of their environments seem to support word learning. The prosodic features of connected speech and infants' early speech perception abilities help them identify utterance and word boundaries (Jusczyk, 1997), a skill needed to learn the correspondence between words and their referents and their combining possibilities. It has been suggested that infants operate with a basic theory of physical world (Spelke, 1991) and perceptual primitives (Karmiloff-Smith, 1992). Nonetheless, these early sensitivities may help the infant to sort out both the speech input and the environment and to link the two.

Learning of specific words is dependent on experience and input, especially for content words (Blockberger, 1995). For example, children who are not exposed to the word 'iguana' are not likely to learn this word. More generally, vocabulary comprehension and production seem to be related to overall quantity of verbal input (Hart and Risley, 1995) and exposure to activities believed to facilitate language learning, such as early literacy experiences (Whitehurst, 1997). Although the hypothesis that the way caregivers speak is essential to language development ('The motherese hypothesis', Furrow, Nelson and Benedict, 1979) has been largely discounted (Gleitman, Newport and Gleitman, 1984), some adult–child interaction characteristics may facilitate word learning (Harris, 1992; Kaiser, Hemmeter and Hester, 1997). For example, some degree of joint attention is necessary for the child to comprehend the adult's utterance, and this may be established by the adult talking about something in which the child is already interested. Contingent responsiveness (partner communication that follows and is related to the child's communication) may facilitate word learning by helping children refine their understanding of the relationships among the speech that they hear, the environment, and their own communicative behaviour (Harris, 1992).

Children seem to be able to take advantage of some early syntactic awareness to learn the meanings of new words (Gleitman and Gleitman, 1992). For example, the structural characteristics of known nouns can give clues to possible meanings of a verb used in the same sentence (e.g. Fisher et al., 1994). Thus children use their emerging syntactic knowledge to learn about semantics, known as 'syntactic bootstrapping'. It has also been suggested that children's semantic and real world knowledge can help them learn some of the syntactic properties of new words (Karmiloff-Smith, 1992). For example, a new word referring to an action is likely to be within the syntactic category verb (e.g. Pinker, 1984). Thus semantic knowledge may help children learn about syntax, 'semantic bootstrapping'. In addition to these processes, constraints on word learning, at least for object names (Golinkoff, Mervis and Hirsh-Pasek, 1994; Markman, 1992), seem to make vocabulary acquisition a more manageable task for young children. Although the specific nature of these constraints is not uncontroversial (Merriman and Tomasello, 1995), it seems that the meanings that children might consider for new words are not completely open but seem to be restricted to a limited range of possibilities. For example, children seem to be aware that a new object label usually refers to a whole object rather than just one part (Mervis and Bertrand, 1993) and that novel object labels refer to unknown objects rather than known objects (Merriman, Marazita and Jarvis, 1995).

Children usually have a production vocabulary of several single words before they begin to make two-word combinations (estimates vary, but Paul, 1998, suggests 50 words). Emergence of word combinations is typically associated with a rapid increase in expressive and receptive vocabulary size (Paul, 1998). Some characteristics of a caregiver's behaviour seem to facilitate use of utterances of increasing length and syntactic and semantic complexity (Kaiser, Hemmeter and Hester, 1997). For example, use of social routines (familiar and limited social contexts) may permit increased attention to structural characteristics of adults' speech. Modelling provides examples of sentences and expansions present slightly more complex restatements of child utterances. These types of adult inter-active behaviours may encourage syntactic production by children.

Whether infants with severe physical impairment have perceptual and cognitive biases similar to those of typically developing infants is an open question. If these early sensitivities are present initially, their develop-mental paths may diverge from those of typically developing children due to differences in physical and perceptual experience with the environ-ment. Distorted or reduced sensory input and limited movement may increase the difficulty of sorting out and linking auditory and visual stimuli. Further, it may be difficult for both infants and caregivers to estab-lish joint attention when child behaviours are easily misinterpreted. Use of a graphic sign display disrupts typical joint attention behaviours because both partners need to look at the display as well as at the objects and activ-ities in the environment. Word learning may be slowed or limited as a consequence of these differences.

Children with motor impairment may experience reduced verbal input due to their own limited verbal output and atypical non-verbal communi-cation behaviours (Blackstone, 1997). Many authors have reported that interaction patterns in conversations involving individuals using graphic communication systems differ from those in which both partners use speech (e.g. Kraat, 1985; Light, Collier and Parnes, 1985a), and tend to be characterized by more passive communication and few utterances by the individual using the graphic system (Paul, 1998). Early literacy activities, believed to be an important language learning context especially for children with limited speech, may also be reduced and may differ qualita-tively for these children (Light and Kelford-Smith, 1993) due to their diffi-culties in responding and the increased time required for personal care (Crowe, 1993). Syntactic and semantic bootstrapping processes and word-learning constraints may not be well developed as a consequence of these differences.

Children with severe physical impairments may acquire smaller vocab-ulary (even in comprehension) than those of typically developing children due to reduced vocabulary learning opportunities. They may acquire the vocabulary size needed to support combinations too slowly or too late to support the transition from the one-word stage to the use of combina-tions. The limited vocabulary available on graphic sign displays and the altered interaction patterns may not facilitate adults' use of modelling and expansion at a level that could be useful to the child.

Interventions that focus on acquiring a large vocabulary may facilitate grammatical learning by providing the 'critical mass' of vocabulary needed to initiate grammatical analysis processes and use of word combinations. Intervention practices such as multiple single-topic displays, aided language stimulation, and large-vocabulary displays may be helpful for word learning because a variety of vocabularies can be introduced. These strategies may support grammatical acquisition as a result of increased vocabulary knowledge and as a benefit of increased opportunities for adult communication partners to provide modelling and expansion.

Joint attention may be an important skill to establish, not only for its communicative value and its contribution to word learning, but also as a way of facilitative graphic sign learning. For example, Hunt-Berg (1998) found that children learned new pictures more quickly when joint attention to the target object was established prior to saying the word and pointing to the corresponding picture. Syntactic and semantic bootstrapping processes may be important to establish due to their potential benefit to vocabulary acquisition through comprehension experiences. Although it is not obvious how such processes could be targeted specifically in intervention, this may be one way in which picture-book reading is helpful for early language development. It could be speculated that repetitious spoken and visual input may help children sort out structural and semantic features that can be used to support learning of novel words.

Discussion

Models of development and the potential obstacles in grammatical knowledge acquisition for children with motor impairment who need graphic systems discussed above seem generally consistent with current thinking on brain and language development, although the relationships among language learning experiences, brain mechanisms, and language development clearly require much additional exploration and research. Acquisition of grammatical knowledge takes place in the brain. Constraints on grammatical knowledge acquisition, whether specifically linguistic principles and parameters or domain general learning processes (e.g. Braine, 1988), must be ultimately expressible in terms of brain mechanisms (formation of synapses, layers and regional connections, and timing of growth and pruning) (Elman et al., 1996). Knowledge is viewed as a set of distributed representations that support behaviour, that is 'fine-grained patterns of cortical activity, which in turn depend on specific patterns of synaptic connectivity' (Elman et al., 1996, p. 364). Constraints on development could shape mature representations of grammatical knowledge and processing mechanisms for comprehension and production (e.g. working memory, connections between representations, Bishop, 1997), but could not pre-determine that specific knowledge content would be learned universally. Nonetheless, linguistic processing could become isolated from other types of processing over time even if learning is initially domain-general (Karmiloff-Smith, 1992).

The fact of development provides a way of conceptualizing learning of very complex behaviours and knowledge representations from minimally specified structures (Elman et al., 1996), consistent with the models discussed briefly above (Clark, 1995; Karmiloff-Smith, 1992; Locke, 1997). Children do not attempt to sort out all aspects of the environmental language from the beginning. Limited processing capacities focus them on certain aspects of linguistic input before others. Modularity, or isolation of linguistic processing (e.g. Fodor, 1983), may be a consequence of development rather than pre-specified or innate (Karmiloff-Smith, 1992).

Timing of stimulation relative to brain development seems critical, although regulation of timing is not fully understood. The same input may have different effects (or non-effects) on the immature brain, and therefore on the knowledge representations acquired, when presented at different points in development. This has been demonstrated repeatedly in experimental studies of animals. Language research with deaf individuals who have learned language at different points during their lives (Mayberry, 1993, 1994) has highlighted that appropriate input within a certain time frame seems essential in acquiring full grammatical competence. In typical development, points of linguistic transitions seem to be correlated with brain development. For example, the vocabulary spurt and onset of two-word combinations is believed to coincide with a period of rapid increase in synapses within and across cortical regions (Elman et al., 1996, p. 289). If appropriately timed input is not provided or the typical developmental pathway is blocked, however, the plasticity of the brain may permit development through alternative pathways (Bleile, 1998; Elman et al., 1996; Karmiloff-Smith, 1997; Neville, 1997). Some children achieve what appears to be normal or typical grammatical behaviour through routes that are known to be atypical, for example because of documented neurological differences (Karmiloff-Smith, 1997).

If children with motor impairment who need graphic systems acquire grammatical knowledge of the spoken environmental language through atypical developmental paths, there may be subtle differences in speech comprehension when probed, even in children who achieve 'behavioural mastery' (Karmiloff-Smith, 1992, 1997). Fine-grained analysis of comprehension of grammar would be needed to detect subtle distinctions in performance. It would be of interest to know whether some of the grammatical comprehension difficulties seen in children with language impairment, such as difficulty with hierarchical structures, dependent relationships and under-specified sentence constituents (Bishop, 1997) may be found in children who use graphic systems. Such comparisons could provide a context in which to examine theoretical questions regarding the nature of language disorder. For example, similarities in grammatical features found to be problematic across children with very different underlying conditions, like neuromotor impairment and language impairment, could be interpreted as evidence that the difficulties noted reflect particularly vulnerable aspects of grammar and may suggest that similar intervention strategies may be helpful. Differences, in contrast, could suggest that the language comprehension difficulties, if any, of children who use graphic systems reflect their particular developmental course. Alternative intervention strategies may be more appropriate in that case.

Whether language intervention strategies should focus on variables believed to facilitate the normal language acquisition process or should focus on alternative teaching strategies has been a matter of debate in the field of augmentative and alternative communication (see Baker, 1998, and Rowland, 1998, for a summary of some of the issues). The importance of timing in brain development suggests that intervention strategies based on typical language development variables may be most effective only within the typical developmental time frame. If the relevant milestones have not been achieved in a timely manner, more overt teaching strategies may be needed. Brain plasticity suggests that alternative paths of development may be promoted if the typical one is not available. Although statistics show that a large proportion of individuals with motor disabilities related to brain damage such as cerebral palsy have some degree of intellectual impairment (Love and Webb, 1996), normal range and high levels of achievement by some individuals (e.g. Willard-Holt, 1998) support the claim that language difficulties are not a necessary consequence. It may be equally important to study variables that have contributed to the success of these individuals as well as variables believed to hinder development in individuals whose mature abilities are more limited.

In establishing priorities, it may be useful to recognize whether variations between learning an alternative language form and what is achieved in the typical developmental situation represent differences or deficits. Whitehurst (1997) proposed three distinctions regarding comparisons with typical spoken language communication. When applied to augmentative and alternative communication, these distinctions would suggest varying levels of concern for intervention, prevention and research priorities. Some observed contrasts may be comparative differences only, with no associated value judgement. Comparative differences will always be present, just as there are comparative differences between dialect and language groups, and may not be a cause for concern. For example, use of non-speech mode may represent a comparative difference from spoken communication, if there is social acceptance of its use in the individual's environment. If so, changing the communication mode itself would not be a priority for intervention. Other dissimilarities may represent competitive deficits on variables that have cultural or social value. For example, independent communication seems valued in Western cultures, and may be one factor involved in successful social integration for individuals who use graphic systems (McNaughton, Mann, Harrington and Harrington, 1988). Reduced independence in communication may therefore represent an intervention issue. Even greater emphasis would be placed on differences judged to represent absolute deficits that would result in a disadvantage independent of cultural setting. For example, reduced or atypical grammatical knowledge acquired by individuals with motor impairment who need graphic systems, if such differences are documented in research studies, might be considered an absolute deficit that would constitute a risk factor for spoken language comprehension, development of graphic language production, and literacy activities for academic, leisure and employment purposes.

Although the language learning experiences of children with motor impairment who need graphic systems may present obstacles to acquisition of grammatical knowledge, language intervention for individuals who require alternative communication systems indicates belief in the possibility of changing the current environment to reduce or eliminate unfavourable effects of earlier experience, which is itself a result of interactions among internal and environmental variables. A deeper understanding of the variables that have an impact on grammatical knowledge acquisition for children who use graphic systems will lead to more effective interventions to facilitate the development of beneficial contexts for social–cognitive and lexical learning that will clarify the language learning task and support grammatical knowledge acquisition as a consequence.

Chapter 6
Reflections on the Development of Alternative Language Forms

JUDITH D. OXLEY AND STEPHEN VON TETZCHNER

The preceding chapters in the present section bring together diverse lines of research that, nevertheless, hang together through several important themes. First, they raise theoretical issues that are basic to the understanding of the language acquisition processes of users of alternative communication systems. To understand this process, there must be agreement upon answers to the classical questions of how language is best defined, and under what conditions a set of behaviours may be considered language. Second, the papers address the specific problems of how language learned through atypical ways and atypical forms may provide insight into language development in general.

The use of graphic representations as a primary system of communication raises special challenges to current understanding of language realization in this modality. This issue has already been addressed in the field of manual sign language development. There is no longer any dispute that national sign languages constitute language proper, complete with modality-specific grammatical systems. These languages convey meaning equivalently, but not as direct recoding of the spoken form. Thus, they can be seen as independent of their spoken counterparts. Currently, however, there is no cultural graphic language that is completely independent of spoken or manual sign forms. Across the world, a number of different graphic signs systems exist, such as Picture Communication Symbols (PCS), Compic and Pictographic Ideographic Communication (PIC) (see von Tetzchner and Jensen, 1996b; Lloyd, Arvidson and Williams, 1998). These systems are analogous to hybrid systems of manual signs, such as Signed Norwegian (Norges Døverforbund, 1988) and Signing Exact English (Gustason, Pfetzing and Zawolkow, 1980), which attempt to recode spoken language into a manually signed equivalent; that is, one with manual markers for spoken morphology and so forth. Hence, one may consider graphic communication systems cited as derived forms of spoken language that solely consist of recoded spoken expressions in a graphic mode, directly or indirectly. The lack of correspondence between spoken input and graphic output is not in itself evidence against such recoding, only against a simple transformation which maintains isomorphy.

The acquisition problem becomes more complicated by the fact that some children develop graphic communication prior to developing spoken language. Clearly, these children are not necessarily recoding anything. In these cases, one may be inclined to attribute the graphic communication a status similar to deictic gestures in normal development of spoken language, but this is defied by the word-like quality of the way graphic signs are used. They appear to be more similar to symbolic than to deictic gestures, and applying deictic status to graphic productions may be mistaken. In typical development, spoken words and symbolic gestures seem to appear at almost the same time (Iverson and Thal, 1998), and first graphic signs may be accorded a similar status. Moreover, graphic sign production may demonstrate structure in the absence of spoken and manual language comprehension (von Tetzchner et al., 1998). In addition to supporting the possibility of non-dependence of graphic language upon spoken language, this finding would also undermine the foundation of intervention aimed at developmental augmentation, which may consist of both simultaneous and total communication. Both strategies are based on the principle that language may develop in different forms, and that these forms support each other. In fact, in cases where speech follows manual or graphic sign use, these modes are primary from a developmental perspective. Moreover, they may be primary because of deficits in the individual child's capacity to comprehend spoken language and the ability to learn another mode.

Describing development

Development is a process of change over time that comprises all aspects of functioning and is the result of an interaction between biological and environmental conditions. According to the orthogenetic principle of Heinz Werner (1948), development is positive, and comprises more complex organization, greater differentiation, and so forth. For all species, development implies a higher degree of self-reliance and independence of the parents. Children exhibiting typical language development rapidly use more words and more complex morphosyntactic structures to enable them to displace their talk from the immediate setting and decrease their reliance on parents for interpretation. Thus, language production serves as a window to development.

However, it is not at all clear how an emerging grammar should be described for children acquiring alternative language forms. The traditional approach has been to use the grammar of spoken language to evaluate developmental status, but the validity of this approach is questionable. One obstacle to the traditional approach is the observation that morphosyntactic structures seemingly not based on spoken language have been demonstrated in users of manual and graphic sign systems (Smith and Grove, Chapter 2, this volume; Soto, Chapter 4, this volume). These structures may be regarded as evidence of emerging or distinct grammars; or alternatively for strategies that compensate for the lack of vocabulary and grammatical markers corresponding to spoken language. In other words, differences need not reflect deficits.

An obstacle to descriptions of the developmental courses of alternative language forms is uncertainty with regard to the reliability of the units that are used. Surprisingly, descriptions of manual sign production sometimes fail even to distinguish between the meaning of the manual sign used, including pronominal reference by means of its location, and the meaning that may be understood from somebody indicating something in other ways, for example pointing at an object (e.g. Goldin-Meadow and Mylander, 1990). This emphasizes the need for describing both the intended meaning of an utterance (i.e. hypothesized or verified), and the form of its actual expression, together with the gloss of the expression. The basic notations suggested in von Tetzchner and Jensen (1996b) and used in this section may be helpful in achieving this goal.

There are problems related to the identification of utterance boundaries, and whether utterances are structured vertically or horizontally (cf. Scollon, 1976; von Tetzchner and Martinsen, 1996). This can be hard to do with manual sign language, but it is even more complicated with multimodal messages. In order to apply, for example, mean length of utterance (Brown, 1973) as a measure of language development, reliable guidelines for segmenting multimodal utterances is imperative. Also 'word order' descriptions are hampered by problems related to segmenting multimodal utterances into 'words', or even recognizing that a multimodal combination is a structure. Similar problems have been evident in descriptions of simultaneous production of two or more manual signs (Klima and Bellugi, 1979). In the case of communication board users, one may have to decide whether the utterance should include manner or path of pointing, in addition to the actual object of the point. When addressing these problems, some of the lessons from the development of descriptions of the morphosyntax of manual sign may prove helpful.

Finally, as long as the parameters of development of alternative communication systems remain obscure, it is impossible to appraise the impact of special learning experiences on language acquisition, and hence to use typical development of atypical language forms as a model for intervention.

Representation and communication mode

Children can learn the meaning of graphic signs in two ways: implicitly and explicitly. During their acquisition of graphic signs, children may learn the signs' meanings implicitly through dialogue and situational cues in the environment, where the relevance of any given feature or combination of features to a particular setting is a crucial factor. The process is somewhat analogous to the process of fast-mapping, in which children draw inferences about the meaning of a new word from the immediate context (Pinker, 1982). However, unlike graphic signs, spoken words are typically not iconic; that is, onomatopoeia rarely is available to cue a word's meaning (Grove, 1997). By contrast, most designers of graphic communication systems have utilized iconic semantic features in the graphic representations used to refer to categories of objects, actions or other states of affairs (Oxley, 1996). The contribution of iconicity to learnability is much discussed, and is generally claimed to be a facilitating factor (Fuller and Lloyd, 1997), although its actual function in the communication process is still obscure.

The iconicity apparent in most graphic communication systems has led to questions about the underlying referents of pictographic systems. Interpretations of the sign SIT from PCS have been presented to illustrate this problem of reference (Smith, 1996b; Smith and Grove, Chapter 2, this volume). This graphic sign depicts a stick-figure person seated on a chair (Figure 6.1). According to Smith and Grove, one may ask whether it refers to concrete elements (person, chair), to the relationship between the elements (on), to the action of the actor (sit), or to temporal aspects of the action setting (sits, is sitting). It is also possible that the sign form actually conveys all of those elements simultaneously. This analysis seriously questions the validity of the practice of allocating traditional word classes to pictographic graphic signs. It is also worth noting that these possible aspects of meaning are all both iconic and conventional and arbitrary, but the very fact that questions about the meaning or use of a sign tend to be related to the sign's form indicates that the pictographic information is taken literally rather than conventionally (e.g. 'on' may be depicted via reference to a light switch, clothes on a person, or one object or person situated on something). The fact that the PCS system sometimes has different graphic signs for different senses of the same spoken word may be taken as further evidence for a bias toward literal interpretation of the sign's form; that is, that the PCS system is independent of the corresponding spoken word that is indicated by the written gloss, a vestige of the system's original design. A valid question is how conflicts between gloss and graphic connotation are resolved by users and communication partners.

One may note that PCS dictionaries without written glosses have recently been produced to address a growing public demand. It may be that this demand is driven in part by conflicts between gloss and meaning, and by a wish to use the possibilities of the graphic medium more fully.

Children may also be taught a sign's meaning explicitly as a translation of or code for a spoken word (Martinsen and von Tetzchner, 1996; von

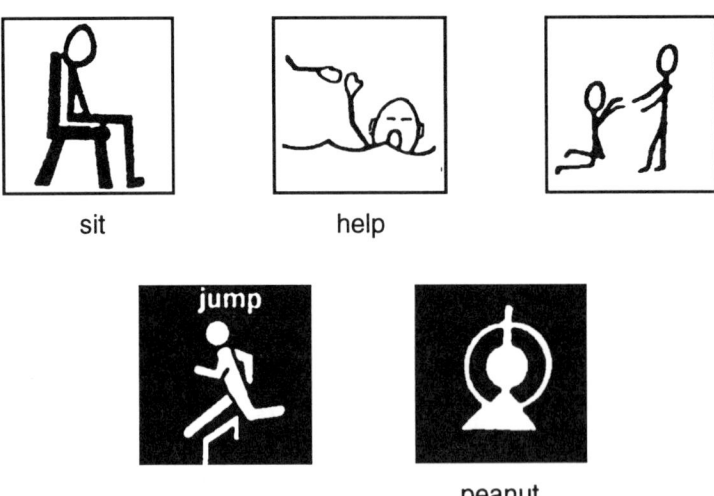

Figure 6.1. PCS: SIT, HELP1, HELP2; PIC: JUMP; Lexigram: PEANUT.

Tetzchner et al., 1996). Neither approach is dependent on iconicity, that is, pictographic similarity. Studies involving associative learning by speaking children seem to indicate a positive effect for iconicity (see von Tetzchner and Martinsen, 1992). On the other hand, the studies of Romski and associates using the non-iconic Lexigrams have also demonstrated considerable success (Romski and Sevcik, 1996). However, it should be noted first, that these Lexigram studies include communication aids with artificial speech, and second, that the intervention was not very successful for the children with poor comprehension of spoken language, indicating that the project applied explicit rather than implicit teaching. Moreover, it is possible that the children with limited comprehension of spoken language would have done better with a more iconic communication system; that is, one in which the form of the signs inherently cued their meaning. This method would assume that the children could detect the cues, understand them, and use them strategically to aid comprehension (Oxley and Norris, in review).

Iconicity may not, however, always be helpful. People in the environment may be so attentive to what they consider the prominent iconic feature that it limits the number of different contextual interpretations. If pictographic signs are interpreted literally by the user, the partner, or both, iconicity may make acquisition harder. As with other contextual cues, the principle of relevance applies (Sperber and Wilson, 1986). Children using photographs or pictographic communication systems must learn which features of the picture are relevant and therefore deserving of their attention. The PIC sign JUMP illustrates this point. It depicts a man jumping, and in order to use pictographic information as a relevant cue to meaning, the child must somehow learn to ignore the man figure and focus on his action. Moreover, whether the graphic sign is treated as linguistic or non-linguistic may depend on the ability to ignore the iconic element to some extent. Iconic features must be treated in a conventional or symbolic manner rather than as elements of a picture.

Considering the restrictions that typically apply to graphic vocabulary size, it would be parsimonious and creative to vary the aspects employed. The relevance of a particular aspect of the graphic sign would depend on context. Changes in the ability to segregate and use different aspects of the signs productively (both literally and metaphorically) may well be an important constituent of the acquisition of graphic language. It is not known when children using graphic communication are able to decompose a whole picture into meaningful elements or how this skill proceeds developmentally. Moreover, the features children are capable of extracting are limited by their developmental status, which tends to make them vulnerable to contextual distractions (Oxley, 1996). Note that relevance, like deixis, is a dynamic phenomenon. Although pictographic signs are themselves static representations, usually of a selected set of attributes, interpreters are subject to the influence of ever-changing contextual cues that tend to alter their disposition to detect certain features. This characteristic is particularly true of young children whose representations lack the stability of their adult counterparts.

The research into speech and visual processing by adherents of parallel distributed processing and connectionist models tends to support the view that relevance is dynamic. At some level in the brain, certain features of the stimulation are apt to be amplified or attenuated according to contextual probabilities, so that the information made available to conscious reflection is altered in a predictable way (Elman et al., 1996). This model is helpful in understanding how it is that an iconic graphic sign may be subject to multiple interpretations. The potential flexibility of purely pictographic communication (unconfounded by written glosses or voice output) should be a useful property, enabling one sign to fulfil many roles. However, this flexibility may be greatly compromised when the domain of its reference is reduced by a gloss, or accompanying voice output. This point reinforces the importance of a fundamental question concerning the nature of pictographic sign referents (spoken words, real world referents, ideas, etc.); that is, whether the learners infer meaning from the picture, or impute meaning to it, similar to how patterns of speech sounds and hand shapes and movements are categorized with the help of meaning in normal signed and spoken language development (cf. Smith and Leinonen, 1992). An investigation into the possibilities of graphic communication may lead to the discovery of a potential for advanced linguistic communication (Soto, this volume), or to the more pessimistic view that graphic representations can never function as independent language, only as a secondary form derived from speech or manual sign (Hjelmquist, 1997, Chapter 3, this volume).

Related to these issues is the question of whether there exists a strategy or strategies specific to the graphic mode that would be 'natural' for the interpretation of expressions in this mode. In the speaking community, numerous conventions are used to add meaning to static pictures. They include deliberate use of perspective (depth, close-up, distance, varied angle of observation, etc.), figure–ground contrast, shading, highlighting of outlines or portions of outlines, colouring, conventionally accepted notations for movement, spatial relationships between elements, and so forth (Mineo Mollica and Peischl, 1997). These conventions may influence the interpretation of the message communicated by someone using picto-graphic representations to communicate. One may speculate what a truly graphic language mode would look like if such conventions were actively used. Some conventions might be used to create inflections, similar to the analogue inflections used in manual signs to mark size (for some categories of manual signs, the amplitude of the sign reflects the size of the object referred to, such as SMALL-CAR and BIG-CAR). The hand shape of GIVE may vary subtly according to physical dimensions of the item being given. GIVE-PEN, GIVE-BALL and GIVE-CUP would systematically reflect the various object shapes (Klima and Bellugi, 1979; Martinsen, Nordeng and von Tetzchner, 1985).

However, even if relevant strategies exist, it is not certain that adults who use spoken language, and do not share a graphic language culture, know what the relevant features of graphic signs are, or that there is a set of relevant features. The lack of a language community may be crucial (see below). There is nothing inherently special about the movements of manual signs. It is the users' attribution of conventional symbolic meaning to them that turns them into language. One reason iconic graphic signs may fail to function as language proper may be that they are treated by adults in the environment as pictures instead of elements of meaning.

Syntax and morphology

Acknowledging that graphic signs carry meaning, Hjelmquist (1997) raises the question of whether it is possible to develop a grammar for pictorial-graphic systems. Indeed, both research and anecdotal evidence support this possibility by supplying examples of individuals 'inventing' grammat-ical features to meet pressing communicative needs. There is no obvious reason why the visual structures described above, for example, could not be used to emphasize topics and salient arguments in a way that is analogue to word order in speech. Word order is one tool that enables this process in speech, creating, for example, sentence forms such as clefts, pseudoclefts, passives and declaratives. However, despite the possibilities, some obvious constraints, both real and artefactual, on grammatical devel-opment must be considered.

First, it is acknowledged that the realization of syntax and morphology of graphic systems is connected to their visual properties. Second, structure may be influenced, and even compromised, by the user's motor speed and coordination. Third, structure may be imposed by the forced choices users must make, given the actual availability of graphic signs. The same principle will apply to people with limited spoken and manual vocabularies. Indeed, part of the motivation for the development of a pidgin language, characterized by limited grammar, is lack of shared vocabulary. Thus, a lack of observable linguistic qualities in graphic system use may not reflect a problem of representation so much as problems related to limited vocabulary and literal interpretation and usage.

In *Philosophical Investigations* (1953) Wittgenstein asks: 'What is your aim in philosophy? – To show the fly the way out of the fly-bottle' (§ 309). The spoken language bias of the communication partners of children who use alternative communication systems may influence their interpretations in such a profound and unreflective manner that crucial behaviours are missed due to an expectation that the communicator will indicate a particular set of elements in a particular order. When the order of selection of graphic signs does not follow the expected pattern of the spoken language, the resultant forms may be labelled as error forms and evaluated as impoverished productions. This may be particularly apparent in teaching sessions. Communication partners may provide a slightly more generous interpretation; that is, that perhaps the user is communicating telegraphically (i.e. incompletely) to save time and thus mitigate the challenges to the chronemic conventions of the speaking community. Indeed, communicative competence may be reflected in the sacrifice of form to sustain an interaction (Nelson, 1992).

Parallel to developments within child language in general and sign language development in particular, a different perspective suggests that the 'errors' may not be errors at all, and that the output reflects a unique adaptation to the linguistic means available to the user. For example, it may be redundant to include individual morphological markers for spatial relationships isomorphic to spoken language when those relationships are inherent in the graphic (see above example of the chair). The use of analogical inflections in manual sign languages supports this possibility (see above example of BIG-DOG), and so does the fact that isomorphic manual representations of spoken language have constantly failed to be adopted by deaf communities since L'Epée introduced 'methodological signs' 200 years ago.

It has been noted that communication breakdowns, which are common in aided communication, may increase if users deviate from the word order of the spoken language. In English-speaking societies, for example, confusion arises when a person points first to a modifier, and then to the remaining elements of a sentence. This order of operations has resulted in confusion about which element of the sentence the modifier was supposed to be modifying. There is also evidence that rather unexpected factors may influence word order, such as the positioning of the items on a communication board. It follows that in these cases, repositioning items may reduce the problem. One possible convention that may increase effectiveness is to indicate question and exclamation marks before the utterance, like in Spanish text, to prepare the communication partner for the type of sentence that is coming. Similar strategies may be found in British Sign Language, where 'bracketing' with question signs like WHY is used to indicate scope.

Last, it should be noted that descriptions of unusual syntax have not dominated graphic language development; rather, it has been a complete lack of syntax (i.e. reliance on single-sign utterances) that has been noted. Typically speaking children have 15–50 words before they start to combine words into a grammar, and it has been suggested that one possible reason for the lack of multi-sign utterances is that motor-impaired children who use graphic signs do not have enough 'volume' to move on to the next step of combining signs (see Sutton, Chapter 5, this volume). However, it has also been observed that children with graphic vocabularies that greatly exceed 50 words have been found to use mainly single-sign utterances. This finding suggests that the hypothesis of 'volume' may be insufficient to account for their failure to develop use of multi-word utterances in the same general sequence as their speaking peers.

Pre-linguistic forms of graphic communication

Another theme concerns the identity of immature forms of graphic modalities. The development of the phonological system proceeds as children hear spoken language and produce vocalizations in the form of babbling, through vocables, word approximations and words (Ferguson, 1978). Children play with syllable shapes, alliteration, segmentation, and so forth. It is possible that babbling plays a transitional role in speech development by automating the production of speech. It is recognized that babbling reflects infants' experimentation with the sound system of a language; the building blocks of speech. There is no doubt that children's brains gradually adapt to the particular sounds pertinent to their speaking environment (Aslin, Juszyk and Pisoni, 1998). Segmentation of the speech stream is also implicated in this brain work.

Petitto and Marentette (1991) describe immature patterns of manual signing that parallel babbling and which they have termed 'mabbling'. Boyes-Braem (1973) and McIntire (1977) have described childish hand forms produced by young children acquiring manual signs. Children who have early access to artificial speech seem to use their communication aids for play and experimentation. The question is whether users of graphic communication systems have access to similar immature forms, or use the graphic forms they have been provided in a manner similar to babbling; that is, some type of 'grabbling' that reflects young children's active experimentation with the elements of a graphic system that are made available to them. Moreover, if grabbling exists, one may ask what kind of experience may facilitate a transition from picture-graphic grabble to graphic language. Another possibility is that many graphic system users get the system at such a late stage that babbling is no longer functional (von Tetzchner, 1997). This is a question that may be answerable by practitioners who are responsible for providing communication to very young children who need graphic systems.

Related to the question of grabbling is whether parallels to the reciprocal imitations often seen in child–adult interactions may be found in dyads with children using graphic communication, and what forms such interactions may take. The seminal research of Selma Fraiberg (1977) on caregiver–child interaction is particularly relevant to this discussion. She was the first to identify clearly the particular forms used by blind infants as exploratory behaviours and pre-symbolic communication. She also recognized that caregivers required training first to detect the relevant behaviours, and next to react appropriately to them. As one moves toward earlier introduction of tangible and pictographic signs for young, non-speaking children (or children at risk), it is imperative to understand the mechanics of an object-based and picture-based graphic mode. For example, young children have problems understanding the symbolic function of an object, that is, that it represents something other than itself.

Reading skills

One aspect of phonological development is its link to the acquisition of reading skills. Babbling and sound play in the development of typically developing children continue into rhyming and other activities that may enhance phonological awareness and sound segmentation. Hjelmquist and colleagues (Hjelmquist, Chapter 3, this volume) have been pursuing research into the latent and observable phonological development of non-speaking children, with the goal of establishing its relationship to learning basic reading skills. Provided that access to an articulatory level of representation is a necessary condition for learning to read and spell, the question is how to provide similar experiences for children without the ability to articulate. Creative use of speech synthesis appears to be the most appropriate strategy. A further complication is that children with very poor articulatory skill may actually experience interference in their developing phonological system of representation.

From a complementary perspective, recent research comparing literate and pre-literate (i.e. those who are illiterate due to lack of education) has demonstrated large, significant differences in their ability to recognize spoken nonsense words, without similar differences in their ability to recognize meaningful spoken words (Castro-Caldas et al., 1998). PET scans displayed differences in cerebral functioning during the two tasks, and thus indicated that learning to read and write during childhood influences the functional organization of the adult brain. The implication for people who cannot speak may be that their development of phonological skills both influences their acquisition of reading, and is itself influenced by the individuals' failure to acquire reading skills. In the study by Castro-Caldas and associates, the recognition of meaningful spoken words was not influenced by literacy. However, it seems likely that the learning of new words in circumstances with few contextual cues to meaning may be more difficult for non-speaking children, who either lack reading skills or have poor reading skills, than for typically speaking and reading children.

The language culture

A recurring issue in discussions of language acquisition is the role of a cultural environment in enabling people to acquire a formal system of language (Nelson, 1996). The lack of parents and other caregivers who use the same language form and imitate significant, potential communicative forms of non-speaking children may be particularly detrimental to language acquisition. The importance of role models to the language learning process has been established through studies of caregiver scaffolding that assists typically speaking children in moving to greater linguistic complexity. Scaffolding techniques by deaf caregivers have also been richly documented, whereas equivalent research for children who use alternative communication systems is lacking. Populations include both children whose uptake is primarily spoken language, and children with limited comprehension of spoken language whose output includes use of graphic signs. The interpretative role of caregivers has been implicated in the overinterpreting of selected behaviours into conventional ways of achieving particular communicative acts (Ryan, 1977; von Tetzchner and Martinsen, 1992).

Characteristics of competent models might include fluent use of graphic signs, comparable dependence on them for communication, and use of comparable methods of access. These models may include adults who use various forms of graphic signs, photographs and pictures. In addition to competent models, children need competent scaffolders; that is, people who understand how best to accomplish language facilitation within the target mode. Scaffolding strategies for beginning manual signers have been shown to differ according to the fluency of the parent in signing; thus, deaf mothers scaffold their deaf children differently and more effectively than the hearing counterparts. Such experienced users are hardly ever available to young users of graphic signs, who never learn as apprentices. It is always adults with their main competence in spoken language and orthographic text who must serve as models, and modelling usually only happens within structured teaching situations. For the evolution of functional graphic language conventions, communities of users – even on a temporary basis – may be more useful than working committees of natural speakers.

Well-formed linguistic utterances of manual sign language exist, complete with modality-specific systems of morphology, syntax and 'phonology' or cherology (Bulwer, 1644; Klima and Bellugi, 1979; Siple and Fischer, 1991). However, hearing persons typically do not grow up in the environments where sign language is in common use, that is, deaf communities. In some sense, the input these users receive is – at best – comparable to pidgin languages: the lexicon is derived from a manual sign language or system, while the syntax and morphology are drawn from the spoken language. More often, as amply demonstrated by Grove, Dockrell and Woll (1996), there is no consistent syntax or morphology in the signing output of people in the environment. The availability of language models is even more limited for children who use graphic communication systems. There is no natural all-purpose language that has pictures as its basic elements, except for written forms like Chinese that are derived from and function as a supplement to the spoken language. This means that children who acquire manual and graphic signs have to invent their own language structure. This may be a difficult but, to some extent, feasible achievement for children with good cognitive skills. However, for children with cognitive impairments it may be unobtainable.

The pidgin analogy may be extended. Pidgin languages are typically established in limited settings, usually to facilitate trading. Research on creole languages shows that children developing language in the context of spoken pidgin expand the use to other settings and create their own syntax and morphology. However, the language situation for such children is very different from that of children who use manual and graphic signs. Their actual use of language may be less restricted than trading pidgins, but significantly more limited than creoles (von Tetzchner, 1985, 1996).

The realization of syntax and morphology of manual sign languages is intimately connected to their visual, motor and kinaesthetic properties. Information is presented both sequentially and simultaneously. Two lines of research investigating use of graphic and manual signs suggest that children learning to communicate with these forms, but without a cultural environment to support them, appear to be creating creole-like language: users of PCS and manual signs change word order from the one canonical to their spoken-language environment; and manual signers appear to be inventing modality-specific morphology that resembles features of formal sign language.

Sociocultural influences may also be important for compensating for the asynchrony between receptive and expressive language. Several authors suggest that large numbers of experiences prepare a foundation for linguistic development (Locke, 1995; Nelson, 1986, 1996). It very likely that children who acquire alternative communication systems have less preparation of this kind than other children.

Concluding comment

The issues raised in the present and the preceding chapters of this section on language development document some of the small and fragmented bits of theoretical and empirical knowledge that have been gained in recent years. However, these reflections emphasize that the old questions remain unresolved and that many new questions need to be addressed. The greatest achievement to date in understanding the acquisition and use of different alternative communication systems appears to be a better grasp of the problem in the form of a frame of reference. Now it seems possible that researchers and practitioners may be able to use this frame of reference to begin to put the pieces together and solve the alternative language acquisition puzzle.

Acknowledgement

The present chapter comprises some of the issues that were discussed during the symposium on language development. The collaborative effort of the symposium and the participants' shared ownership of the ideas discussed are acknowledged. However, the present authors are responsible for the interpretations and perspectives presented here.

Section II
Natural Language
Processing

Chapter 7
Language Processing Techniques and Resources for Communication Aids

STEFAN LANGER, SHERI HUNNICUTT AND
MARIANNE HICKEY

Introduction

This chapter summarizes activities in natural language processing concerned with augmentative and alternative communication (AAC) applications, and AAC applications that use non-trivial natural language processing (NLP) techniques. First we present a short state of the art for the intersection of the two research fields, including the results of the first two workshops on NLP for AAC in Dundee and Madrid including related publications.

Within the last decade, the face of research on natural language processing has changed. One major tendency is the increased orientation towards robust techniques that can be used for real applications. The increased availability of electronic text has led to a quest for practical solutions to process unrestricted text and to a greater consumer interest in NLP applications such as reliable machine translation, text summarization, automatic indexing and dialogue systems. This quest for real-world applications has also led to an influx of statistical techniques into research on language processing.

The second development is closely related to the first. Recent years have seen the emergence of comprehensive language-related resources, such as large corpora and broad coverage electronic dictionaries. Some of these resources are freely available, and some are even distributed on the Internet.

Until recently, AAC applications did not receive much attention in NLP, nor did AAC research follow closely developments in NLP. Beginning in 1996, however, there have been several activities and publications for the purpose of exchange and collaboration between the two research fields.

Workshops

The first workshop on NLP for AAC was held at the Applied Computing Department at the University of Dundee, September 1996. The second workshop on the same subject took place at the conference of the European Chapter of the Association for Computational Linguistics/ Association for Computational Linguistics in Madrid, July 1997. The third workshop took place at the research symposium after the 1998 ISAAC conference in Dublin.

Publications

Some results of the first workshop and additional papers on NLP and AAC have been published in a special issue of the *Journal of Natural Language Engineering* (4(1)). The proceedings of the second workshop have been published (Copestake, Langer and Palazuelos-Cagigas , 1997). The results of the Dublin workshop are presented in the chapters in this section.

The results of the workshops and the publications indicate that NLP and AAC can both benefit from an exchange of ideas and techniques. In the following survey, we outline the state of the art, including summaries of the results from the workshops in Dundee and Madrid. We include the outcome of the presentations as well as interesting systems that have been described in other publications which were not presented at the workshops. We distinguish between systems that can be used to build unique messages, message generation systems, including word prediction devices on the one hand and systems that are used to access a set of pre-stored messages on the other.

Linguistic techniques in communication aids

Message generation

The best-known message generation systems in AAC are word prediction systems integrated in a voice output communication aid (VOCA). Word prediction is one of the most used techniques to ease (and sometimes to accelerate) communication for non-speakers. It has been reported that users of word prediction programs achieve keystroke savings of up to approximately 50% (Higginbotham, 1992). No further improvement seems to be possible with the common statistical techniques that mostly rely on word n-grams:sequences of n adjacent words in a text.

Results from research in computational linguistics can play a role for further increase in keystroke savings and lower cognitive load by including syntactic and semantic features in the prediction process, or through advanced statistical treatment (e.g. Markov models, neural nets) by training the system with suitable syntactically tagged corpora. Statistical information on categories of words can be added to the traditional bigram and trigram techniques that operate on word forms, or a system can rely on grammars and conceptual modelling to predict well-formed utterances, i.e. utterances that comply with the linguistic knowledge provided. The research reported to date concentrates on English. As noted in the chapter by Palazuelos et al. (Chapter 9, this volume), however, differences among languages such as the number of possible inflections, compounding conventions and morphologically encoded grammatical agreement within phrases can have a large influence on keystroke savings. Whereas for non-inflectional languages, such as English, the simple techniques in current use can be said to have good results, this is not true for all languages. Garay-Vitoria and Abascal (1997) show that, for the Basque language, the use of standard word trigrams or bigrams for word prediction leads to unsatisfactory results because each word can have too many different word forms. The authors demonstrate that morphological analysis is essential to achieve satisfactory keystroke savings.

A common method of linguistic prediction is to include information about n-grams of syntactic categories. This improves the treatment of words that rarely occur in the input or in the training corpus. A system that uses statistics on syntactic tags, in addition to statistics on word forms, has been described in Tyvand and Demasco (1993). At Dundee University a model of English language syntax has been used to improve the performance of a predictive word processor (Swiffin, Arnott and Newell, 1987; Arnott, Hannan and Woodburn, 1993). Palazuelos-Cagigas, Godino-Llorente and Aguilera-Navarro (1997) report that, for Spanish, the inclusion of syntactic tags improves the performance of their word prediction system.

The KOMBE project developed a prototype word prediction system that relied entirely on grammatical and semantic rules, instead of on statistical data (Guenthner et al., 1993a,b, 1994). All continuations of sentence beginnings offered by the system obeyed the syntactic rules of the system's grammar and the restrictions described in the conceptual module. A prototype of KOMBE was implemented for German and French. Currently there are plans to use the approach for building a language exercise system for autistic children (Godbert et al., 1997).

A very promising possible further development of word prediction systems is the use of research into statistical NLP, especially related to corpus research and to language modelling used for speech recognition (Beeferman, Berger and Lafferty, 1997). The extraction of linguistic knowledge from corpora, for use in the word prediction system Profet, has been carried out at the Royal Institute of Technology (KTH) in Stockholm. To achieve this, a new database has been constructed from two large Swedish corpora – a 150 million-word text corpus and a one million-word grammatically tagged corpus (Ejerhed et al., 1992). The algorithm that accesses this database utilizes two Markov models to compute the probability for any word in the corpus to be the next word in the text (Carlberger, 1997). Another use of statistical methods is found in a neural net design that has been used by researchers from Spain and Scotland to improve substantially the prediction of word classes for a prediction algorithm (Palazuelos, Aguilera, Ricketts, Gregor and Claypool, 1998).

Apart from word prediction it is possible to think of other, more sophisticated ways to assist speech-impaired users in the message building process. One possible approach is language generation from reduced input such as key words or telegraphic messages. This is the concept used in the Compansion project at the University of Delaware (Cushler et al., 1996; McCoy, 1997). Message generation involves high level NLP – the system has to make a choice between several expansions, add endings to words and ensure a well-formed syntactic structure. The Compansion system uses syntactic and semantic knowledge to expand telegraphic input from the user into well-formed English sentences. The project in which this work is being done has been going on for a number of years. The researchers are currently investigating the system's practicality by integration of the device into a commercial communication aid. Results of this evaluation study are presented in McCoy and Hershberger (Chapter 10, this volume).

Another approach to message generation, constructing full sentences from sentence templates, is outlined in Copestake (1997). In general, although generation approaches have problems coping with disambiguation of multiple results, they seem very promising in the long term for the development of new communication aids.

Closely related to language generation is the translation of symbol sequences into natural language. This is an area of AAC research where techniques from computational linguistics are indispensable. In NLP, research on machine translation has made good progress during recent years and, although commercial systems are still far from perfect, they are now being widely used.

In symbol- and icon-based communication aids, translation from symbol sequences to natural language allows users to communicate with partners who are unable to understand the symbol language. Primitive systems of this kind simply translate each symbol into a word but, in many cases, the output is grammatically unacceptable, and is sometimes not even understandable. Research projects have investigated more sophisticated symbolic to natural language translation techniques. In 1986, a system was designed at KTH in Stockholm to translate Blissymbol sequences into well-formed Swedish, English, French and Spanish sentences (Hunnicutt, 1986). Similar programs were developed later on, among them a French system for the automatic interpretation of iconic utterances proposed in Vaillant (1998).

Language processing techniques in message retrieval

The requirements for message selection systems are quite different from message building systems. Here, the higher level organization of communicative structure becomes more important than syntactic and morphological microstructure. Contributing to the study of higher levels of communication is the area of discourse structure which has been studied within the NLP research field, especially in conjunction with the construction of natural language dialogue systems (*Computational Linguistics* vol. 23(1) was entirely dedicated to this subject). However, there has not been a great deal of scientific exchange between research in discourse structure in the NLP arena and research in AAC.

A useful starting point for the design of a communication aid is to look at theories produced by sociolinguists and psycholinguists on how natural speakers communicate using speech. Todman and Alm (1997) show that it is possible to apply models of conversation in order to introduce efficient message selection and prediction into the augmentative communication system TALK. The authors concentrate on the question of how a model of speech production described by psycholinguists can be used in the design of new AAC systems. They give an outline of a model that links approaches to AAC, pragmatic aspects of natural conversation and AAC user goals which is based on experiences with communication aids and their users. The model represents an attempt to provide a coherent descriptive framework within which the various research strands can be accommodated. The application of this approach to the pictographic system PICTALK is described in File and Elder (1997). Todman, Alm and File (Chapter 8, this volume) present the underlying theory of TALK and PICTALK and the results of evaluating both systems.

In AAC systems based on message selection, special consideration of the way in which humans organize their knowledge is necessary to provide methods of structuring texts in such a way that users will have rapid access to them. At least two research systems explicitly rely on such an approach. SchemaTalk (Vanderheyden, 1995) uses a hierarchical schema approach (Schank and Abelson, 1977; Schank, 1982) to organize messages in a database. Trials with the research prototype have shown that this type of organization simplifies access to the messages. SchemaTalk works with a text-based interface and requires literacy, whereas ScripTalker, also partly based on the schema approach, has been designed for illiterate users (Dye et al., 1998). The interface for the ScripTalker prototype organizes the messages in a virtual town, where the user can go from one building to another. When entering a building, the user is presented with a scene associated with it, such as a restaurant interior, and messages are associated with objects in the scene. For example, in a restaurant setting, utterances might be activated by mouse-clicking on a glass on the table, the menu or the bill. The second phase of research on ScripTalker has just been completed and the communication aid is now commercially available.

All the message retrieval systems described in the previous section need the user, or a caregiver, to organize the message database in order to provide efficient access to messages. This type of system requires a high cognitive effort to enter a message and to retrieve messages. In order to select a particular message, the user not only has to be aware of its existence in the database but also has to remember the access route. Serious retrieval problems can result if there is a large pool of messages, especially for those that are not used frequently. These considerations have led, within the WordKeys project (Langer and Hickey, 1997, 1998), to a different approach to message retrieval for AAC systems, which is based on recent research in intelligent text retrieval. In this prototype communication aid, messages do not have to be organized manually. The system automatically indexes any new message and stores it, with its index, in a database. The index is built from the word forms, their lemmas and morphological bases. Messages can be retrieved by typing in one or several index words or by using words with similar meaning to the index words. The system relies on a large lexicon to find semantically related words, such as synonyms and hyponyms (subordinated words such as puffin to bird), for the query expansion. In this way, the user does not have to remember the exact wording of a message, or any access route. If he or she enters a key word, this will, in most cases, lead to the message or messages required.

Other communication aids

So far, this survey has considered voice output communication aids. An associated field of research is concerned with devices that help users with language impairment to understand written or spoken language. Devlin (1997) describes work on a system that simplifies newspaper text for aphasic users who have difficulties in understanding complicated sentence patterns. The algorithms make use of techniques also used for automatic abstracting and the implementation of simplified languages in the NLP field. A large lexicon is used to find appropriate synonyms for words that are difficult to understand and complicated sentences are simplified to a syntax that is easier to parse for the user. Research on this system is continuing within the PSETT project.

Text simplification and summarization methods from NLP are also used to produce TV subtitles for Japanese, in an approach described in Wakao et al. (1997).

For persons with motor disabilities who are not able to use a keyboard, man–machine communication can be difficult. The commercial introduction of speech recognition has provided an avenue for these persons to use a computer, giving them access to word processing, spread sheets,

Internet and many other facilities that are only available to computer users. Carlberger (Chapter 12, this volume) shows the role of grammars and lexicons in such a system, which uses speech input to control a knowledge-based engineering program, allowing motorically disabled designers to continue work in their profession.

Evaluation of novel techniques in AAC systems

One critical question concerning the application of novel techniques in word prediction is whether they improve the performance of the system. Palazuelos-Cagigas et al. (Chapter 9, this volume) argue that it is necessary to standardize evaluation procedures in order to answer this question.

Evaluation of techniques for AAC devices is best done in a realistic communication setting. However, this type of evaluation is often not feasible because of the lack of time, resources and evaluation subjects. Copestake and Flickinger (Chapter 11, this volume) show how logged data is used to quickly evaluate new ideas for prediction algorithms. Ahlsén and Strömquist (Chapter 13, this volume) present ScriptLog, a tool for logging comprehensive data on the writing process of an individual. The collected data can be used for diagnostics, but also for evaluation purposes. Such methods are necessary to ensure performance improvement during the development of any one system, and are also crucial in making comparisons among various systems.

Acknowledgement

Research for this chapter has been partly funded by the EU through the Training and Mobility of Researchers (TMR) fellowship programme. The authors want to thank the participants of the two workshops on NLP for communication aids. This chapter would not have been possible without their presentations and their contributions to the discussions.

Chapter 8
Modelling Pragmatics in AAC

JOHN TODMAN, NORMAN ALM AND PORTIA FILE

A model for AAC evaluation

The design of AAC systems to facilitate socially effective conversation for people who are unable to speak is a difficult task and it is unlikely that any system will be entirely satisfactory. It is important that the strengths and weaknesses of such systems are evaluated against relevant criteria. They are most likely to be amenable to such evaluation when they have been designed with explicit attention to specific, as well as general, social goals that users may be helped to achieve when using them. Specific goals that have motivated design features of an AAC system lead directly to meaningful criteria against which the effectiveness of the system may be judged. Specific goals may also be conceived as subgoals contributing to the achievement of broader social/personal goals.

There is an unfortunate tendency to confuse linguistic competence, an ability to generate a grammatically correct unique utterance for every occasion (e.g. Chomsky, 1965), with communicative competence, whatever makes an interaction work from the point of view of mutual goal achievement (e.g. Hymes, 1972). The question of how best to design AAC systems to help users to achieve their social goals requires consideration of pragmatic features of natural conversation that 'make it work' in this sense. For example, if it is found that mutual enjoyment of social, interactional (as opposed to transactional) conversation is enhanced when control of topic direction alternates between partners (Cheepen, 1988), an AAC system that aims to promote the goal of enjoyment of social interactions should seek to facilitate approximate equalization of control of topic direction (Todman, Alm and Elder, 1994). Similarly, if it is found that lengthy unfilled pauses tend to result in negative attributions regarding social competence (McLaughlin, 1984), an AAC system that aims to promote the goal of attracting positive attributions should seek to reduce unfilled pauses to a minimum (e.g. Todman and Lewins, 1996).

Viewed in this way, pragmatic features of natural conversation provide another level of subgoal to be considered in the design of AAC systems and thereby constitute 'first-step' criteria against which systems may be evaluated. They are not of value in and of themselves, but as means to an end. It will not be enough to demonstrate that an AAC system makes it possible for a user's pre-utterance pauses to be shorter than previously. Satisfactory evaluation also requires that changes in pause times are shown to be related to better achievement of user goals, such as enjoyment or creating an impression of social competence (e.g. Todman, Lewins, File, Alm and Elder, 1995).

Focusing on one pragmatic feature and one goal at a time will, however, tend to provide a distorted, probably over-optimistic evaluation of an AAC system. A particular approach to AAC design, such as an emphasis on the pre-storage of phrases, may be very successful in terms of reducing pause times and fostering enjoyment in introductory social conversations. It may, however, be less successful when it comes to the pragmatic importance of uniquely tailored responses for the achievement of a goal such as developing a long-term relationship. For this, an approach that emphasizes support for precision in phrase generation may seem more appropriate. Evaluation of an AAC system should include consideration of how effectively it supports those goals for which its design features may seem to create problems, as well as those goals that its design features are directed toward (e.g., Todman, Elder and Alm, 1995; Todman, Rankin and File, in press). Of course, it is not possible to consider a full range of pragmatic features and short- and long-term goals in any one evaluative study. Rather, what is needed is a theoretical framework within which aspects of evaluation that are focused on in different studies can be accumulated to build up a balanced overview of strengths and weaknesses of an AAC system, providing impetus to further development.

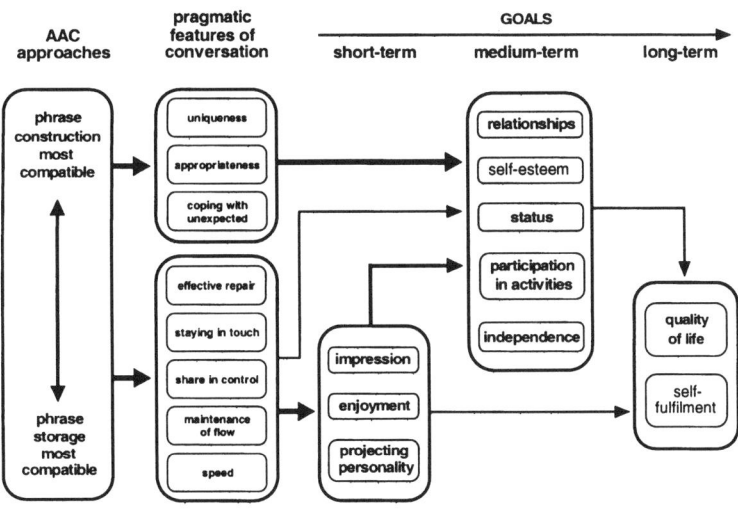

Figure 8.1. A model for AAC evaluation linking design approaches, pragmatic features of conversation and user goals.

The model illustrated in Figure 8.1 is an attempt to provide a theoretical framework with the features alluded to above. The arrows in the model represent suggested links, some of which have received a measure of support from the results of evaluation studies, but most of which remain hypotheses to be tested in further research studies. The model was developed (Todman and Alm in Copestake, Langer and Palazuelos-Cagigas, 1997) in the context of the TALK/PICTALK family of AAC systems. Some of the implications for design and evaluation with respect to those systems will now be discussed. This is done in the hope that these illustrative examples of the evaluative usefulness of the model will stimulate debate on the extent to which the model, or some variant of it, may be useful in relation to the design and evaluation of other AAC systems.

TALK: A text-based system

This model emerged from the work done on the TALK prototype (Todman et al., 1994). This was a communication system designed to experiment with the introduction of new ways to produce natural topic flow in an augmented conversation. A description of the features of TALK will be helpful at this point, in order to make clear the aspects of the model which TALK embodied.

Earlier work had already established the usefulness of users having available ready-made opening and closing remarks, and quick 'backchannel' phrases (Alm, Arnott and Newell, 1992). In trials of a system which had only these features, a number of brief conversational encounters proved possible to enact. In terms of the model proposed, the prototype was in the *phrase-storage* category, and attempted to provide the pragmatic features of *effective repair*, *staying in touch*, *share in control*, and *speed*. The *maintenance of flow* feature was not relevant, since the system only helped the user to perform opening and closing and give feedback to another speaker.

In evaluating the system, measures of conversational rate were taken, transcripts of the sessions were coded using a categorization of speech acts, and the participants' subjective judgements of the conversations were obtained with questionnaires and interviews. The rate measures showed users achieving 19 to 54 words per minute. Both the number of speech acts performed by the user, and their variety, increased when they used the system. This related to the pragmatic goal of *share in control*, and was a likely factor in the *impression* which the user was able to create. The questionnaires and interviews showed a more positive view of the interactions by both participants when the prototype was used, in all three short-term categories: *impression*, *enjoyment* and *projecting personality*. The one negative point made by the subjects in this evaluation exercise was that the system was quite limited in its operation, and did not assist in the central, topic-discussion part of a conversation. The pragmatic feature which needed addressing was *maintenance of flow*, which the subsequent TALK system attempted to provide.

The successful features developed with the earlier prototype were included within the TALK system design, which is shown in Figure 8.2. On-screen buttons allowed the user to easily access opening and closing phrases (such as: Hello, How are you; I'm fine; I'll speak to you using this computer; Well – better be off; Bye for now) and to produce a range of quick backchannel remarks which were random choices made from the categories: I see (*Uh huh*), Please say more (*More*), *Agree*, *Disagree*, Don't know (*Dunno*), *Thanks*, Please wait while I find the next thing to say (*Wait*), May I interrupt (*Interrupt*), That's good (*Good!*), That's bad (*Bad!*), *Yes*, *No*, Mistake there – will say again (*Oops*).

Two new features were developed for the TALK system. In an attempt to provide the user with the ability to carry out topic discussion, the system stored a large amount of conversational material. The user accessed this, not by traditional hierarchical or keyword search methods, but by means of a set of conversational perspectives. It was hoped that these would provide a better way for the user to maintain the flow of a conversation. The perspective buttons can be seen on the left of the screen. They fall into three groups. The *Me–You* buttons allow the user to move back and forth between texts related to themselves and texts related to the person they are speaking to. For instance, if the topic is holidays and the user has just described their plans for the summer, if they press the *You* button, texts might appear such as 'What are your plans for the summer?'. The time perspective buttons at the bottom allow the user to move between texts relevant to the *Past*, the *Present*, or the *Future*. The set of perspective buttons in the middle represent aspects of the topic: *Where*, *What*, *How*,

Me	Greet	Stories	Storage	Switch	Finish	Ques	F'back
You						Sympa	Hedge
	Our first house was in Carnoustie	Most of my childhood we lived in Dundee	I was away at college in Motherwell for two years			Saying	Sorry
Where							
	I don't remember it at all	We lived mainly in Charleston and Menziehill	It was really different living on the west coast			Uh huh	More
What						Agree	Disagree
How	Carnoustie is well known for its golf course	I really liked living there	I like the west coast of Scotland better than the east			Dunno	Thanks
When						Wait	Interrupt
Who	The first flat I had on my own was at Blackwood Court					Good!	Bad!
Why						Yes	No
	It was a real adventure living on my own for the first time					Oops!	Random
Past						Repeat	Quit
Present						Edit Last	
Future						Edit Text	Go Edit
							Speak

Figure 8.2. The interface for the TALK system.

When, Who and *Why*. Using these perspective buttons, the conversation can be guided through and across topics in a natural-seeming 'step-wise' manner, which is what is required of successful conversational topic flow (Jefferson, 1984).

A second new feature added to TALK was the ability to make comments which were quite context sensitive, and yet were often repeated. These were in contrast to the quick-fire comments already provided, which needed to be a bit blander and more multipurpose to work in differing contexts. The first versions of TALK provided no means of creating unique text during a conversation, as a means of testing the possibilities of such a system to its limits. By adding the context-sensitive comments, the system could to some degree address the desirable pragmatic features of *uniqueness, appropriateness* and *coping with the unexpected*. Of course, supplying the user with the ability to make unique text would meet these requirements, but there is a serious time-penalty which must be paid in return for this flexibility. The interface shown in Figure 8.2 does in fact have a *Go Edit* button which takes the user to a text creation tool. However, as noted, if this takes too long, then the user has not been offered much help. The context-sensitive comments were provided in six categories, which were derived from experience in using the system without them: *Questions, Feedback, Expressing Sympathy, Hedges, Common Sayings* and *Apologies*.

The TALK system has been evaluated against a number of the pragmatic goals it is intended to assist, and evaluations are continuing with two users in particular. Conversational rate was improved quite markedly over users' existing methods of communication; rates of 60 words per minute and better being achieved consistently by one user; and participants' ratings of enjoyment increased with conversational rate (Todman and Lewins, 1996; Todman, Lewins, File, Alm and Elder, 1995).

The performance of *repairs, staying in touch* and exercising *conversational control* all looked very promising from the evaluation sessions, but definite conclusions await a more detailed analysis.

In order to test the success in maintaining conversational flow, and also to gauge the perceived quality of the conversations generally, transcripts were made of conversations held using TALK and also of conversations on the same subject between two natural speakers. Raters were asked to judge the quality of the conversations from the transcripts, using the categories of the conversation's naturalness, cohesiveness, fluency, balance, liveliness and friendliness. The content of the computer-aided conversations was rated significantly higher ($p < 0.001$) than that of the unaided samples (Todman, Elder and Alm, 1995). This finding came as something of a surprise to the researchers, since the purpose was to establish whether conversations using pre-stored material would simply be able to equal naturally occurring conversations in terms of quality of content. A plausible explanation for this finding is that naturally occurring talk is full of 'messy' features which listeners, using their ability to infer what the speaker is intending to say, tend to discount. Pre-stored material is selected because, by its nature, it may be of particular interest, and it is expressed more carefully than quick flowing talk. It may therefore appear more orderly and dense with meaning than natural talk.

PICTALK for children

The PICTALK system (File et al., 1995) is based on the TALK system but is intended to support the casual conversation of people who not only cannot speak but who also are unable to read. In fact, TALK/PICTALK are a whole family of systems in which the TALK system is the most powerful and most complex. Where TALK uses text to indicate the content of utterances that the user can choose to speak (using a speech synthesizer), PICTALK uses pictures and labels. Content utterances in PICTALK are also stored within an organizational framework that is designed to enable their prompt retrieval in 'real-time' conversations. Again the screen is divided into three major sections, with perspectives to select specific content on the left, the selected specific content phrases in the middle and general purpose comments on the right. In PICTALK, however, the detailed design of the system is constrained by the need to limit the complexity of the system to that suitable for someone who is either very young or who has learning difficulties.

At present, the PICTALK system is being developed to facilitate social conversation by young children or by older children who have learning difficulties. When considering how to design and evaluate the system, it is

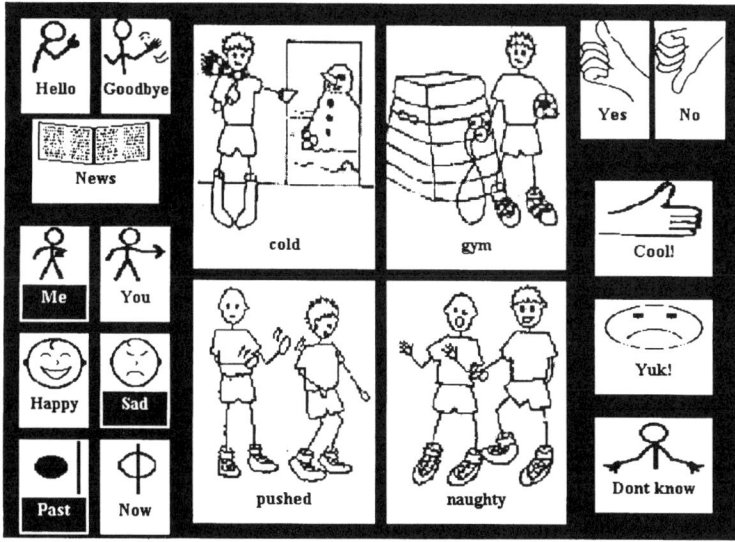

Figure 8.3. The interface for the PICTALK system.

necessary to consider what pragmatic features are required to support the children's social goals. The model outlined in Figure 8.1 is for cognitively able adults and is likely to require modification to meet the social goals of children. For example, children certainly are interested in enjoyment and in making an impression but they are perhaps more likely than an adult to achieve these at a pragmatic level by making outrageous comments. Despite the discomfort that carers and professionals may feel about including such utterances, it may be particularly important to allow children to have them available in order to learn when their use is acceptable. Such utterances can be easily accommodated in the comment section of PICTALK.

Comments can fulfil other pragmatic functions such as initiation to get attention (e.g. 'Hey!') and repair when something has gone wrong (e.g., 'Oops' or 'What?'). McTear's (1985) examination of the pragmatics of children's conversations suggests that children use pragmatic devices for such purposes. Further, Ball et al. (1998) have reported that generic utterances such as these make up 48% of pre-schoolers' utterances. A current research project is investigating how to select a few such comments and then train children to use them effectively in conversation. Different comments need to be tried out to determine which the children can use to support the intended pragmatic functions and, more importantly, whether they contribute to achieving the desired social goals.

Pragmatic features to grab attention and to retain control may be more relevant for children than those for sharing control because sharing in control may be less important for children, whose conversations are more egocentric. Some theorists, notably Piaget (1959), have suggested that children are more egocentric than adults in all aspects of social relationships, including conversations, which is usually taken to mean that they respond less to the listener's perspective. While later work has suggested that the level of egocentrism which is in general exhibited by young children may not be as great as suggested by Piaget (e.g. Selman, 1980), nevertheless the ability to make this type of social adaptation is not fully developed for some years and children therefore may be less responsive to their partners (McTear, 1985).

This egocentrism of children's conversations might make it easier to improve the conversation speed by predicting the next utterance the child might wish to use because the child's next move in the conversation may depend more on the child's last utterance, which is known by the system, than on the partner's last utterance, which is not known. It may be a matter of selecting an appropriate perspective within the PICTALK framework rather than a specific utterance because, having selected the perspective, usually any of the available items will do. From McTear's (1985) work, it seems plausible that children may be able to recognize a suitable utterance as appropriate if it were suggested, even if they are unable to recall and locate it. The ability to produce appropriate utterances at a reasonable speed seems as important for PICTALK users as for TALK users, though the pragmatic function may not be to *share control* so much as to *stay in control* in order to get attention to promote the social goal of making an *impression*.

It is necessary to evaluate the effectiveness of PICTALK for supporting these pragmatic features of *staying in control* and increasing the *speed* of the users' conversation. The role of these pragmatic features for promoting the children's social goals must also be considered. For example, achieving increased speed in this way or retaining control may interfere with other social goals such as *developing relationships*. The possibility of a positive relationship between conversation *speed* and creating a positive *impression* for child PICTALK users, such as has been found for adult TALK users, needs to be tested for child users. There is evidence that higher social status and more success in relationships are achieved by children who make comments relevant to ongoing activities rather than drawing attention to their own interests (Hazen and Black, 1989).

PICTALK also has design features that are intended to support the social goal of *independence* by allowing the user a limited but manageable control over the utterances available for a particular conversation. Phrase construction is very difficult for people who cannot read. However, the user-editing facility does allow the user to prepare the PICTALK system for a particular conversation by replacing unwanted items with an item from a small set of pre-prepared alternatives. Users can try out the speech associated with each button before selecting the button that they wish to include in their system. To increase user independence, this user-editing facility could be extended to allow users limited access to a database containing a large number of previously stored alternatives. Again, it would be necessary to evaluate whether the provision of a facility for controlling the content available for a conversation improves the child's sense of *independence* and *self-esteem*.

Chapter 9
Considerations on the Automatic Evaluation of Word Prediction Systems

Sira E. Palazuelos-Cagigas, Santiago Aguilera-Navarro, José L. Rodrigo-Mateos, Juan I. Godino-Llorente and José L. Martin-Sánchez

Introduction

During the last few years, much effort has been put into improving the quality of evaluation methods used in speech and natural language processing. Several initiatives have emerged to develop reliable assessment methodologies for robust information extraction, text retrieval, speech recognition systems, etc., and although general guidelines for natural language processing systems assessment can be found, there is still no standard for word prediction systems evaluation. In this chapter we present some of the problems found in evaluating and comparing different word prediction systems, mainly due to lack of standardization and evaluation resources, and some ideas towards the goal of solving these problems, by using automatic evaluation procedures and significant metrics.

Evaluation plays a crucial role in systems development, since it gives rise to objective performance measurements, allowing comparisons between systems or accurate measurements of the improvements (if any) due to new techniques or theoretical or algorithmic approaches. In order to achieve meaningful results, the evaluation process needs to be very carefully designed, selecting suitable parameters that accurately represent system performance, and the methods applied to determine the values of such parameters.

During the last few years, we have witnessed considerable activity in the field of natural language processing (NLP) systems assessment. The evaluation of NLP applications, commercial or experimental, is playing an increasingly important role, both in the academic and industrial natural language environments (Lehmann and Oepen, 1996). Researchers, engineers, managers and end users need specific tools and guidelines to measure and assess the quality, progress, improvement and suitability of the current applications with respect to intended use.

Projects such as TEMAA (Thompson, 1994), EAGLES (Eagles Group, 1995 and Gibbon, Moore and Winsky, 1998), and the TSNLP (Lehmann and Oepen, 1996), are three good examples of the vast effort made in this area. The general idea behind all of them is to establish a generally applicable framework for the evaluation of NLP products. The main results of the above mentioned projects are approaches such as the Parameterisable Test Bed (Thompson, 1994), the application and extension of already existing standards in software engineering to NLP systems (Thompson, 1994 and the Eagles Group, 1995) and the development of guidelines for test suite construction, maintenance and application.

From these projects, as well as exhaustive documentation and solid theoretical foundations, actual and practical applications have been developed, such as evaluation guidelines and resources, for example, for spell checkers, spoken language systems and writing aids.

In this chapter various ideas related to specific aspects of the evaluation of word prediction systems are discussed. Little effort has been made toward publishing in this area: therefore this paper intends to offer a general perspective on the problems that arise when facing such a task, while showing some meaningful considerations on metrics and approaches to be considered.

Most of the discussion below has its origin in the evaluation stages of the VAESS project (Palazuelos-Cagigas and Aguilera-Navarro, 1996) and subsequent work developed at the Royal Institute of Technology (KTH) (Carlberger, 1997), Dundee (Palazuelos, 1998) and our laboratory (Palazuelos-Cagigas, Godino-Llorente and Aguilera-Navarro, 1997).

Word prediction applications: users and user interfaces

Generally speaking, a word prediction application attempts to determine which word a user is typing or is going to type, before he or she types it completely, that is, at the same time the user is writing. The predicted words are shown on the screen, so that, if the desired one is included in that list, the user can select and insert it in the text, avoiding the need to type the rest of the word.

Word prediction may be useful for several kinds of users, and its effects depend on their particular characteristics, needs and linguistic and motor skills. On the one hand there are users with different degrees of physical problems, from slow typists to people who have to make a great effort to write, or who are not able to use a conventior al keyboard (switch users). In this case, users benefit from the keystrr ke savings, which means a reduction in the physical effort needed to enter the texts.

On the other hand, people with linguistic problems may also take advantage of word prediction, for example, dyslexic users or persons with other linguistic impairments, children, and people learning a second language. These users may have difficulties in writing properly, and grammatical guidance may be a great help, supporting them in entering text with better linguistic structure. Word prediction can also reduce the number of spelling mistakes, because these users may be able to recognize and select the desired (correctly spelled) words when they are predicted. Studies on the effects of word prediction for users with linguistic problems can be found in Carlberger (1997) and Magnuson (1998), for example.

Some users find more important qualitative than quantitative effects, and the use they make of word prediction will be highly dependent on subjective reasons (such as whether they find it pleasant to use). Additional benefits of word prediction may be higher motivation and interest in writing, independence (in communication aids), confidence, and quality/quantity of the generated texts (more correctly spelled words, better intelligibility and longer texts) (Morrison and Martin, 1998).

The user interface of the applications will be very different, according to their goals. For example, applications for persons with severe motor problems are based on matrix scanning, with the predicted words included in the keyboard simulator. Applications oriented to help keyboard users consist of a small menu containing only the predicted words that can be selected with a combination of keystrokes (such as the function keys).

This wide range of goals, users and interfaces complicates the comparison between word prediction systems, because the performance measurements may be different for each particular task, user and implementation detail. The common factor in all these systems is the use of a word prediction engine, which is the part taken up in this paper, although some comments on user and user interface considerations are also given.

Our aim is to measure the quality of a word prediction system as a natural language processing tool. It is assumed that better prediction will result in better performance when incorporated in a user application. Evaluation of the word prediction algorithm alone avoids introducing factors which might vary among different interfaces or different users. User-centred evaluation is very important for systems development, because it provides subjective opinions plus objective measurements of the system's behaviour as a whole, but this is beyond the scope of this chapter. The effect of the user interface should also be minimized, if not eliminated, by using measurements independent of it.

Automatic evaluation of word prediction systems

Performance evaluation in general is aimed at getting information about certain parameters of a system that allows one to compare systems (evaluation between systems), different generations of the same system, or even the same system under different conditions (diagnostic evaluation), depending on the evaluator's specific role as user or developer. In our case, different parameters of the word prediction, such as keystroke savings and prediction coverage, will be measured in order to evaluate its quality.

Even when not every evaluation parameter can be automatically extracted (for example those involving user aspects and effects of mistakes), automatic test procedures are preferred. Two of the main advantages of automatic evaluation procedures are the possibility of using test corpora large enough to produce statistically valid performance figures, and the possibility of repeating the experiments under the same or different conditions. The evaluation objectives should be defined exactly, so that valid comparisons/interpretations of the results can be made. Different situations can be studied.

On the one hand, the prediction system as a whole can be evaluated, with all its information and extra acceleration procedures: such as automatic addition of white space, capitalization of the first letter after a full stop and suffix prediction. This will be particularly interesting for users, because it will provide information on the performance of the whole prediction algorithm. Subsets of the system features could be evaluated, to measure the effect of each one individually.

On the other hand, the quality of the word prediction can be evaluated by itself, isolated from other prediction features such as suffixes. This is especially important for developers, for example. In this case, there are two possibilities:

- Evaluating each word prediction system with all its specific information (such as different dictionaries, training sets and statistical and grammatical information), or evaluating it with subsets of this information. This will allow the evaluator to determine whether the use of a particular dictionary or certain combination of methods gives rise to better results.
- Establishing the training information, to test the performance of the word prediction methods in particular conditions. This is very important in diagnostic evaluation (for developers), to compare the intrinsic performance of several techniques under exactly the same conditions. If this test is run in different systems, each one a combination of different word prediction methods, it will be determined which combination is the most efficient under certain conditions. For example, comparing systems based on word bigrams and word trigrams, with dictionaries generated from the same text; the results with large texts may show that the most efficient prediction method is the use of word trigrams (or n-grams with a large n), but, if the training set is not very

large, word bigrams (or n-grams with smaller n) may be better, because of the reduction of the sparse data effects.

In each case, some of the system features vary, but the rest of the test conditions (such as test set and language) will remain unchanged, as will be shown in the next sections.

Factors for consideration

When evaluating word prediction systems, very different results may be obtained depending upon the test conditions and the actual implementation, because several factors not directly related to word prediction quality may influence them. In order to make valid performance comparisons, those factors should be controlled, or, at least, their effects taken into account (Palazuelos-Cagigas and Aguilera-Navarro, 1996). In the following sections, these factors are enumerated and their effects explained.

The differences among the languages

Differences may be found when doing a comparison of word prediction systems in several languages, due to the specific characteristics of each one. First of all, the effect produced by the same prediction method in each language may be different. In the second place, some of the methods applied for a particular language may not be feasible or may not make any sense in the others. For example:

- The different behaviour of verbs in English and Spanish: verbs in English have from three to five different forms, and, in Spanish, each verb (regular or irregular) has up to 53. This makes the prediction of verbs in Spanish very difficult, producing a large increase in dictionary size, or in the prediction algorithm complexity, depending on the method chosen to handle it.
- In German, a very common method for generating new words is the concatenation of words. Some of the consequences in the word prediction mechanisms are: it makes words much longer, so many keystrokes are saved if one of them is predicted; the composed words can be predicted 'component by component', which is impossible for other languages; it increases the training complexity, because a segmentation process is needed to determine the components to include in the dictionary. In case this is not possible and whole compound words are considered, the number of different words appearing in the texts is larger, the dictionary size increases, and also the probability that words are not included in it.

There are language-specific features (not present in other idioms) that can help in the prediction process, such as morphologically encoded grammatical agreement between the article and noun in Spanish, which is not present in English.

Training and test corpora

The selection of the training and test corpora to be used in the system is one of the key factors to be considered: their careful design is essential, as system performance will depend heavily on them. In this section, some factors to take into account in the text selection are presented.

One of the parameters to decide upon is the size of the corpora. As in any NLP application, as much text as possible should be used, in order to obtain accurate and reliable models in the training stage, and statistically valid performance measurements in the tests. However, using large texts for evaluation can lead to unrealistic results. Take, for example, the case in which learning capabilities are included in the prediction. If very long texts are used with the adaptive prediction mechanisms, high levels of adaptation will be reached, producing good results. However, users will never write texts as long as these, so the adaptation level reached in the evaluation will never be obtained and the performance in the real case will certainly be inferior. In automated laboratory tests it is possible, of course, to use as much data as are available.

The problem of using small corpora is that they may produce results highly dependent on the text and with little statistical significance, although this effect may be reduced if they are very carefully selected, with linguistic judgement. If only a small corpus is available, it can be split into several parts. The algorithm is then trained with all the parts except one, and that one is used to test the system. The process is repeated several times, leaving out different parts, and finally averaging the results. In general, strategies involving the execution of tests with several medium-sized texts are preferred, finally averaging the results.

In case of evaluation in user's conditions, training and testing corpora should be generated from texts entered by the user (logged data), totally adapted to his/her writing style. These are very difficult to obtain, especially large corpora for all the languages (except possibly for English) and confidentiality issues are usually involved. It should also be taken into account that logged texts will be over-adapted to a particular user. Further considerations on the evaluation of word prediction using logged data can be found in Copestake and Flickinger (1998a).

Degree of agreement

Another key factor is the degree of agreement between the training and test sets: they must be completely different. Measurements taken with test corpora that overlap the training texts are not valid. Additionally, the limit should also be defined for considering the training and test corpora as being too closely related to lead to valid results. Great care must be taken when comparing different systems when they have been trained with different databases, considering the agreement between training and test material. If one of the systems is trained with data closely related to the application domain of the test material, it would outperform a system trained with data not so closely related (even when the latter uses better prediction methods). This is especially important when testing whole systems, in which the training corpora are not established.

Prediction features

In this section several prediction features which may influence the system performance to different degrees will be presented.

One of the more influential factors is the number of predicted words shown simultaneously to the user. Obviously, with more predicted words offered, fewer keystrokes are needed, because the desired word appears sooner, thus obtaining better performance results.

The maximum number of words shown is related to user considerations: in practice, too many words cannot be presented to the user at the same time. Several persons in the word prediction community have observed that most people can observe five words at a glance. This number keeps the right balance between extra cognitive load required and time saving: if more words are shown, the user needs more time and effort to read them when searching for the right one, making the prediction counter-productive (unless the user decides to ignore it). Of course, for automatic word prediction evaluation in laboratory conditions any number of words can be used.

Some systems use suffix prediction when word prediction fails. This method is quite effective with new words, because it includes the most frequent endings. It should be decided whether this feature is included in the statistics, depending on the desired test: comparing systems with all their features, or only specific prediction methods. Regarding the maximum number of suffixes to set, the same considerations as with the maximum number of predicted words should be taken into account.

Other system features

There are more techniques, which, strictly speaking, may not be considered prediction methods, but may accelerate the writing process when included in a system, thus influencing the performance results. For example, the automatic inclusion of white space and autocapitalization of the first letter after a full stop reduce the number of keystrokes needed to write the text, or the automatic elimination of the rejected words (if a word appears in the menu several times and it is not selected, it will be assumed that it is not the desired one, and it will not be shown again while predicting the current word). As with suffixes, it should be decided whether these techniques are included in the evaluation or not.

It is also quite common that not only the prediction is evaluated in tests, but also the interface of the system into which it is integrated. For example, if the system has switch input with automatic scanning, the number of keystrokes is the number of times the user has to press the switch (two keystrokes/letter with row/column automatic scanning, one keystroke/letter with linear scanning, etc.).

The use of accelerators can lead to very different results: each time an accelerator is used, an extra keystroke is added to the statistics, reducing the savings in keystroke number, but saving time. With explicit rejection, no keystrokes are needed to select the predicted word but if the system is a window appearing on the screen, accessible with the normal keyboard, the keystrokes are from the keyboard.

As stated before, the user interface aspect of system evaluation is not emphasized in this paper. Nevertheless, it is a key point in word prediction applications evaluation, as the main target of this research area is improving the communication skills of people with disabilities.

Metrics

In this section, certain measurements that seem to be relevant when evaluating word prediction performance are explained. Every parameter captures certain information about the prediction process, and the selected metric depends on the evaluator's interest.

The parameters that will be explained are keystroke savings, prediction coverage and learning rate. The use of time/speed measurements will be avoided because they are highly dependent on both user and interface design, and the description will focus on measurements that can be automatically obtained from 'standard' text corpora, not dependent upon consideration of the users.

Keystroke based measurements

In this subsection, measurements related to keystrokes will be described. This is one of the main points in word prediction systems evaluation, as these measurements are directly related to physical effort reductions from the user's perspective, especially important for people with physical disabilities.

There are two possibilities: to evaluate the keystrokes a user has to type or the keystroke savings due to the word prediction aid. In the first case, the method is to measure the number of keystrokes a user has to type to enter the text (number of keystrokes before he or she is offered the desired word, plus the number of keystrokes needed to select the word). Depending on the level of detail required, the following measurements may be interesting:

- exhaustive graphs detailing the number of words versus the number of keystrokes needed to write them (the number of keystrokes typed before they are shown plus the keystrokes needed to select it, or the word length (measured in keystrokes, to be consistent) in case the

word does not appear), or
- the average number of keystrokes needed to write a word, that is, in a more compact way. This figure could further be related to the average word length (measured in keystrokes) of the particular language (or corpus), for example, as a percentage, showing the average number of keystrokes typed per word.

The second case is complementary to the one already described. The method is to calculate how many keystrokes the user does not need to type. This can be considered more relevant from the user's perspective, because it actually represents the reduction in effort the user obtains when using the word prediction system.

The formula to calculate the percentage of keystroke savings is:

$$\text{Savings (\%)} = 100* \frac{\text{Keys}_{woWP} - \text{Keys}_{WP}}{\text{Keys}_{woWP}}$$

where Keys_{woWP} is the number of keystrokes needed to write the text without word prediction, and Keys_{WP} is the number of keystrokes needed to write the text using word prediction.

It is important to note that up until now the measurements are based on keystrokes, but corpora are composed of characters. Therefore, some kind of relationship between keystrokes and characters needs to be derived, in order to apply objective keystroke measurements. This relationship is dependent on the user interface and may not be the same in different systems, so the number of keystrokes per character should be standardized. For example, with a conventional keyboard, one character is equivalent to one keystroke (two if the character is capitalized, or has an accent); in systems based on row–column matrices scanning, two keystrokes per character are needed, and four in the case of capital letters.

A unique equivalence list should be provided, because keyboard layouts vary according to the language. As a proposal, the number of keystrokes per character could be similar to the one using a conventional keyboard (with English keyboard layout):

1 keystroke per lower-case character (even if there is an accent)
2 keystrokes per capital character (even if there is an accent)
1 keystroke per number
1 keystroke per sign which does not need to use the Shift key: these are:
   , . ; –] # = \ / [\
2 keystrokes per sign which needs the Shift key: these are:
   ! £ $ % ^ & * ( ) _ + { } @ < : | v ~ >

1 keystroke per selected word. If the system needs more than 1, it should
   be reported, because it can substantially affect the final result. It would
   also be very good to include both measurements
4 keystrokes per other character

Finally, it should be pointed out that some of the features mentioned in
the section 'Other system features' should also be considered when
producing these figures, and must be explicitly indicated. For example,
the final white space in the word should be included in the length, as it is
automatically added when the word is selected, constituting an important
part of the keystroke savings.

Prediction coverage measurements

In general, prediction coverage can be defined as the number of words
correctly predicted, taking into account several factors that play a crucial
role in the performance results. The idea is to evaluate to what extent the
test corpus is covered by the prediction capabilities of the system. These
measurements are more important for dyslexic users, for example. Even
when they are not able to write every word correctly, they may be able to
recognize and select them in the menu, increasing their whole text quality,
and probably quantity.

It is considered that a word has been correctly predicted if at least one
character (and probably a white space) is saved. The measurement that is
made here is the number or the percentage of words predicted in the text.

In case grammatical information in the training and test sets is available, similar measurements can be made for grammatical coverage,
counting the number or percentage of categories correctly predicted, to
evaluate the accuracy of the linguistic module.

Generally speaking, the following factors should be considered, as they
influence the prediction coverage results:

- the number of different words in the training corpus;
- the number of different words in the test material;
- the language perplexity or entropy, because in languages with higher
  perplexity the prediction complexity is larger (for example, languages
  in which words have many different forms);
- the grammatical coverage. Where grammatical knowledge based on
  rules is applied, very different results may be obtained using texts with
  different levels of agreement with the rules. A metric for this grammatical coverage should be defined, possibly related to the percentage of
  sentences that follow the existing rules;
- the agreement between the test material and the system dictionaries,
  which can be measured as the number or percentage of words in the
  test texts that appear in the dictionaries. Note that it may be different
  from the number of words actually predicted due to two reasons: if the
  system learns, each new word will be written only once, and

subsequently it will be predicted, and short words may be typed before they are predicted, even though they are in the dictionaries.

Learning rate

Another important measurement is the learning rate, which consists of evaluating the learning speed of the prediction system as a measurement of the adaptability/flexibility of the prediction system. This is accomplished by computing the keystroke reduction at regular intervals throughout the input of a text, and representing a plot with the keystroke savings versus the number of words. In systems with learning capabilities, the keystroke saving improvement throughout the text can be observed (Claypool et al., 1998).

Proposal

In this section, a proposal is outlined for making automatic tests to obtain as much useful information as possible. On the one hand, it will be very interesting to have performance results valid for a comparison. On the other hand, knowing the best performance of the systems (with all the dictionaries, suffixes, grammatical information, extra features, etc.) will make it possible to look for reasons for the differences in the results (or the lack of them). This will probably provide clues for future directions, showing the effects of changing prediction parameters, or using different methods.

The idea of automatic performance evaluation has been previously proposed to a certain degree of specification, with the name of Parameterisable Test Bed (PTB) in Thompson (1994). Our proposal is rather far from the general framework under PTB's foundation as yet, our approach being much more limited in extension. However, further generalization will be carried out in the future, adopting all of the PTB's formulation requirements.

Nowadays, an automatic evaluation tool exists for nearly every prediction system, with different degrees of complexity and flexibility, and totally associated to the system where it is integrated, with its user interface peculiarities, specifically prepared for the kind of experiments each developer is interested in.

Our proposal stems from the need to implement a tool to evaluate only the word prediction, a tool that will automatically perform the whole evaluation process, not dependent on the user interface, flexible, and more general and complete than the already existing tools. We have attempted to make it as general as possible, although it may be used in a more summary form in case there is an especially interesting subset (for example, text coverage evaluation using only the 'X' dictionary and a particular prediction technique). The following steps should be carried out as automatically as possible for every single experiment (Gibbon et al., 1998):

- Evaluation set-up, in which the values of the parameters for the evaluation are established: language, training and test sets, maximum number of predicted words, number of keystrokes associated with each character, desired results.
- Training procedures, in which the system is trained with the pre-defined training sets and the knowledge sources are extracted (dictionaries, rules).
- Test procedure: to perform the test under the established conditions.
- Scoring: generation of the results files according to the measurements to be done.
- Analysis: analysis of the results files, comparison between results of different experiments, or with the theoretical limits (for example, maximum keystroke savings with a particular prediction method for a particular test).
- Reports generation. The reports which are generated would be complete enough to allow replication of the experiment, and extensive enough to help in the assessment process. For example, they should include at least the following information:
  - values for the input parameters;
  - values of other system features that may influence the results (such as number of suffixes);
  - parameters of the corpora: corpora length, average word length, percentage of common words, etc.;
  - results of each experiment.

It may be interesting to evaluate the actual performance limits. This involves the execution of at least two additional experiments: the first would aim at determining the theoretical maximum performance for a particular prediction method. For example, to evaluate the maximum performance of grammatical methods, an experiment should be performed in which the part of speech of the following word is always the correct one. The second would determine the lower limit for a particular test set which involves running the experiment without applying word prediction.

Sets of experiments may also be defined: each experiment may be performed several times under different conditions, such as several test texts, with certain training texts, with the system's own dictionary, including and excluding particular features, for different languages. If a common prediction interface is defined, and is used by the evaluation tool and the prediction systems, only an evaluation tool will be needed, and exactly the same experiments could be performed with different prediction systems.

Conclusions and future work

In this chapter the need for a standard for the evaluation of word prediction systems has been outlined, according to the current international efforts on standardization of evaluation and assessment processes in NLP tools. Some of the specific problems and factors to be taken into account when facing the evaluation of word prediction systems have been described. Several metrics to evaluate the performance of these systems have been introduced, and finally, a proposal for automatic evaluation of word prediction systems has been outlined.

We by no means consider our proposal to be a thoroughly tested approach. It is a first attempt towards presenting ideas, guidelines and recommendations, and the first step towards starting a detailed discussion with experts in the field. The final goal is the development of a globally accepted evaluation framework for the word prediction research community. We are confident that efforts in this direction are worth the time devoted to them, and could probably boost advances in our area, in the same way that standardization of evaluation approaches did for the spoken language community in the past.

We have actually implemented some of the ideas shown in an automatic evaluation tool for a word prediction aid in Spanish. Major work needs to be done in refining the ideas, measurements and procedures outlined above, especially in those aspects related to the user-centred and user-interface-centred evaluation.

Acknowledgement

The authors would like to thank Alice Carlberger and Sheri Hunnicutt for their valuable comments and suggestions during the preparation of this chapter. This work has been supported by Comunidad Autónoma de Madrid, in the project 'Predicción de Palabras, Aplicación a la Ayuda de Discapacitados y a la Enseñanza de Lenguas'. Ref.: CAM 07T/0010/1997.

Chapter 10
The Role of Evaluation in Bringing NLP to AAC: A Case to Consider

KATHLEEN F. MCCOY AND DAVE HERSHBERGER

Introduction

Evaluation of prototype augmentative and alternative communication (AAC) technologies is a very difficult task for several reasons. Among these are the difficulties inherent in evaluating a 'partial' system – i.e. one whose focus is on a single aspect of an overall system. For example, for several years, we have been applying natural language processing (NLP) techniques to the field of AAC in order to develop intelligent communication aids that attempt to provide linguistically 'correct' output while increasing communication rate. Our focus has been on the processing and system knowledge required in order to expand the user's input. The outcome motivating this project was primarily rate enhancement. While a research prototype was developed at the University of Delaware based on an NLP technique we called COMPANSION (because it takes a COMPressed message and through expANSION, converts it into a well-formed sentence), its practical deployment and outcome evaluation faces several difficulties. These are primarily because the focus of the technique was on processing, but an evaluation requires, and is dependent on, an entire device (i.e. input interface, processing and output interface). We include an informal experiment which allows a partial analysis of the technique. While such experiments are unable to shed light on possible outcomes of system use, they do validate some assumptions and point out differences among users from different populations.

In continuing our investigation of how COMPANSION might be incorporated into a viable AAC device, a joint project between the University of Delaware and the Prentke Romich Company was undertaken to investigate the possibility of incorporating COMPANSION into a viable communication device for a particular population. The development methodology for this project includes ongoing evaluation of subcomponents of the system and tailoring of the system processing to the specific population through a data collection and analysis effort. A portion of the collected data has been set aside for testing purposes.

There has been a great deal of discussion about outcomes in AAC – and indeed the measurement of the outcomes of various AAC methodologies with various populations of AAC consumers is a very important research question. One must recognize, however, that a particular instantiation of an AAC prototype device consists of many different components. In addition, there are several different dimensions along which outcomes can be measured. This chapter can be viewed as a cautionary note about drawing too strong a conclusion about (either positive or negative) results of evaluating outcomes of a particular AAC methodology. In particular, not only must one identify what kinds of outcomes are of interest, one must also decide which component of the system is responsible for the outcome results.

In a research setting we often conceive of an idea – generally pertaining to just a portion of an AAC device. However, in order to test the efficacy of this idea, an entire system must be instantiated. One is then left with the question of which component of the system is responsible for a particular evaluation result.

In this chapter, we first abstractly describe the components of an AAC system and discuss trade-offs concerning decisions made with respect to these various components. Next we discuss different kinds of measurable outcomes that a particular AAC device may have on a user and indicate how a device may have an unexpected positive outcome along some dimension that was not originally planned for. We then describe the particular research prototype whose intention was to demonstrate the feasibility of a particular natural language processing methodology, and point out the difficulty in evaluating the prototype system. We then describe the informal experiment which can be used to validate implementation. However, in order to evaluate outcomes of using the processing methodology, a full system must be developed with a particular population of users in mind. We describe our efforts toward this end with emphasis on our methodology for incremental testing of subpieces of the prototype, and tuning the processing to the particular target population. Hopefully this methodology will indicate various kinds of deficiencies in subpieces of the system which could be remedied before the complete system is evaluated.

Computer-based augmentative and alternative communication

A traditional computer-based AAC system can be viewed as providing the user with a 'virtual keyboard' that enables the user to select items to be output to a speech synthesizer or other application. Such a device can be thought of as consisting of four components: (1) a physical input interface providing the method for activating the keyboard (and thus selecting its elements), (2) a language set containing the elements that may be selected; in the language set we must consider what the items are (e.g. letters, words, phrases), and how the items are organized for selection (e.g. letters in alphabetical order or with most frequently selected letters in front), (3) a processing method which may consist of several levels and is responsible for creating some output depending on the selected items, and (4) an output interface (e.g. a speech synthesizer) which provides feedback to the system user and/or to his/her communication partners. All of these elements must be tailored to an individual depending on his/her physical and cognitive circumstances and the task they are intending to perform.

For example, for people with severe physical limitations, access to the device might be limited to a single switch. A physical interface that might be appropriate in this case involves row–column scanning of the language set that is arranged (perhaps in a hierarchical fashion) as a matrix on the display. The user would make selections by appropriately hitting the switch when a visual cursor crosses the desired items. In row–column scanning the cursor first highlights each row moving down the screen at a rate appropriate for the user. When the cursor comes to the row containing the desired item, the user hits the switch causing the cursor to advance across the selected row, highlighting each item in turn. The user hits the switch again when the highlighting reaches the desired item in order to select it. For users with less severe physical disabilities, a physical interface using a keyboard may be appropriate. The size of the keys on the board and their activation method may need to be tailored to the abilities of the particular user.

Notice that the components of the AAC device are not independent of each other. Consider that the language set low-level processing method may influence the language elements that make up the selectable items. For instance, suppose that the low-level processing in the system consists of word prediction where the system attempts to predict the desired word on the basis of the first several letters. Then the language set had better contain elements that enable the user to select a predicted word or to continue typing out one letter at a time, and these items should be organized in such a way so as to make the selection decision easy. Thus in measuring outcomes, suppose that a word prediction system (a processing method) is evaluated and appears to be ineffective in that it does not raise communication rate. Such a failure may not be due to the processing method at all, but it may rather be the result of choices made with respect to the language set and the way that the user may select a predicted word.

One purpose of this chapter is to point out places where these types of misleading conclusions can be avoided by separation and individually testing various components of the system. For example, in a case where the theoretical keystroke savings of a word prediction system (when measured appropriately) is high but communication rate is not, one might turn to non-processing aspects of the system in order to find the cause. Presumably such testing might decide which component is at fault when a particular evaluation is not optimal.

Consider as well that selection of components for a computer-based AAC device generally has many trade-offs. Assuming a physical interface of row–column scanning, a language set consisting of letters would give the user the most flexibility, but would cause standard message construction to be very time-consuming. On the other hand, a language set consisting of words or phrases might seem more desirable from the standpoint of speed, but then the size of the language set would be much larger causing the user to take longer (on average) to access an individual member. In addition, if words or phrases are used, typically the words would have to be arranged in some hierarchical fashion, and thus there would be a cognitive/physical/ visual load involved in remembering and accessing the individual words and phrases. Each of the choices must depend on the user of the system (i.e. their physical and cognitive abilities) and on the kinds of outcomes desired.

Outcomes

In addition to matching the user's physical and cognitive abilities to the system components, one must also consider the kinds of outcomes that may be important for a particular consumer. Like the trade-off in various decisions concerning the system components, there may be trade-offs in outcome possibilities. By the same token, a system designed with one kind of outcome in mind (e.g. rate enhancement) may show an unexpected positive benefit along another outcome dimension (e.g. literacy enhancement).

The outcome of a particular AAC intervention may lie along several different planes. Consider that an outcome to be measured might reflect the immediate consequences of the device use. Questions here include whether the device facilitates:

- faster communication;
- better ability to express oneself;
- fewer keystrokes;
- more fluent (natural) conversation;
- more natural interactions;
- longer turns;
- positive perceptions of communicative competence.

One might also consider more long range consequences of the device use. Questions here include whether the device has a positive effect on:

- interaction;
- literacy skills;

- turn-taking skills
- socialization;
- personal opportunities because of improved communication abilities;
- the user's communicative competence.

Finally, one might consider some questions about the practical usability or non-communicative aspects of device use. Questions here include whether the user:

- has more enjoyment using the device;
- wants to use the device;
- participates more in conversations when using the device;
- participates less in destructive behaviour after the device is introduced.

Notice that a negative outcome evaluation could be the result of several different things. For example it could be:

- the physical user interface is not appropriate;
- the 'editing' facilities provided in the language set are not sufficient for the task;
- the language set itself is too complex;
- the processing method requires too much cognitive load;
- the processing method does not provide a good match with the user's style;
- improper training or instruction.

Thus, care must be taken when drawing conclusions about outcomes both in terms of the importance of one kind of outcome over another and in terms of determining the true sources of an evaluation result.

New technique: processing evaluation

In this chapter we focus on some of the results from a research project that has been ongoing for nearly 10 years. The beginning of the research culminated in the development of a processing technique known as COMPANSION. Because the COMPANSION project was focused on processing and did not consider the other components of an AAC system, a full evaluation of the technique was not possible. Instead, the technique was informally evaluated through a simulation experiment (described below). Through this experiment several challenges with bringing the technique to a full AAC system were uncovered. Subsequent to this, the team at the University of Delaware joined up with a team from the Prentke Romich Company. The expertise of these two teams lies in different parts of the total AAC system. We describe our current research effort with emphasis on our methodology for testing system components in isolation (with respect to a particular user population). In this way we hope to tailor the processing methodology, the language set and the physical interface to facilitate positive outcomes. The testing methodology (mixed in with the development effort) has the potential for saving a great deal of time.

A large research effort at the University of Delaware resulted in the development of a technique that could expand telegraphic sentences into full sentences (Demasco and McCoy, 1992; McCoy et al., 1989, 1994). The technique, termed COMPANSION, was an effort that concentrated on the processing phase of an AAC device. Other researchers developed systems with similar goals (e.g. Hunnicutt, 1986; Reich and Shein, 1990). The processing phase itself is rather complicated and requires a great deal of information to be associated with the lexical items (words) that can be selected by the user.

The processing model underlying COMPANSION was implemented in a prototype system, but little effort was placed on components of the system beyond the processing component. An assumption of the system was that the input interface to the system would be word-based. That is, each word of input would take a (basically) constant amount of time (regardless of how many characters were in the word). We call this constant amount of time a keystroke. Word endings (e.g. +s plural or +ed past tense) would require an additional keystroke to select. No more specific assumptions about the physical interface or language set were made.

Thus the focus of the research was on a 'black box' which took the words input by the user and expanded them into full sentences to be output via an output interface (e.g. print or a speech synthesizer). COMPANSION potentially increases the communication rate by requiring fewer words to be selected (since it requires just the content words of the desired utterance to be input) and by eliminating the need for selecting morphological endings.

As an example of the kind of processing that could be done, consider the following example handled by the prototype research system:

Input: think red hammer break John
Output: I think that the red hammer was broken by John.

Evaluating the technique

A problem facing the evaluation of the COMPANSION technique was that an AAC technique such as COMPANSION cannot really be tested in isolation: it is a high-level processing technique and all other components of the system must be designed and implemented in order to actually test a processing technique. Moreover, once an entire system is implemented, one runs the risk of negative evaluations being a result of a mismatch between the technique (or user) and the choices made for the other system components.

Upon further inspection, we decided to run some experiments that we felt might help evaluate the coverage of the technique itself. In the COMPANSION technique a primary emphasis was the inclusion of a sophisticated semantic knowledge base and numerically-based heuristics for reasoning about relative word roles. For example, the system might take a set of input such as: '<apple> <pear> <eat> <john>' and generate 'An apple and a pear were eaten by John'. Note that in order to generate such a sentence the machine had to recognize that <apple> and <pear> were the things being eaten (recognizing a conjoined theme), and that John was doing the eating. In addition, appropriate determiners (e.g. 'a') were added (but not to proper nouns such as John), and the appropriate passive construction was used (requiring the past tense form of 'be' and a past participle ending on the main verb) in order to maintain the input order selected by the user.

One kind of evaluation one can do with such a technique is to evaluate the inferencing methods of the technique. To accomplish this, we need a methodology for deciding the specific functionality (i.e. the input/output requirements an optimum COMPANSION system should exhibit). Ideally, we would like our system to act like a familiar human partner does. Thus, our initial evaluation attempted to uncover interaction patterns that occur between an AAC user and a familiar listener. Our analysis emphasized the types of linguistic transformations performed in translating word sequences to sentences.

Method

Pilot data were collected by transcribing videos originally recorded in conjunction with Hans van Balkom. Adolescent students with cerebral palsy described pictures in a children's book to their primary speech therapists, using their own manual symbol charts. Four such adolescent–therapist dyads were videotaped and analysed.

Each student was instructed to describe the pictures as if telling a story to younger children. The therapist was instructed to repeat each word as it was selected by the student, paraphrase the sentence when it was completed, and then ask the student for confirmation that the paraphrased interpretation was correct. A single camera was used to videotape both the student and the therapist. Students took between 11 minutes and one hour to retell their stories.

Results

Some interactions consistent with the COMPANSION approach

Standard COMPANSION

Some interactions with the therapist followed the 'standard' operation of the COMPANSION system.

S: \<girl\> \<make\> \<in\> \<pan\> \<egg\> \<breakfast\>
T: Girl will make the eggs in the pan for breakfast.

Here the therapist has added tense, and determiners. In addition, the plural form of 'egg' was chosen. Though not indicated by the student, the plural form may have been chosen using default knowledge (that people generally eat multiple eggs for breakfast) or it may have been the result of extra-linguistic information (e.g. the picture being described at the time). Notice that the preposition 'for' was also included in the expanded message. This addition required reasoning about the semantics of the input sequence. For example, breakfast was the 'reason' for making the eggs and should be introduced with a *for* preposition.

Word order changes

An assumption of the COMPANSION system has been that the words will be given to the system in the same order that they should be output in a sentence. However, some of our analysis reveals that the therapist sometimes did not follow the word order initially given by the student. The above example falls into this category: the eggs and the pan have been switched in the therapist's output. Consider the following example as well:

S: \<boy\> \<table\> \<dusting\> \<grandmom\> \<floor\> \<sweep\>
T: Boy is dusting the table and the grandmom is sweeping the floor.

Notice that in this instance the student is not following a standard subject–verb–object ordering of the words. The therapist changes the order to follow standard English word order (it is not obvious how to form an English sentence while keeping the word order given by the student).

Agent inference

The COMPANSION system expects that a user might omit an agent when referring to him/herself. An agent might also be omitted if it was obvious from context. This behaviour was also found in our analysis. Because the story was about a boy and a girl, students sometimes did not specify an agent, yet it was inferred by the therapist:

S: \<wash\> \<clothes\>
T: They are washing clothes.

Verb inference

Another assumption of the COMPANSION system is that the main verb may be left out in some situations (particularly when the main verb is either *have* or *be*). We have argued previously that a system must have the ability to reason about which verb is most appropriate in the given situation. Our default rule (i.e. if there is an animate agent and an inanimate object, then the verb 'have' should be inferred) is consistent with examples found in the transcripts. Consider the following, where both the agent ('they') and the verb ('have') have been inferred.

S: <toys>
T: They have toys.

Conjunctions and possessives

Students sometimes left out conjunctions in the pilot study. This occurred both at the sentence level and in both subject and object positions in the sentence:

S: <boy> <girl> <made> <bed> <up> <in> <morning>
T: The boy and the girl made up the bed in the morning.

The inference of when a conjunction is necessary is complicated by the need to indicate possessive information correctly. The following example contains an inferred possessive.

S: <boy> <girl> <girl> <clothes> <my> <mother>
T: They're giving their clothes to their mother.

This example is interesting in that it points out several of the difficulties inherent in inferring when a possessive is needed. Note above there was both a conjunction (<boy> and <girl> combined to 'they') and two possessives. A possible possessive rule might require that if you want a possessive followed by a noun, just put the two items next to each other (e.g. <girl> <clothes> for 'the girl's clothes'). Note here <girl> <clothes> was translated as 'their clothes' as if <girl> was now 'standing for' the combined agent. However, this strategy was not followed for the second possessive (the strategy would have resulted in <girl> <mother> being used). Rather the student chose the first person possessive pronoun, 'my', to indicate the recipient in the message.

It is not clear in the data how much of the therapist's interpretation was influenced by the picture book itself. Nonetheless, this example raises important questions about how to determine when a possessive form is desired.

Some interactions beyond the scope of current technology

Dropped word (in interpretation)

In some instances the therapist did not include words given by the student in the interpretation even though they often contributed to the intended meaning. Consider:

S: <two> <table> <in> <table> <dining> <room>
T: There were things on the table in the dining room.

Notice that table occurs twice in the student's input, but only once in the interpretation. In some sense, the student's input is 'linguistically' sound. He is saying two things about a table (a) there are two things on it, and (b) the table is in the dining room. If these two assertions were stated as two separate sentences, then 'table' would occur twice. However, as a single sentence there is a way to combine the thoughts without repeating 'table'. Compare this example with the possessive case above for an illustration of the difficulty in distinguishing this case from that of a possessive.

Other times the dropped word did not contribute to the meaning:

S: <girl> <look> <at> <to> <boy>
T: The girl's looking at the boy.

Replacing a word (not included in interpretation)

In some instances the therapist ignored words selected by the student, even though there was no obvious indication from the student to ignore the word.

S: <girl> <help> <clothes> <up>
T: Girl clothes up. She's hanging the clothes up.

Note that in the above example <help> does not occur in the output. The example also shows a case where a new verb has been inferred (probably from the extra-linguistic context).

More complicated verb inference (adding or replacing a word)

In some instances the therapist inferred a verb which was not actually included in the input:

S: <boy> <girl> <up> <table> <for> <lunch>
T: OK. They're setting up the table for lunch.

Discussion

A study such as that described here has some advantages, but also raises some questions. Presumably it gives us insight into the limits of a proposed technique and indicates what we should strive for in an implementation.

What this study does not tell us is whether or not the technique is effective or whether an entire, usable system that uses the technique can be built. In addition, it is likely that different populations of users will use different linguistic structures in their expression. Even here we must take care in the conclusions drawn. For instance: we do not know what prior knowledge led to the therapist's interpretation. For instance, since both participants saw the pictures, did prior knowledge of anticipation play a major factor in determining the communicative intent? For example, inferring 'they' as the subject instead of 'I', 'he', 'she' etc. would be much easier while looking at a picture of two people. This same sort of thing is likely to occur when a familiar listener and an AAC user have shared knowledge concerning a situation.

We do not know what kind of interaction between a machine and a user might be appropriate. In the experiments the students were performing a task given to them by a therapist. If the therapist misinterpreted their intent, would they be willing to try to 'correct' the therapist or would they be content that an acceptable answer had been provided? This may be different when a non-speaking person initiates communication in order to convey information to a person.

We do not know whether the telegraphic speech is a result of 'intentional' omissions (due to a conscious decision on the AAC user's part or due to their language abilities) or whether selections to create fully grammatical forms were not available on the system. In other words, were articles, conjunctions, etc. omitted to increase rate, omitted because the individual did not know how to use them properly, or omitted because those words did not exist on their communication board and therefore could not be generated? We should draw different conclusions (and perhaps different kinds of interventions) depending on which of these was the case.

Thus this experiment gives us some insight, but the development of a specific system for a specific task is ultimately necessary. Since during this development many decisions may affect the ultimate usability of the system, one must (1) choose a specific population, and (2) tailor all system components to individuals to ensure system usability.

Joining forces: expertise from several places

The University of Delaware and the Prentke Romich Company (PRC) joined forces in order to develop a prototype system that used the COMPANSION technique and contained all of the other system components. In order to be able to tailor all of the system components, we focused on a single target population and attempted to build system components that would be appropriate for this population. At each stage, individual testing of components has been an important step.

Target population

In considering a target population we looked for a group of users who would be likely to produce telegraphic input, would benefit from the expansion of that input into full sentences, and that could be counted on to use a fairly limited number of words and linguistic structures. This was crucial because the COMPANSION technique requires a lot of information on each word and must understand all sentence structures. We chose to consider a young population of users who have cognitive impairments that affect their expressive language ability. Whether a child with cognitive impairments is verbal or non-verbal, their expressive language difficulties may include the following (Kumin, 1994; Roth and Casset-James, 1989): (1) short telegraphic utterances; (2) sentences consisting of concrete vocabulary (particularly nouns); (3) morphological and syntactical difficulties such as inappropriate use of verb tenses, plurals and pronouns; (4) word additions, omissions or substitutions; and (5) incorrect word order. While such children may have the ability to functionally communicate their needs and wants, intervention to assist them in their language production should be beneficial both from a social and an educational perspective.

In developing a device geared toward this population, several issues must be dealt with. Here we focus on three to emphasize our processing methodology:

- lexical access – what is an appropriate method for providing such a user with access to the lexical items that they wish to communicate? This includes language set and physical input interface.
- verification of user input/output assumptions – what kind of input will this population produce and what expansions are reasonable?
- user interface issues – what kind of interface is necessary for a user with cognitive impairments to be able to access the system? Crucial here is the user's ability to sift through the expansions provided by the system and select the one they desire for output.

Lexical access: Communic-Ease Map™

PRC has a great deal of expertise in the area of physical input interfaces appropriate for a wide variety of users. In addition, it has provided effective language sets coupled with low-level processing to provide users with a mechanism for outputting desired messages. In fact, PRC has expertise in providing lexical access to the population under study. The speech output communication aids that PRC designs for commercial use incorporate an encoding technique called semantic compaction, commercially known as Minspeak® (a contraction of the phrase 'minimum effort speech') (Baker, 1982, 1987). The purpose behind Minspeak® is to reduce the cognitive demand as well as the number of physical activations required to generate effective flexible communication. It uses a language set (i.e. a set of selectable items) consisting of a relatively small set of icons that are rich in meaning and associations. These icons can be combined to represent a vocabulary item such as a word, phrase or sentence, so that only two or three activations are needed to retrieve an item. This small set of icons thus allows access to a large vocabulary which is stored in the device. Since they are rich in meaning, icons designed for MinspeakR can be combined in a large number of distinct sequences to represent a core lexicon easily.

The Minspeak® language set and processing was first utilized with PRC's Touch Talker™ and Light Talker™ communication aids (which united different physical interfaces with the icon encoding). With these Minspeak® systems, if icons on the overlay remain in fixed positions, once learned, they allow the individual using the system to find them quickly and automatically. This automatic processing was facilitated by the design of pre-stored vocabulary programs known as Minspeak® Application Programs (MAPs™). In these programs a large vocabulary is pre-stored in a well-organized fashion using a logical, paradigmatic structure that greatly facilitates learning and effective communication.

One of these MAPs™, Communic-Ease™, contains basic vocabulary appropriate for a user chronologically 10 or more years of age with a language age of 5–6 years. Communic-Ease™ has proven to be an effective interface for users in our target population, providing access to approximately 580 single words divided into 38 general categories. Most of these words are coded as two-icon sequences. The first icon in the sequence (the category icon) establishes the word category. For example, the <SKULL> icon indicates a body part word, the <MASKS> icon indicates a feeling word, and the <APPLE> icon indicates a food word. The second icon denotes the specific word. For example, <MASK> followed by <SUN> produces the word 'happy'; <APPLE> followed by <APPLE> produces the word 'eat'.

In addition to the words which are accessed via the icon sequences, Communic-Ease™ contains some morphology and allows the addition of endings to regular tense verbs and regular noun plurals. However, to accomplish this, additional keystrokes are required. It is also possible to spell words that are not included in the core vocabulary.

The Communic-Ease™ MAP has proven to be an effective means of communication for individuals in our target population. Thus this MAPTM implemented on PRC hardware has provided a physical input interface, the portion of the language set necessary for selecting vocabulary items, and a low-level processing technique which allows users within the target population to functionally communicate. However, users tend to produce telegraphic messages consisting of key word sequences. Thus they would likely benefit from the addition of COMPANSION-like processing.

Design methodology: user-centred design

Notice that the Communic-Ease™ MAP and the PRC input/output interfaces are proven useful for the population under study. We take these components, but must ensure that the remaining components are appropriate for the user population. Some issues we must handle include:

- What is the range of input structures the system must handle?
- What are the appropriate expansions of that input (and how can the machine be programmed to output a set of appropriate expansions)?
- What additions must be made to the language set to provide appropriate selection and editing facilities?
- How should the language set be organized?
- What kind of interface will allow effective use of the system?

Our methodology in this collaborative effort is to design a system that is geared toward the specific user population. Thus, we have set out to validate our assumptions about the user input and output requirements and to tune the user interface (i.e. editing, language set organization and physical interface) to the population. Our system input/output functionality has been determined by a collection of transcripts from Communic-EaseTM users. We have collected both raw keystroke data (so that we can establish the range of input we expect from the population) and keystroke data from videotaped sessions where interpretations of the keystroke data are provided by a communication partner. These data allow us to ensure the output from the system is in fact appropriate.

Collection of such data has allowed us to:

- validate expected sentence structures;
- validate the expectation of limited vocabulary;
- validate input assumptions.

In addition, we plan to validate our interface requirements on the basis of iterative user testing. The interface will be developed so that it can be customized to the specific needs of particular users.

User interface issues: user-centred design

Envisioned system

The envisioned system combines the PRC Liberator™ system (which provides both a physical interface and low-level processing) that runs a modified Communic-Ease™ MAP (which provides a standard vocabulary and its access method) and an intelligent parser/generator (which provides the COMPANSION-like processing). The input from the user will be through the Liberator™ keyboard (most of whose keys contain the icons which are transformed into words via the Communic-Ease™ MAP). The user will receive feedback through an Interface Display. Part of the Interface Display looks much like a standard Liberator™ display (e.g.

showing selected icons and words). An additional area of the Interface Display will show the transformed sentences which the user may select to be 'spoken' by the system. The user may ask the system to speak the sentences through a private audio channel in cases where he or she is unable to read the display.

The Liberator™ Overlay/Keyboard accepts user input via a variety of methods (e.g. direct selection), and can also limit user choices via Icon Prediction. With Icon Prediction only icons that are part of a valid sequence are selectable. The user selects icon sequences that are transduced into words or commands according to the Communic-Ease™ MAP. In normal operation, icon labels and the transduced words are sent to the Interface Display to give the user feedback (words may also be spoken incrementally).

In the proposed system, these components are supplemented with an intelligent parser/generator (IPG) that is currently under development. IPG is responsible for generating well-formed sentences from the user's selected words and is a simplified version of COMPANSION. IPG also provides further constraints on the Icon Prediction process. For example, if the user selected 'I have red,' the system might only allow icon sequences for words that can be described by a colour (e.g. shoe, face).

IPG encodes a set of transformations for expanding sentences input by the user. These transformations have been motivated by our study of transcripts collected from current Communic-Ease™ users. Using these transcripts, the processing of the system can be tuned to handle the kinds of constructions common to this particular population.

Interface issues: isolation and testing

Beyond the basic operation described above, there are a number of interface issues that need to be resolved before a completed system is developed. These issues are being explored in early interface prototypes with iterative user testing. For example, one question with the interface concerns the method with which users select the desired expansion when the system comes up with several possibilities. The particular user population poses several challenges; they most likely cannot read, and may not be able to remember what they desire if several possibilities are presented to them.

Our methodology here includes building a prototype interface (using our intuitions from knowledge of the target population) and then adjusting the interface through user testing and further interface development. This interface testing need not be done in the context of this particular system. Rather a 'simpler' task will be given (e.g. a game) to test the feasibility of the interface components. In this way we hope to isolate interface components from the cognitive demands of the entire system.

For instance, one important aspect of the system operation is selecting the desired expansion from a list of possibilities calculated by the system. We have implemented an interface which provides for selecting from a list which is presented to the user both visually and auditorily. The system 'scans' through the list one at a time, highlighting the list item and speaking the item through a private auditory channel. The user may select the desired item at any time during the scan. The interface is designed flexibly. The number of items to select from, the speed of the scan, and the method of selection may all be customized by changing some system parameters.

Rather than testing this interface in the context of the whole system (which may be confusing for a user), the interface testing is planned in a simple 'game' situation. In the game the user will have to select the correct item from a list. In this way the selection and presentation parts of the interface may be tuned to the user in isolation from the rest of the system. Other aspects of the interface (e.g. the editing functionality, the presentation layout) will be developed in a similar manner.

Development methodology: verifying user input/output assumptions

The prototype system combines the PRC's Liberator™ platform and Communic-Ease™ Map with the current-generation intelligent parser/generator. In the implementation the Liberator™ will function primarily as the user's keyboard and a tablet-based portable computer will contain the parser/generator and function as the Interface Display. The two systems will be connected via an RS-232 or IR link. This strategy allows for rapid initial prototype development.

Our project methodology is to develop and test the robustness and usability of the system in phases. The parser has been developed in C++ and is being refined and tested as other parts of the project progress. A core grammar has been created and is being revised and enhanced to handle a larger variety of structures. Current lexicon efforts involve expanding the number of entries beyond the basic Communic-EaseTM vocabulary and adding the necessary semantic knowledge. The first version of the Windows-based user interface has recently been completed and is now being evaluated internally.

Several evaluations of the completed prototype system are planned. For instance, a theoretical evaluation of the grammar coverage is ongoing. As has been stated, we have collected key selections from current users of the Communic-Ease™ MAP. In some situations, we also have an interpretation of those keystrokes provided by the communication partner in a videotaped session. These video sessions have been transcribed and aligned with the keystroke data. While some of these data are being used to develop the grammar, we have set aside a portion to be used for testing purposes. These test data will allow us to test the system's grammar in several ways.

First, the robustness of the grammar can be tested by determining the number of completed input utterances found in the collected data that can be handled by the grammar. Second, the appropriateness of the grammar can be tested by determining how often the grammar's output matches the interpretation provided by the communication partner in the video sessions. Because we have much more keystroke data than transcribed video data, we also plan a test of grammar appropriateness by comparing the output of the grammar with that generated by a human faced with the same sequence of words.

In addition to the theoretical grammar testing described above, we also plan an informal evaluation of the usability of the system. We plan to iteratively refine the interface by doing usability studies of our prototype with current users of the Communic-Ease™ Map. One aspect these studies may shed light on is whether or not users in the population under study can in fact select their desired sentence when a list of possibilities is presented to them.

Conclusions

Evaluation of a new AAC methodology is a very difficult task. A complete AAC system consists of multiple components – all of which must be tuned to particular users. In evaluating outcomes, care must be taken to determine appropriately which component must be updated. Any one of the system's components may be responsible for a negative outcome and one must take care that conclusions drawn are not too broad. In addition, a negative outcome may be the result of poor training or not enough practice on the system. Not only this, but the outcomes themselves contain a great deal of variety. For instance, a system initially conceived as a rate enhancement technique may end up having a positive effect on literacy skills.

Here we focused on the development of one particular project and have discussed the notion of separate evaluation of subcomponents and ongoing evaluation in conjunction with the development.

Past efforts have allowed us to take some components which have already proven useful for this population. For instance, we know that the target population is already accustomed to the access technique, the vocabulary, and the language encoding system of the Liberator™. We have described ways of testing subcomponents (e.g. the processing sophistication of IPG). However, new issues come up in integration which require further attention. These include questions such as: 'How cognitively disorienting is the additional information provided by the system?', and 'If additional information is provided, how should it be presented?'. Questions such as these provide avenues for further work.

Acknowledgement

This work has been supported by a Small Business Research Program Phase I Grant from the Department of Health and Human Services Public Health Service, and a Rehabilitation Engineering Research Center Grant from the National Institute on Disability and Rehabilitation Research of the US Department of Education (H133E30010). Additional support has been provided by the Nemours Foundation.

The authors would like to thank Arlene Badman, Patrick Demasco, Clifford Kushler and Christopher Pennington for their collaboration on the project. In addition we thank John Gray for his discussions and implementation of many of the C++ aspects of the system, and Marjeta Cedilnik for her work on the grammar (and transformation rules).

Chapter 11
Evaluation of NLP Technology for AAC Using Logged Data

ANN COPESTAKE AND DAN FLICKINGER

Introduction

The aim of this chapter is to illustrate an approach to evaluating NLP techniques for use in research on AAC systems. Evaluation of NLP technology in general is a notoriously thorny issue (for a summary of approaches see Sparck Jones and Galliers, 1995). However, our immediate goals are relatively restricted. First, we are currently primarily interested in evaluation up to the level of research prototypes: thus rather than looking at complete systems, we are using formal and informal evaluation techniques to compare the performance of different NLP algorithms on the same task, and also to screen possible NLP techniques for their likely utility in tackling problems in AAC. Evaluation of techniques in isolation is much simpler than evaluation of complete systems, since it involves looking at specific criteria relevant to particular aspects of performance. Second, our current aims in evaluation are primarily internal (that is, directed at development within a project) rather than external (allowing comparison between sites). We will return to some of the issues involved in extending this work to external evaluation at the end of the chapter.

In what follows, we will first describe the methodology we adopted for data-logging, then discuss how the logged data was used to evaluate prediction algorithms. The techniques used in the prediction experiments and the results obtained have been reported previously (Copestake, 1996, 1997), so our purpose here is to discuss the use of logged data in more detail and to evaluate its advantages and disadvantages. We then describe more informal evaluation using logged data as a way of looking at recurrent conversational situations and some additional information revealed by audiotaping experiments. We will conclude with a discussion of how our data-logging methodology might be improved, and the role data-logging plays within a wider evaluation context.

Data collection methodology

The experiments described make use of data collected from JL, who has been using a prototype AAC system that was developed at the Center for the Study of Language and Information (CSLI) as his main communication aid. JL has lost speech due to amyotrophic lateral sclerosis (ALS or Lou Gehrig's disease). The prototype system comprises software designed to aid text input to a text-to-speech generator (JL uses an external DecTalk). The system runs on a standard laptop while still allowing the use of other software (email, Web browser etc.). It incorporates word prediction, based on word frequencies trained dynamically on the user's input, and also a small number of user-defined fixed phrases, accessible via dedicated keys. A much larger set of fixed phrases is available via a menu interface, but we will not discuss this here, since JL does not use this facility. More details about the system are given in Copestake (1996, 1997). We have logged JL's data for about three years. During most of that time, his condition was relatively stable, and he was able to enter text by operating a keyboard with one finger, with numeric keys used to select prediction menu options.

Initially we simply logged the text that was passed to the speech synthesizer for output, using a format of one utterance per line. We also logged commands to the synthesizer, such as changes in rate and volume. It became apparent that we also needed information about the timing of each utterance, so later versions of the logger included time-stamps. The most recent version of the logging software also records data from the prediction engine at the points at which a menu item was selected. For example:

16:41:07::{8,w,ill}{8,,it}{5,,to}{2,tr,ansfer}{6,the,n}{5,the,se}{2,fi,les}
{5,,to}{7,n,ew}{0,co,mputer}16:42:31::
i will use it to transfer these files to my new computer

This indicates that the utterance was begun at 16:41:07 and finished at 16:42:31 (i.e. the rate was about 8.5 words per minute, although we cannot tell whether JL was typing continually or not). Some words were typed in full (I, use, my). In other cases the prediction menus were used: for instance w was typed but will was then selected from the menu (key 8), it was selected before any letters were input, and so on. Selecting *then* was presumably an error, corrected to *these*. The menu ordering was set up so that the preference order on selections was 0,9,8 etc., rather than 1,2,3, because JL was operating the keyboard with his right hand, and the higher digits were therefore more accessible. JL had the option to turn off data-logging if a conversation was particularly sensitive; however, he very rarely used this.

As we will discuss below, this data-logging was not perfect – for instance, it would have been useful to collect data about every keystroke (although this would have been difficult to implement). However, as we will describe in the next sections, it gave us a good basis to compare prediction algorithms and also to decide which NLP techniques appeared to be the most promising avenues for research for this type of AAC.

Experiments on word prediction

Measuring prediction performance

Though prediction is only ever a small component of an AAC system, evaluating prediction algorithms is non-trivial. There are multiple dimensions on which we might measure performance of algorithms. The primary one concerns the accuracy of the prediction – this is normally expressed in terms of keystrokes saved compared to typing the full utterance. Of course, this is only an approximation to the ultimate criteria, which are saving of time and effort on the part of the AAC user. Even if we assume that all aspects of the user interface layout etc. are kept constant when comparing prediction algorithms, keystroke saving will not correlate well with speed/effort saving if the overhead of making the selection differs significantly between algorithms. Prediction is only useful in circumstances where text entry is relatively slow or where the input is somehow artificial and therefore difficult to reproduce correctly, for instance when entering lengthy commands to a computer (see, for example, Darragh and Witten, 1992).

For the case of someone like JL with advanced ALS for whom movement is very restricted and very tiring, it is reasonable to suppose that the cognitive overhead of using a menu is relatively low compared to the effort of entering a keystroke. As we will discuss in more detail below, JL usually took the option of using the prediction menu when it gave the desired word. Therefore keystroke saving is a useful criterion and we use the following metric:

$$(1- \frac{\text{keystrokes + menu selections}}{\text{keystrokes needed without prediction}}) \times 100$$

For example, choosing table after inputting 't' 'a' would give a score of 50%, since a space is automatically output after the word.

Using logged data in a prediction testbed

The prediction testbed uses logged data to train a statistical prediction algorithm and then tests its performance on a fresh set of data. Following standard practice in NLP, we used a 90%/10% split between training and test data. We should emphasize the importance of keeping the training and test data completely distinct. It is invalid to assume, for instance, that a prediction engine with a sufficiently large lexicon would cover all words in a test set and that it is therefore legitimate to acquire the word-list from the test data, since no matter how large the lexicon, there will still be unseen tokens in any reasonably sized unrestricted test set. For instance, Brown et al. (1992) report that an almost 300 000 word vocabulary contained fewer than 90% of the distinct tokens in the Brown corpus. Most prediction systems will operate with a much smaller vocabulary, so the unknown word problem is proportionally more significant.

The basic assumptions behind the use of logged data in training and evaluating prediction algorithms are:

- the logged data will be more representative of the type of text a user wishes to input than any corpus could be;
- the prediction algorithms can and should adapt to a user's data.

Clearly this is not true of all possible uses of prediction: if the system is designed to help a child with spelling or language difficulties, for example, it should correct errors rather than reinforcing them. However, for a user without language problems, prescriptivism is generally inappropriate.

When using the testbed, we make the initial assumption that we have a 'perfect' user: one who always chooses the prediction menu item when it is available. Discrepancies between predicted and actual results are discussed in the next section. One major advantage in using the testbed methodology is that we can implement algorithms very quickly, without too much concern for robustness or for issues such as memory usage. A system that is to be used daily by someone with ALS has to be very reliable, even if it is only a prototype, and this greatly increases the implementation time needed.

In the prediction experiments we reported in detail in Copestake (1996, 1997), we used 26 000 words of text (around three months of JL's data). We did not use an external lexicon as a source of words, although in one experiment we did use external corpus data in order to provide part-of-speech tags for the collected word list. An algorithm based simply on word frequencies constructed from the training set and dynamically updated during processing of the test set gave 45.3% keystroke saving with a menu size of 10. Adding the best performing adjustment for recency increased this to 46.5%. We also experimented with taking context into account using n-grams: part-of-speech bigrams based on JL's data gave 49.0% keystroke saving. However, there was a decrease in performance when using part-of-speech bigrams derived from a text corpus. Thus the text corpus did not provide a good model for the AAC data even at this very abstract level.

Based on these evaluations, we changed the CSLI prototype to incorporate the recency metric. We did not, however, add the syntactic bigram technique. Although it might have produced some improvement in actual performance, the testbed experiments showed that this would not be very large, and the increase in code complexity meant that it would have been relatively costly to implement robustly and to maintain. It therefore did not seem to be the most promising place in which to expend implementation effort.

Actual vs. theoretical performance of prediction

The figures given above are for theoretical performance of prediction with a 'perfect' user. Clearly, even with someone like JL, who regards prediction as an essential component of an AAC system, actual results will not be as good. A user may miss a predicted choice, or inadvertently select the wrong menu item. Comparing prediction algorithms for their theoretical performance is only valid if their ranking with respect to actual performance is the same. This will not be universally true: in particular, techniques which result in changing menus are not directly comparable with systems with static menus, and systems with large lexicons which give more menu choices may be more confusing than systems with smaller lexicons.

To some extent, we can use JL's logged data to compare actual and theoretical performance of the algorithm implemented in the CSLI system. Consider the following example, which was logged using the version of the CSLI prototype that adjusted predictions based on recency:

11:55:48::{0,ta,ke}{9,tr,ay}{7,o,ff}{0,a,nd}{8,pl,ug}{1,,me}{4,w,ith}{7,,t he}{8,ext,ension}11:57:53::
take tray off and plug me in with the red extension cord

Here 56 keystrokes would have been needed without prediction. JL actually took 32 keystrokes, compared with the theoretical performance for the algorithm of 26 (with the frequencies that were in effect at the time that this sentence was logged). Based on a manual evaluation of a small fraction of the logged data, this is a reasonably representative example: on average the actual keystroke saving was around 80% of the theoretical saving. Obviously this figure will be very dependent on the user and the user interface, and will also be affected by changes in the algorithm. For instance, even though the prototype's algorithm and the more complex algorithm mentioned above used the same word list, and both involved menus which could change, they are not completely comparable, since the menus are less predictable in a more context-dependent system.

In principle, it should have been possible to check automatically the actual performance against the theoretical performance, by running the prediction algorithm in the testbed on the logged data so that it was in the same state as the actual system, and comparing the 'perfect user' simulation against the actual choices. In practice, too many variables crept in for this to give accurate results. The prediction order in the simulation did not always exactly match that recorded for the running system, because the testbed did not include all the data which were going into the running predictor. This occurred when JL used the predictor to compose email (he did not wish us to log his email). Since the frequencies were adjusted dynamically, and also affected by recency, the scoring of words that had been used in email messages was higher in the logged data than it was in the simulation. (The manually calculated figures above were obtained by looking at data collected from close to a point where we had downloaded the predictor frequencies, so should not be too affected by this source of error.) Furthermore, JL sometimes used cut and paste to input text, and this was not recorded. Comparing actual and theoretical performance was not our primary aim in carrying out data-logging, but if we had been attempting to evaluate user interface designs, for example, this sort of problem would have been very serious.

Advantages and disadvantages of logged data for evaluating prediction algorithms

To summarize, based on our experiments, we see the following as the main advantages and disadvantages of using logged data to evaluate prediction algorithms.

Advantages

- Logging allows the collection of more realistic data than can be obtained from existing corpora.
- Compared with collecting data in an experimental setting, data-logging involves very low overhead for the quantity of data obtained.
- The same logged data can be used in batch mode for multiple experiments in order to tune prediction algorithms.

Disadvantages

- Logged conversations must be treated as confidential, so cannot be widely distributed.
- In order to collect data from a user over an extended time period, it is necessary to have a cooperative user and an implementation that is robust enough for everyday use.
- There is a danger of developing systems that are over-adapted.
- Simulating the performance of prediction techniques by running in batch mode does not allow for effects of the algorithm on ease of choice of menu items.

Conversational situations: logged data and audiotaping

In contrast to the formal evaluation of variations on prediction algorithms discussed in the previous section, we have also used the logged data informally, as a way of pre-screening possible NLP techniques for further investigation. Designing prototypes by introspection into the nature of the sort of conversations that an AAC user might want to have has obvious flaws as a research methodology. While the ideal situation would be to construct prototypes, which could be evaluated by representative users, this can be very expensive. By using logged data from an AAC user, we can get some idea of how important particular phenomena are and whether an NLP technique might be worth applying. We have also been looking at various corpora of spontaneous speech, since the logged data are limited by the capabilities of the AAC prototype.

For instance, one possible technique for improving prediction might be to classify words by subject area so that once a topic is identified (automatically or by the user), those words can be preferred. However when we tried to simulate this technique, using an existing manual classification of some of JL's vocabulary, we found no improvement in performance (actually there was a slight degradation). Examining the collected data more closely, it became apparent that it was relatively unusual for there to be a clear classification of sentences in terms of the concepts we were using. In the cases where there were clear topics, the sentences only used a tiny proportion of the topic-specific vocabulary, and most of the words in the sentences were not topic-specific. For instance, a conversation might be about Wimbledon, which could be classified under the topic 'sport'. But the great majority of the sports vocabulary would not be used in the sentences about Wimbledon, and most of the words in a sentence about Wimbledon would not be specific to the sports vocabulary.

We therefore decided that identification of topic was not a likely route for substantial improvements in word prediction. Furthermore, this experience suggested to us that constructing topic-based templates or partial utterances was not very promising either, at least as a technique for facilitating a major proportion of the conversation. The logged data, and experience with speech corpora, suggest that when a conversation is 'about something' the topic will be too specific for it to be likely that useful phrases can be constructed in advance, by someone who does not know the AAC user.

Semantic concept classification is clearly sometimes useful in AAC, for instance as a way of aiding retrieval of pre-stored messages (e.g. Langer and Hickey, 1997) or of creating customized vocabulary for particular users in special situations (e.g. for school use, when the topic of a lesson is known in advance; Sinteff, 1998). Also some situations are sufficiently important that a topic-specific set of words and phrases would be useful, even if those situations only account for a small proportion of the AAC user's time. Interacting with a doctor might be one such case. But even in this situation it appeared to us that it would be more promising to provide tools that aid the AAC user or a helper to prepare for the conversation, rather than to build specific topics into the system.

However, examination of the logged data does reveal some patterns which we believe we can usefully exploit. For instance, a large proportion of the collected data consist of requests that someone performs some action on JL's behalf. A large proportion of these requests are concerned with routine needs and can be dealt with by user-defined fixed phrases. But there are also many cases where the request concerns a non-routine action: mending something, helping with a computer problem, asking some third party about something, etc. The vocabulary concerning the topic of the request is not predictable, but there are conventional ways of making requests, which we can exploit, and also likely ways in which the dialogue will proceed. Since we only have one side of the conversation, and are lacking information about the context, there is no way of being sure what is going on, but we can assume that a sequence in the data such as:

please ask Jim to come over tomorrow
thanks

indicates that the interlocutor agreed to the request. In contrast, in:

please mail the letter
hall table

the second utterance is likely to be a clarification, probably about the location of the letter. We discuss how we are attempting to exploit this sort of convention in dialogues in Copestake (1997).

One thing that becomes apparent when looking at logged data is how repetitive they can appear in tone and style. In JL's data, for example, requests for action are usually expressed as imperatives, normally preceded by *please*. This is, of course, also something that people interacting with AAC users and AAC users themselves comment on. We believe there is considerable scope for varying phrasing according to parameters such as politeness, without very much extra work on the part of the AAC user, again because of the high degree of conventionality.

Because of the one-sided nature of the logged data, we tried audio-taping some of JL's conversations. This did not provide us with nearly as much data as we would have liked, because at the point we carried out the taping, JL was contributing far fewer words to conversations than he had been. However, taping did make evident many aspects of the interaction that we could not have discovered from data-logging alone. One of the most significant was that it became apparent that it was frequently very difficult for JL to break into a multi-participant conversation, even after he had composed some text. The problem was partly the volume of the DecTalk synthesizer – although this can be set to be quite loud, changing volume requires some intervention on the part of the user and a volume that would be adequate to be guaranteed to be overheard over a loud conversation would be unpleasant under other circumstances. The other problem is timing: breaking into a conversation effectively requires that the timing of the interruption be very precise, which is problematic if the utterance is being made by a text-to-speech synthesizer. We hope to investigate ways in which we might alleviate these problems by using speaker identification technology in order to allow the volume and precise timing of an utterance to be controlled automatically. Another interesting observation was the extent to which JL was using his computer resources and the Internet as part of his interaction with visitors, particularly by playing music from Web sites and by showing people Web sites that he had found. A promising line of investigation would be to see if this sort of interaction could be integrated into an AAC device (see Copestake and Flickinger, 1998).

Conclusion

As we discussed in the introduction, the evaluations reported here are purely internal. One of the problems that we have found with work on prediction is that there is no accurate way of comparing our results with those reported by other groups, partly because of the lack of a common test corpus. Ideally, data logged from a user of an AAC device would form a component of such a corpus but confidentiality is clearly a problem. One area for future work is to see whether some of the recently distributed speech corpora (e.g. CALLHOME, CALLFRIEND) have sufficiently similar properties to AAC data that they could be used as a realistic common testbed.

In addition to the functionality of the current version of the data-logger, there are at least two facilities that we would aim to incorporate into any future system:

- Data should be encrypted as they are logged, for security on the user's machine and in data transmission. If the data are being used for routine testing of a statistical prediction technique, it may not be necessary for the experimenter to ever look at the unencrypted data.
- Ideally, logging should cover all keystrokes, menu choices etc. and also identify actions such as text cut-and-paste, so that accurate measurements of user input can be made. The state of the word prediction system (i.e. word frequencies etc.) should be automatically dumped at

regular intervals. This would allow automatic compilation of information of statistics about the use of the AAC system.

The techniques we have described, which are based on data-logging are, of course, only part of a full evaluation process. The collected data have proved invaluable to us as a resource in this early stage of our research on AAC, both as a way to allow us to make more informed choices as to the sort of NLP techniques which might be most promising, and as a way of evaluating slight variations on the well-established techniques of word and phrase prediction. There are other aspects that we have not discussed in detail here. For instance, our proposed cogeneration technique makes use of an extensive grammar of English, and the logged data provide us with one source of information from which to construct test suites to allow us to ensure that the grammar has adequate coverage. However, the ultimate test has to be user evaluation of a full prototype system.

Acknowlededgment

We are very grateful to Greg Edwards who implemented the CSLI AAC system and the data-logger described here. We would also like to thank Ai Kato, who conducted the audiotaping experiments and transcribed the results. Mistakes etc. are the responsibility of the authors. This material is based upon work supported by the National Science Foundation under grant number IRI-9612682.

Chapter 12
Grammar and Lexicons for a Speech-interfaced Knowledge-based Engineering Program (ICAD)

ALICE CARLBERGER

Introduction

This chapter describes an interface for augmentative and alternative communication with a vocational tool rather than with other human beings. Central issues are the recognition of numbers, the word classification system used by the speech recognizer class pair grammar, and the creation and training of Nparse, a probabilistic grammatical-phrase parser. A preliminary comparative study involving testing of recognition with versus without a class pair grammar and recognition with two class pair grammars of differing granularity are presented.

The tool itself, ICAD, developed by Concentra Ltd, is a knowledge-based engineering (KBE) system, which efficiently integrates geometric and graphical information with design methodologies, textual rules and catalogue information. The use of KBE systems has enabled a dramatic increase in productivity compared to pen-and-paper engineering (Bickley and Hunnicutt, 1993; Burnett et al., 1991). With ICAD, drawings can be created in two ways: either line by line or through rules that create a generic model from which drawings can be generated. The first method is used for one-off drawings, the second for drawings that can be reused, with or without modifications (Bickley, Hunnicutt and Lamel, 1993). Typical applications are architectural layouts and the configuration of heating and wiring systems or automotive and aerospace components. ICAD is used by Boeing, British Aerospace, Jaguar, Lotus, and hundreds of other companies in the United States, Europe and Japan.

Traditionally, KBE software has been accessed step-by-step via commands on a keyboard in conjunction with a pointing device such as a mouse, joystick, trackball or tablet. However, in recent years, voice has been explored as an alternative method of access in such systems (Bickley and Hunnicutt, 1993; Bickley, Hunnicutt and Lamel, 1993; Bickley et al., 1993). In the ENABL project (ENabler for Access to Computer-Based

Vocational Tasks with Language and Speech), a speech user interface for Swedish is under development for ICAD (Carlberger, 1998; Carlberger et al., 1997b). The purpose is to allow engineers who have lost the use of their upper extremities due to an accident or illness to continue, restart or start a technically challenging job commensurate with their training, skills, and any previous level of remuneration. For these individuals, it seems that the expressiveness and flexibility of natural language in the form of speech could constitute a viable, natural and efficient substitute to manual input devices. Support for this view is found, in Ball and Ling (1995) (among others), who suggest that speech might be a convenient means of specifying an overall task in one or a few sentences. Further support is found in a study conducted by Hugunin and Zue (1997) which suggests that, with the right design, speech-based interfaces could significantly enhance a human being's interaction with the computer compared to standard desktop application interfaces. However, at the same time, Hugunin and Zue point out the inherent risk for misrecognition of the user's utterance as well as the potential for such errors to become catastrophic.

The three-year EU-funded ENABL project started in January 1996 and is a cooperative effort between Concentra Ltd and Sheffield University in England, and Enter Rehabilitation and the Royal Institute of Technology (KTH) in Sweden. The first two applications (demonstrator systems) will be the design of wheeled toys and cardboard boxes, respectively, by two Swedish engineers in their late twenties with spinal cord injury. The first engineer still possesses some manual dexterity and will be using the speech interface in conjunction with a pointer. He has no previous experience of wheeled-toys applications. The other engineer has no use of his upper extremities and will be using the program exclusively by voice. He has been designing and constructing cardboard boxes for several years with a sip-and-puff device.

This chapter focuses on the development of the ICAD speech user interface lexicon and grammar, including a probabilistic grammatical-phrase parser, class pair system for the speech recognizer, and training and test materials for the speech recognizer and parser. Central issues are word classification and the recognition of numbers, compounds and user-defined names. Comparative studies of recognition with versus without a class pair grammar and two class pair grammars of differing granularity will be presented. Throughout the chapter, the words 'command', 'sentence', and 'utterance' will be used interchangeably. Likewise, the terms 'subject' and 'speaker' will be substituted for each other.

Speech user interface overview

The guiding principle for the work in the ENABL project is to create a generic, reusable and robust platform for a speech user interface, which can be updated and adapted for specific needs. This principle calls for the development of a general structure that is application- and user-independent. A number of modules, such as the recognizer (Ström, 1997), parser (Carlson and Hunnicutt, 1996), and ICAD, are doing specific processing and the interaction between them is handled by The Broker, developed at KTH (Lewin, 1997 and Sjölander et al., 1998). The speech user interface, also under development at KTH, is shown in Figure 12.1. When a spoken command has been detected, it is first analysed by a robust speaker-independent continuous-speech recognizer, which relies on phonetic and semantic information from the lexicon and word sequence information from the functional-grammatical class pair grammar. The output from the recognizer is then fed into the parser, Nparse, which splits the command into simple grammatical phrases, using an n-gram grammar in conjunction with grammatical feature information from the lexicon. Nparse also looks up any ICAD action tag associated with a content word in the lexicon. The parser output is then passed on to ICAD, which performs an action according to its interpretation of the action tag or sequence of action tags. Examples of actions are the resizing of an object or its positioning according to coordinate specifications.

Acoustic training of the speech recognizer

To cover various voice types and dialects, 25 male and 25 female speakers, reading approximately 60 sentences each, were recorded. Speech was recorded at 16 kHz with 16 bits per sample. The effective recording time per speaker averaged 4 minutes, resulting in a total of 203 minutes. Due to the lack of publicly available engineering speech corpora, a mixed database of manually screened phonetically balanced newspaper sentences and sentences from a natural-language script for constructing a hinge in ICAD was used. Basic user interface commands were included.

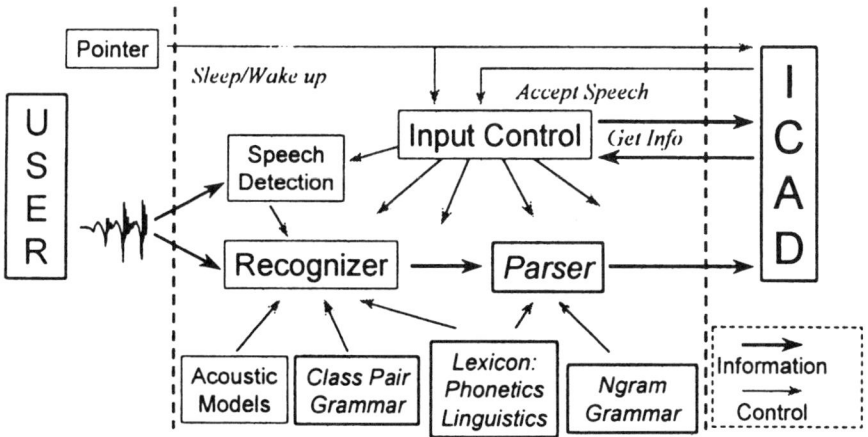

Figure 12.1. Speech user interface.

The readings were then hand-checked for accuracy and marked for extra-linguistic features such as lip smacks, hesitations, repetitions and pauses.

Speaking to ICAD

A primary goal of the ENABL project is to allow the user to interact as naturally and efficiently as possible with the program, as this is expected to enhance his productivity. Commands were created manually within the project, for training and testing of the system, in the following manner. Two Concentra engineers converted keystrokes and mouse clicks and sequences of these into realistic natural-language commands, which were translated into Swedish by a Swedish linguist in consultation with the engineers. The commands were then modified with linguistic data elicited in the ICAD user training.

An important aspect in the ICAD user training was to collect speech and language data to be used during the process of design of the speech recognizer, the speech user interface and the two demonstrator systems. A training engineer travelled weekly to the wheeled-toys application user's residence to work with him, and a large part of the training was directly applicable to the user's work. A Wizard-of-Oz training protocol was used to elicit suggestions for words and phrases that the user would prefer, based on the user's technical background, vocational task and short-term memory. These suggestions were incorporated into the Swedish commands, which were then examined for appropriateness and accuracy by two Swedish mechanical-engineering students.

Functionally, several types of commands can be distinguished in ICAD. These are illustrated in Figure 12.2 with one or several speech command samples for each type.

Most commands turned out to be verb-initial and no longer than five words. Therefore, this was chosen as the preferred format. The length preference, however, does not apply to mathematical formulae and commands containing numerals. Likewise, the verb-first predisposition does not pertain to coordinate specifications or if-then rules.

As the two users start using speech-interfaced ICAD in their work, it is expected that they will have further opinions about phrasing and wording. Therefore, user interaction will be studied and the system modified based on these observations. In particular, the specification of coordinates and the use of inflections, compounding and object naming will be studied. Although it is expected that users will not vary the form of spoken commands greatly once they learn ways that work, it is necessary to ensure that the system understands commands that are natural from the user's perspective. Part of the evaluation of the system will include convenience and cognitive load for the user, and efficiency of the user's design work. Furthermore, throughout the project, a team of speech pathologists monitors the voices of both users.

Functional Command	Example Speech Command (Swedish)	English Translation
Line-by-line construction	Rita en cirkel.	Draw a circle.
Textual rules	Om . . . Så . . .	If . . . Then . . .
Number specification	Sätt höjden = 35, 50.	Set height = 35. 50.
Basic user interface	Dela vertikalt.	Split (screen) vertically.
Menu selection	Visa trädkommandona. Välj . . .	Show tree commands. Choose . . .
Database search	Hitta billigaste handtaget i databasen.	Find cheapest grip in database.
Object viewing	Visa ovanifrån i ruta 1.	Show top view in Window 1.
2D object manipulation	Centrera plattan. x = 2. y = 0,	Center plate. x = 2. y = 0.
3D object manipulation	Rotera handtaget 45 grader runt x-axeln.	Rotate grip 45 deg around x-axis.
Mathematical formulae	x2 = y2 + z2	x2 = y2 + z2

Figure 12.2. Command types according to function.

Class pair grammar

Due to the lack of corpus material, a class pair grammar, rather than a bigram grammar, was used. A non-hierarchical word classification system was created through abstraction from a large, unstructured set of commands. The class pair grammar was then generated through machine analysis of a representative subset in conjunction with functional-grammatical class look-up in the lexicon. It includes 12 classes of numerals representing 60 basic digits, from which all other numbers can be derived by the system. This is an important part of the grammar, since numerals are notoriously difficult to recognize by phonetics alone.

To reduce the number of distributional anomalies in the class pair grammar, word sequences with expected high frequency have been entered as single lexicon entries with underscores linking the constituents. They must be treated as single units both by the class pair grammar and the parser. Examples are the prepositional adverbial phrases 'från vänster' (from the left) and 'från höger' (from the right), which have been classified as VIEWTYPE by analogy with single words like 'ovanifrån' (from the top) and 'underifrån' (from the bottom). They are all treated as adverbs by the parser.

Study

A preliminary comparative study of speech recognition with three class pair grammars of differing granularity has been carried out, the hypothesis being that finer grain yields better recognition. (In the rest of this chapter, the concept 'class pair grammar' will simply be referred to as 'grammar'.)

Grammar 1 contains one single class, which means that there are no restrictions on what word is allowed to follow another word. That is to say, Grammar 1 is really the absence of a grammar, but, for pragmatic reasons, in this study it is called a 'grammar'. Grammars 2 and 3, on the other hand, are real grammars. The former consists of 74 classes of three kinds: (1) truly functional-grammatical (e.g. TREE_VERB), (2) strictly functional (e.g. COLOUR) or (3) strictly grammatical (e.g. NOUN). (The strictly grammatical classes are residual classes, which, it is hoped, can be divided or dispersed into new or existing classes, once more data on how users actually speak are obtained.) Grammar 3 contains 84 classes and differs from Grammar 2 only in its sensitivity to definiteness. For instance, the word 'vinkeln' (the angle – in Swedish, the definite article is morphologically encoded as a suffix on the noun and adjective) is classified as INPUT_NUM_DEF in Grammar 3 but INPUT_NUM in Grammar 2. The two grammars contain no other inflectional classes, apart from the genitive (e.g. PART_GEN).

First, seven subjects (five males and two females) were recorded reading approximately 60 commands each, the commands varying in length from 1 to 12 words and many of the longer commands containing numbers. The recordings were then run through the recognizer, once with each grammar, yielding both sentence level and action level n-best lists. (Each content word has a unique action tag, except for synonyms and forms inflected for definiteness.)

For each speaker, the number of utterances with an incorrect top hypothesis was counted.

Across all three grammars at both sentence and action level, the best recognition results are obtained for the two female subjects, S5 and S3. The reason for this is not apparent. Conversely, S6 exhibits the worst results, possibly due to a larger number of word-internal pauses and hesitations compared with the other subjects. Table 12.1a and Figures 12.3a (sentence level) and 12.3b (action level) show error rates in table and graph format with subjects in order of performance.

The fact that both Grammars 2 and 3 yield significant reductions in error rate compared with Grammar 1, both at the sentence and action levels, illustrates the importance of grammar in recognition. It can be seen, in Table 12.1b, that error reduction ranges from 51% to 88% at the action level, and from 40% to 78% at the sentence level. Figures 12.4a and 12.4b show the error reduction provided by Grammar 2 over Grammar 1, and by Grammar 3 over Grammar 1, respectively. A less uniform distribution is shown in Figure 12.4c, where Grammar 3 exhibits a reduction over Grammar 2 for all subjects except S5, for which it has no effect; the highest reductions, approximately 20%, are found in three subjects, while two of the others exhibit reductions around 15%. At the action level, on the other hand, Grammar 3 affords no reduction over Grammar 2 for two subjects, and for one subject even increases the error rate, due to an instance of unfortunate interplay of phonetics and grammar. For the rest of the subjects, Grammar 3 decreases the action level error rate by about 10–20%.

Nparse, the grammatical-phrase parser

Nparse, a probabilistic example-based grammatical-phrase parser for speech recognition of general and domain-specific language, is under construction at KTH. The development of Nparse originated as part of the

Table 12.1a. Error rate of recognition without any class pair grammar vs. with two class pair grammars of differing granularity: sentence and action level, respectively.

| | Sentence Error (%) | | | Action Error | |
	Gram1	Gram2	Gram3	Gram1	Gram2
Subject 5	39.0	8.5	8.5	39.0	5.1
Subject 3	44.1	11.9	10.2	42.4	5.1
Subject 7	48.3	17.2	13.8	44.8	8.6
Subject 2	56.6	23.3	18.3	53.3	13.3
Subject 1	63.8	22.4	19.0	62.1	19.0
Subject 4	56.9	25.9	24.1	55.2	20.7
Subject 6	91.4	55.2	43.1	81.0	39.7

Table 12.1b. Error reduction rate provided by two class pair grammars of differing granularity: sentence and action level, respectively.

| | Error Reduction (%) | | | | | |
| | Gram2 over Gram1 | | Gram3 over Gram1 | | Gram3 over Gram2 | |
	Sentence	Action	Sentence	Action	Sentence	Action
Subject 5	78.2	86.9	78.2	86.9	0.0	0.0
Subject 3	73.0	88.0	76.9	88.0	14.3	0.0
Subject 7	64.4	80.8	71.4	84.6	19.8	19.8
Subject 2	58.8	75.0	67.7	78.0	21.4	12.0
Subject 1	64.9	69.4	70.2	72.3	15.2	9.5
Subject 4	54.5	62.5	57.6	59.4	6.9	-8.2
Subject 6	39.6	51.0	52.8	59.5	21.9	17.4

Waxholm Project (Carlson and Hunnicutt, 1995, 1996). The parser allows multiple-word interpretation via a text/word graph system. Four levels of operation are used: top, phrase, pre-terminal, and word. Names of phrases and pre-terminals are assigned by rules that use syntactic, morphological and semantic features. Through these features, words are associated with pre-terminals. Sequences of pre-terminals and phrase nodes then undergo n-gram analysis, and the resulting hypothesis probabilities are calculated as smoothed sums of logarithmic probabilities. The probabilities are then trained by a tree bank, producing a set of n-grams.

For the ENABL project, a parse training corpus was created. Each of the 2800 training commands represents a typical and unique syntax for the ICAD application. Of these, 2700 are frequently used number types consisting of unique configurations of the same 12 basic digit classes used in the class pair grammar, both with and without a class for units of measurement. In the bootstrapping of the parser, the commands were first run through a small, handcrafted set of n-gram sequences. They were then corrected manually to reflect the desired parse for a given input, resulting in a parse training tree bank. Parse trees of the two commands 'Rita under-ifrån i ruta tre' (Draw bottom view in viewport three) and 'Sätt höjden lika med trehundrafem millimeter' (Set height to three hundred five millime-tres) are shown in Figure 12.5.

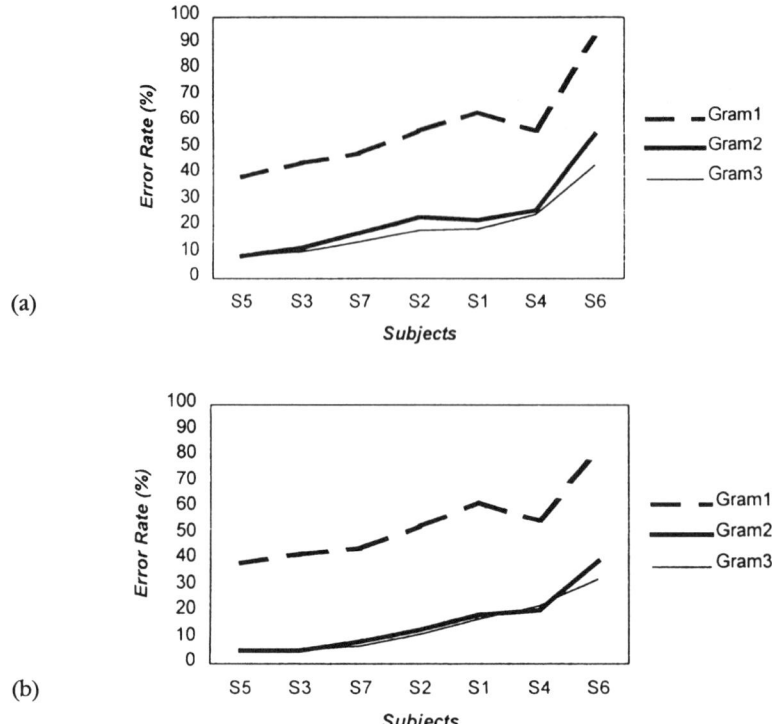

(a)

(b)

Figure 12.3. (a) Sentence level error rate: Grammars 1, 2 and 3.(b) Action level error rate: Grammars 1, 2 and 3.

Lexicons

A 575-word lexicon consisting of general-application vocabulary such as function words, alpha characters, basic digits, units of measurement, operands, geometric shapes, and other technical vocabulary was created. In addition, a 220-word lexicon of vocabulary specific to the wheeled-toys application, containing, for example, tricycle parts, was built. Only inflections of expected high frequency in the application have been included in the system.

Together, the two handcrafted lexicons serve as a base for the generation of the recognizer lexicon and the parse lexicon, whose entries are identical but differ in terms of linguistic information. The recognizer lexicon structure is shown in Figure 12.6a. Field 1 is the orthography, Field 2 a phonetic transcription, Field 3 a tag used by the class pair grammar, Field 4 (if any) a tag used by ICAD to determine an action, and Field 5 (if any) a tag used for disambiguation. The parse lexicon structure, whose entries contain the ICAD action tag followed by grammatical-feature tags, is portrayed in Figure 12.6b.

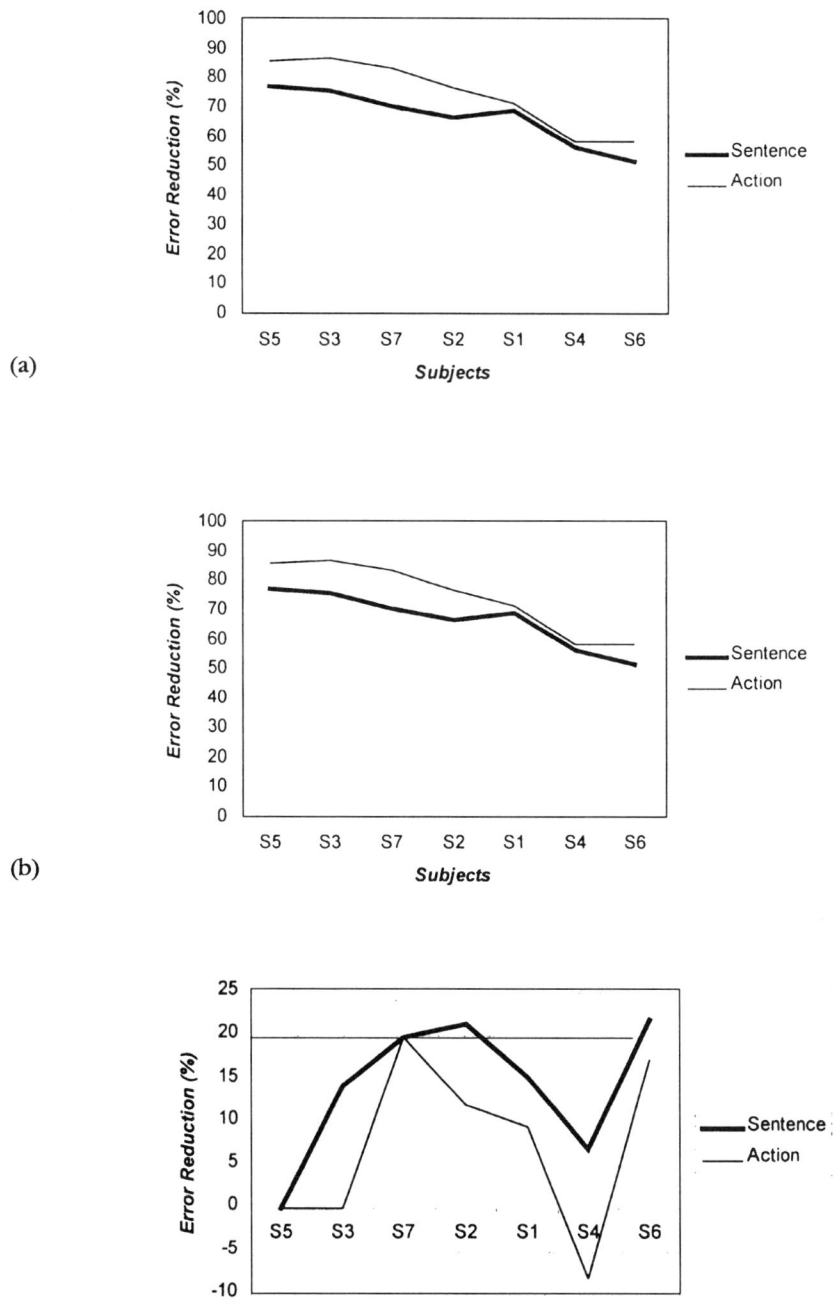

Figure 12.4. (a) Error reduction provided by Grammar 2 over Grammar 1: sentence and action level, respectively. (b) Error reduction provided by Grammar 3 over Grammar 1: sentence and action level, respectively.(c) Error reduction rate provided by Grammar 3 over Grammar 2: sentence and action level, respectively.

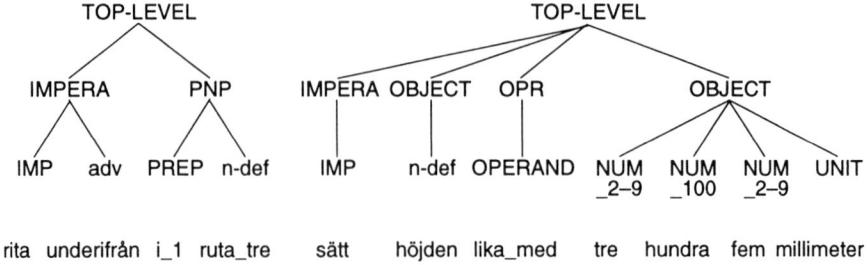

Figure 12.5. Parse trees of the two commands: 'Show bottom view in window 3' (lit. Draw from below in window 3) and 'Set height equal to 305 millimetres'.

billigaste	B'LIGASTE	ADJ_SUP_DEF	CHEAPEST	
bind_ihop	B'IND IH'O:P	LINK	LINK	
blinka_med	BL"INGKA ME:D	BLINK	BLINK	IMP
bläddraren	BL"ÄDRAREON	WINDOW_TYPE	BROWSER	
bläddrarfönstret	BL"ADRARHyF'ONSTRE0T	WINDOW_TYPE	BROWSER	
byt_till	B'Y:T TIL	SWITCH_TO	SWITCH_TO	
böjningsradie	B'ÖJNINGShyRA:DIE0	INPUT_NUM	BEND_RADIUS	

(a)

<billigaste>	"billigaste" ->CHEAPEST A DEF -vara -GEN -PRON -SUPINE -NAME -ACC
<bind_ihop>	"bind_ihop" ->LINK IMP -vara -GEN -PRON V -SUPINE -NAME -ACC AKT
<blinka_med>	"blinka_med" ->BLINK IMP -vara -GEN -PRON V -SUPINE -NAME -ACC AKT
<bläddraren>	"bläddraren" ->BROWSER N -NEU DEF -PL -vara -GEN -PRON -SUPINE -NAME -ACC
<bläddrarfönstret>	"bläddrarfönstret" ->BROWSER N NEU DEF -PL -vara -GEN -PRON -SUPINE -NAME -ACC
<byt_till>	"byt_till" ->SWITCH_TO IMP -vara -GEN -PRON V -SUPINE -NAME -ACC AKT
<böjningsradie>	"böjningsradie" ->BEND_RADIUS N -NEU -DEF -PL -vara -GEN -PRON -SUPINE -NAME -ACC

(b)

Figure 12.6. (a) Speech recognition lexicon excerpt. (b) Parse lexicon excerpt.

Future linguistic work

Certain linguistic restrictions or preferences pertaining to command length, syntax, morphology and synonymy have been imposed to facilitate recognition. Some of these will be removed as the system develops and improves. Moreover, as the ICAD user becomes more proficient, he will undoubtedly find shortcuts in his command syntax as well as the need for new commands. The linguistic components of the speech user interface will therefore need to be updated at regular intervals, and an updating mechanism is currently under development. Part of this work includes optimizing the word classification system, used by the class pair grammar, with a minimum of manual labour. More complex common structures of the general language that would pose a problem for the parser have already been mapped out and solutions proposed.

Compounding, i.e. the forming of a new word through the concatenation of two or more words, is a highly productive process in many languages, including Swedish. An example is 'bokrea' (book sale), from 'bok' (book) and 'rea' (sale). For our purposes, a compound is defined as a concatenation of two words, at least one of which can stand alone, and at least one of which occurs in more than one lexeme or inflection. According to this definition, approximately 25% of the words in the current lexicons are compounds. Most of these are nominal (noun + noun or adverb + noun) and usually consist of a part and a dimension, e.g. 'handtagsradie' (grip radius), 'handtag' (grip) + s [link] + 'radie' (radius). In addition, the majority of the compound components themselves constitute stand-alone words in the system. Therefore, it is desirable to store the components rather than the full compounds in the lexicon. This approach, used in other natural language processing systems as well (e.g. Carter et al, 1996), will be explored along with the possibility of implementing a compounding module. The possibilities of handling object labelling with single-digit-letter sequences within such a compounding system will also be examined.

Acknowledgements

ENABL is a Telematics Application Project supported by the Commission of the European Communities. We gratefully acknowledge the financial support of TIDE (EU), NUTEK, and KTH. Nparse is under development by Rolf Carlson for use in speech technology applications. Researchers involved in the development of the speech user interface are, in alphabetical order, Alice Carlberger, Rolf Carlson, Joakim Gustafson, Erland Lewin and Nikko Ström.

Chapter 13
ScriptLog. A Tool for Logging the Writing Process and its Possible Diagnostic Use

Elisabeth Ahlsén and Sven Strömqvist

Introduction

The aim of this chapter is to present the possibilities of the ScriptLog computer tool for logging the writing process and to discuss how ScriptLog could be used for diagnostic and evaluating functions in the assessment of writing disorders and writing aids. ScriptLog is being developed within the research programme 'Reading and Writing Strategies of Disabled Groups' at the Department of Linguistics, Göteborg University, supported by the Swedish Research Foundation for Social Sciences (SFR). The research programme focuses on studying the writing process and modelling how this process is affected by different types of disabilities, e.g. dyslexia, deafness and aphasia. The assumption is that different groups need partly different types of computer support for writing, depending on the way the writing process is affected.

The research programme has the following aims:

- To develop a research environment for contrastive studies of the writing process in language users with different types of disabilities.
- To develop and test multimedia tools for computer supported analysis of the writing process, tailored for persons with disabilities.

It is associated with European Research Initiative COST A8, 'Learning Disabilities as a Barrier to Human Development' and the Spencer Foundation project 'Developing Literacy in Different Contexts and Different Languages'.

There are five dimensions:

1. Disability: three types of disability affecting writing – dyslexia, deafness and aphasia.

2. The pragmatic dimension: reading and writing in different social activities.
3. The cross-linguistic dimension: typological differences of writing systems.
4. The developmental dimension: processes of reorganization related to disabilities.
5. The multimodal dimension:
   - perception–production
   - speech – writing
   - perceptually driven process of development
   - language disturbance – reading and writing disturbance
   - possibilities for compensation with multimedia support.

The research programme is being carried out in three main steps:

Step 1

- The dimensions: disabilities, pragmatic and multimodal are in focus.
- Data collection and analyses.
- Adult subjects with different disabilities are studied with respect to:
  (a) spontaneous use of writing in everyday situations
  (b) controlled experimental tasks on a computer.
- Basic versions of multimedia tools for data collection are developed, to be modified.

Step 2

- Cross-linguistic dimensions are added.
- Other research groups in Europe are added for cross-linguistic comparisons.
- The multimedia tool is developed for different orthographies.

Step 3

- The developmental perspective is added.
- Pilot studies with different age and language groups are made for dyslexia.

ScriptLog

Concerning computer tools, the research programme has focused primarily on the development of computer software for logging text production for research purposes, i.e. the first of the aims mentioned above. ScriptLog works as an ordinary text editor, with or without stimulus presentation. It has been used for the collection of text data in the form of picture-based story writing where the stimuli are presented by the

Scriptlog (using 'Frog, where are you?' a story which is extensively used in the collection of cross-linguistic language acquisition data). It has further been used in logging text writing representing different social activities (or genres), such as route descriptions, job applications and free narration of an event ('I have never been so afraid').

Data have been collected for children of different ages and for adults, for groups of dyslexic, deaf and aphasic adult subjects and for dyslexic children.

ScriptLog logs all keyboard and mouse events in time. It gives overview statistics automatically:

- total writing time;
- total pause time;
- number of keystrokes;
- number of editings;
- number of pauses according to a pause criterion (e.g. 2 seconds or 5 seconds).

In addition, the program presents the text in different forms:

- the text product (Example 1);
- the text with markings of pauses and editings, according to menu choices (Example 2);
- real-time playback of the keystroke events;
- a log file with all times, screen positions and keystrokes (Example 3).

The log-files can also be exported to Excel for computation of further statistics. A number of specific programs for statistics and visualization of result data are under development.

Example 1

På natten när pojken hade somnat smet grodan ur burken och hoppade ut genom fönstret.
(Translation: In the night when the boy had fallen asleep the frog sneaked out from the jar and jumped out through the window.)

Example 2

```
<SECTION 2><6.95>PÅ <DELETE2><3.70>å natten när <2.48>
p<3.60>oj<2.30>ken  <2.95>h<3.63>ade  fö<4.16>rs<2.55>v
<4.48>unnit<6.60> <DELETE10> <3.18>somnat       <3.05>smetv
<DELETE2> <2.98>grodan <10.68>ur <4.43>b<2.70>urken <8.10>
o<2.36>ch ho<3.10>ppade  <5.05>ut genom fön<14.31>stret
<4.31>.<2.15>
<SECTION 3>
```

Example 3

Table 13.1.

Time	Type	From	To	Key
119.30	9	2	0	<SECTION>
126.25	7	0	0	P
126.90	7	1	1	Å
127.65	7	2	2	
128.90	5	3	3	<DELETE>
129.05	5	2	2	<DELETE>
132.75	7	1	1	å
133.80	7	2	2	
134.71	7	3	3	n
135.78	7	4	4	a
136.21	7	5	5	t
136.35	7	6	6	t
136.85	7	7	7	e
137.76	7	8	8	n
138.03	7	9	9	
138.93	7	10	10	n
139.86	7	11	11	ä
141.00	7	12	12	r

See further Strömqvist and Malmsten, 1998. For another program with similar functions, see Severinsson-Eklund and Kollberg, 1995.

Analysis of writing abilities

Based on the ScriptLog data, together with video recordings, test data and spoken control data, different profiles of problems in the writing process are being developed for the different groups with writing disabilities and for individuals within the groups. Since extensive and detailed data on the writing process of the different groups, together with analysis tools for statistics and visualization of results are available, we expect results that are highly relevant for the application of psycholinguistic modelling of the writing process and of the different disorders of writing.

Analyses are made of the written text products at the sentence, phrase, word, morpheme and letter levels with classifications of types of problems.

Analyses are further made of the dynamic features of the writing process, e.g. pausing (frequency, times, positions, distribution in texts), editings (frequency, distance, types) and the number and speed of keystrokes. (The latter is also used as a reference for the keyboard ability of each individual.)

Comparisons are made between the content, form and production process of speech and writing. Preliminary results show considerable variation between the three groups with writing disabilities. A few examples of the findings are the following.

The *distribution of pauses* is different. For example, dyslexics make many pauses within words, but not many final pauses for going back to check and make long distance editing. Aphasics use extremely long pauses between words and thus have extremely long writing times.

The *use of sentence-like units* varies. Dyslexics very often omit any overt sentence boundaries, such as full stops and sentence initial capitals. The deaf subjects use phrase or sentence-like units, quite often separated by a number of full stops, not always using sentence initial capitals. Aphasics mostly use sentence boundaries correctly; the sentences are, however, sometimes not grammatically correct.

Dyslexics as well as aphasics produce a large number of spelling errors based on *speech-like writing*, i.e., they seem to rely on phoneme-grapheme conversion in their writing. Congenitally deaf subjects have a high production rate and relatively few spelling errors, but several types of grammatical errors. Aphasics produce the largest number of *contextually dependent spelling errors*, i.e. anticipations and perseverations of letters (Ahlsén, 1998; Strömqvist and Ahlsén, 1998; Strömqvist and Wengelin, 1998; Wengelin, 1998a,b).

Scriptlog as a tool for diagnosis and evaluation

The analyses and expected results bring us to the second aim of the research programme, which is the potential use and development of ScriptLog as an analysis tool for clinical and educational purposes. There is a need for a tool of this type, given that suitable instructions for its use can be added.

Such a tool should be able to minimally give a profile of what the main problematic surface features of the writing process are. It could also be extended to provide a tentative interpretation of the profile in the light of a psycholinguistic model of writing. Based on this interpretation it could also suggest possible computer support as well as training procedures to alleviate some of the problems.

Discussion

Two main points of discussion are:

1. The potential use (and misuse?) of ScriptLog as a tool for diagnostic and evaluative purposes in clinical and/or pedagogical contexts.

2. The potential development of a way to use ScriptLog in combination with different types of computer support for writing, such as spell-checking, word prediction and top-down structuring support.

The first question concerns whether it is better just to collect data concerning types of problems in the writing process and list those in a profile, or whether the research results to come, including a model based interpretation of the problem sources, should be employed. In the latter case, we would have a more expert-system like tool, which could also suggest therapy and compensation. The questions are then how much of the analysis and interpretation should be made by a human expert, and who should be allowed to use such a tool. On the one hand, an interpretation of the findings in terms of their causes is clearly more valuable and clinically sound. On the other hand, it probably takes a human expert to use this information in an optimal way.

The second question concerns the development of ScriptLog as a tool for evaluation. Questions of compatibility and combination of different programs are notoriously hard to solve and today there are probably insurmountable obstacles which prevent the use of ScriptLog together with computer supports for writing.

But, nevertheless, it is worth discussing the possibility of combination. If ScriptLog is to be used as a tool for diagnosis and evaluation of the ability to write text, it is a natural expectation that one should also be able to evaluate text writing with the use of programs for writing support. In the first place, this is how, for example, a dyslexic person is most likely to write in everyday life. Secondly, it would then be possible to compare writing without support to writing using different types of support in the same individual. This would, of course, be an immensely valuable application, if it could be attained.

Chapter 14
Some Future Research Directions

NORMAN ALM, STEFAN LANGER AND MARIANNE HICKEY

Introduction

In this chapter we give a summary of the research on natural language processing (NLP) and augmentative and alternative communication (AAC) presented in this section. We also point out some possible future research directions in AAC related to language resources and language processing techniques.

Most of the authors of the chapters presented here are researchers who occupy the middle ground between AAC and NLP. Some are AAC researchers who have moved into NLP in order to improve augmented communication. Some are NLP researchers who see in augmentative communication an interesting and worthwhile application of the knowledge from their field. The chapters cover a number of evaluation issues when dealing with AAC, ways for augmented communication to operate at the level of pragmatics, logging the use of AAC and computer-aided writing systems as a means of providing material for evaluation, making use of this material and problems that can arise with this, using speech recognition to make it possible to drive a complex software package without hand use, and developing protocols to allow valid comparisons between word prediction systems. Themes and issues arising from these papers can be summarized under the categories of models, tools for analysis, and findings.

Models

Two approaches can be taken to augmented communication: generating unique text and using pre-stored text. For generating unique text, word prediction schemes are now in general use. The compansion technique, of expanding compressed input, is under development. Techniques which make use of pre-stored text include selection from a single small list, hierarchical and network storage structures, and attempts at using semantic and pragmatic characteristics of the text itself to aid retrieval.

A model for AAC is suggested which incorporates both message generation and message retrieval and places both in the context of the short-, medium- and long-term goals of communication. Thus message generation, while slow, helps to achieve such pragmatic features as appropriateness and coping with the unexpected. Message retrieval, while not providing unique material, can better achieve the pragmatic features of effective repair, staying in touch, and so on. These pragmatic features in their turn map in differing ways onto such goals as making a good impression, projecting personality and developing relationships.

Tools for analysis

Two tools for analysis were presented in the chapters and also emerged from the discussions at the workshop: automatic logging of an AAC user's output and evaluation criteria.

Automatic logging could produce material which is superior to corpus-based data, being more individual, and more appropriate, given the wide range of different sources needed to produce a corpus. There are confidentiality issues here, however, given the personal nature of much everyday conversation. One solution suggested for this in the workshop discussion was to have researchers who had data derived from logging offer to run other researchers' prototypes with their data, so that the data always remained with them. A potential disadvantage of logged data compared with that derived from a corpus is that the logged data may be too adapted to the individual from whom it was derived, and this possibility must be borne in mind. Examples have also been given of the usefulness of logging written data from people with aphasia, dyslexia and hearing impairment.

Evaluation criteria for word prediction systems and for voice output communication systems were derived at the workshop from the papers presented, and from the discussion which followed.

For word prediction systems it was suggested that the evaluation criteria should include:

- rate;
- keystroke saving;
- cognitive load;
- pleasure in use.

The last category is not a trivial one, having its own value, but also being connected with factors such as motivation and fatigue.

For voice output communication systems the suggested evaluation criteria included:

- rate;
- number and variety of speech acts;
- conversational control;
- effective repair;
- staying in touch;
- maintenance of flow;
- enjoyment of participants.

Findings

A number of findings resulting from the research which has been carried out over the past few years are presented in these papers and were also reported during the workshop discussions.

The importance of taking account of pragmatics in AAC design is now generally recognized, and work based on evaluating prototypes with pragmatic functions bears this out.

The application of complex and processing-intensive computational linguistics to problems in AAC is very difficult. The richness, ambiguity and context sensitivity of natural language is a challenge for all work in this area. However, some progress has been made, in the field of natural language processing in general, and in its application to AAC system improvement. Particular areas which could be improved with mainstream natural language processing techniques are unique text creation and applications of speech recognition.

The usefulness of word prediction as a rate enhancer has been questioned, with the problem of increased cognitive load being highlighted. Very slow typing users can still benefit from word prediction. With some users, keystroke reduction itself is useful, and with others the pleasure in use resulting from seeing that the system is tracking the user's language is significant in helping with motivation and general satisfaction with the system.

The increasing availability of augmentative communication in a wide range of languages has highlighted the fact that word prediction performance is quite language dependent. This, among other considerations, has emphasized the need for an agreed protocol which would allow word prediction systems to be compared with each other. What is needed is a way of eliminating the influence of factors such as the user interface, test texts, language differences, and so on, and to be able to make comparisons between systems on the basis of their predictive techniques alone.

Some ideas for future activities

Data for research purposes

In the last two symposium meetings it has been pointed out by several researchers that there is a lack of suitable corpora for AAC research. For all applications that make use of language processing techniques – even those based on simple statistical means – a suitable corpus for training would be helpful. We see two possibilities for building a corpus:

- Corpus of real messages. Here several problems would emerge:
  – private content versus availability for other researchers – this problem could be partially circumvented by ensuring that the data are given anonymously;
  – a lack of sufficient data sources for building a large corpus;
  – responses from conversation partners are difficult to retain.
- Corpus of newsgroups/chat room/ electronic mail messages. These are methods of communication that are potentially close to AAC in several ways:
  – quick response generation without many formal requirements;
  – casual language;
  – intermediate level between written and spoken language.

The advantages and disadvantages of the two types of corpus suggest that a useful solution would be to build a corpus of real AAC messages that is augmented with additional material from other sources. This would enable statistical systems, which need a large amount of data, to be trained.

Integrating different approaches

Message building systems (typically word prediction) and message selection systems are based on different philosophies. The former emphasize the creative use of language, allowing users to generate new and unique utterances when they are communicating. The latter emphasize the repetition and timing factors in language use, which both play important roles in human interaction, and allow users to reuse conversational material relatively quickly. In everyday conversations, both strategies are used. Natural speakers often recycle whole phrases, as long as the conversation is about subjects they are highly familiar with, but, if the situation requires it, they spontaneously produce unique utterances.

Integrated AAC systems would incorporate both approaches – they would include a message generation module, such as word prediction, as well as an efficient message storage and selection system. NLP techniques can help to build an integrated system that has the advantages of both communication approaches, by automating the storage and retrieval of unique messages that are produced by the user. For example, an integrated system might look like an advanced word prediction system that is linked to a message database, where every message the user produces is stored. Similarity of form and meaning, automatically detected by the system, could be used to group the stored messages and to avoid storing almost identical messages. Spell-checking routines can be used to avoid the storage of messages that contain misspelled words.

For users of symbol, icon or sign languages who are learning to write natural language, integration of that language and natural language in one system, linked by a translation module, could help users to learn natural language (Hunnicutt, 1996).

Making use of speech recognition

Another idea that emerged from the discussions at the workshops was to use speech recognition to process the input of the conversation partner. The acquired information could then be used to help predict the next message required by the user of the communication aid. Speech recognition systems can now cope, with a limited accuracy, with input from new speakers and with continuous speech. Even if speech recognition were kept to the simpler level of recognizing isolated words, or spotting particular words in the partner's speech, these could be used to predict appropriate utterances or to determine the topic of the conversation. An alternative, or additional, approach might be to use the outcome of intonation research to recognize types of speech acts, to predict if a response is necessary and to determine which type of response would be appropriate.

Multilingual systems and message translation

Finally, multilingual systems could be built. AAC users, like everyone else, face the challenge of learning and using foreign languages. To our knowledge, there is not yet a word prediction system on the market that supports easy transition between different languages. Even more interesting seems a system that translates automatically between languages. This is possible with current NLP techniques. If an AAC system were connected to a machine translation module, the non-speaker might have considerable advantages over natural speakers when travelling abroad.

Conclusion

The chapters in this section, the results of the workshops and the publications of recent years show that natural language processing techniques already play an important role in research on communication aids, and we hope that this development is going to continue for the benefit of AAC consumers. Language processing and information retrieval techniques will be used increasingly within AAC devices because they offer substantial potential for further improvements in performance, and there do not seem to be many alternative ways to enhance communication aids. More intelligent AAC devices, which implement language processing techniques, are likely to take more of the cognitive load away from the user, increase communication fluency and help non-speakers to participate more fully in conversations. To conclude, it seems that the transfer of research in language and speech processing into AAC will offer some challenging long-term research perspectives, and that established NLP tools and techniques can offer more immediate benefits in terms of enhancing AAC devices.

Section III
Graphic Symbol Use

Chapter 15
Considerations for Understanding the Nature and Use of Graphic Symbols

Filip T. Loncke and Lyle L. Lloyd

The use of graphic symbols has been the subject of interest within the field of augmentative and alternative communication (AAC) for many decades. In the early years of AAC practice and research, questions such as 'Which graphic symbols have the strongest potential for communication?', 'Which characteristics of graphic symbols enhance their accessibility?', and 'What is the effect of the use of graphic symbols on speech communication?' were raised (e.g. Lloyd and Karlan, 1984; Luftig and Bersani, 1985a). These questions continue to be central discussion issues in the field (Fuller, Lloyd and Schlosser, 1997). However, they have also increasingly become part of broader discussions in a variety of areas and approaches to communication. Characteristics and use of graphic symbols have been discussed as they relate to semiotics (Soto and Olmstead, 1993), classification and taxonomy of linguistic and non-linguistic symbols (Lloyd and Fuller, 1986), and understanding the nature of microgenesis of utterances (Loncke, Vander Beken and Lloyd, 1998). Awareness has grown that a number of factors should be taken into account during the complex decision-making process of selecting graphic symbols for aided communication (Schlosser, Lloyd and McNaughton, 1997). Interestingly, the use of graphic symbols within AAC is leading to a number of fascinating developments and debates on issues such as the existence of 'native users' of graphic symbol communication (Grove et al., 1997; von Tetzchner et al., 1996), representation and semantics ('What does a symbol stand for?') (e.g. Hjelmquist, 1997), the order of acquisition and the interrelation of different representations (Grove and Smith, 1997), and the effect of graphic symbol communication on the emergence and acquisition of literacy (McNaughton, 1998b; McNaughton and Lindsay, 1995).

Need for models and taxonomies

There is currently a search for models that have sufficient power to encompass, explain and predict the major processes involved in the use of graphic symbols. In a chapter dealing with model development for understanding AAC, von Tetzchner et al. (1996) described the need for a model that is, at the same time, general and specific. They noted that the model should be compatible with existing models of general communication, but should also provide a framework capable of accommodating critical AAC characteristics such as the use of multimodal communication and derived forms of language (e.g. concepts encoded into a graphic system). It should also demonstrate the dynamic relationship between linguistic and non-linguistic information processing, and physical, cognitive, interactional and socioeconomic aspects, specific to AAC.

Since the 1980s, models and taxonomies have been proposed for analysing the processing and use of AAC. These models and taxonomies have been explored mainly in search of answers to the following questions:

1. Which features of graphic symbols have a direct impact on the way the symbols are processed?
2. How does the use of graphic symbols affect the pragmatic structure of communication, including initiating, turn-taking, etc.?
3. Is using graphic symbols non-linguistic or is there potential for linguistic processing?
4. How can the use of graphic symbols promote cognitive and linguistic growth and literacy acquisition?
5. How distinctive is graphic symbol communication from other aided and unaided AAC?
6. Are there different types of processing involved in accessing meaning from graphic symbols?
7. Is there a relationship between (a) the level of competence achieved in the processing of different types of graphic symbols and (b) literacy acquisition that can be used to enhance literacy instruction?

Research and clinical issues

Initially, the use of graphic symbols was most significant in direct interactive communication between AAC users and individuals in their environments. AAC users communicated wants and needs and engaged in social exchanges and information transfer by accessing graphic symbols on communication boards. The use of graphic symbols was motivated and encouraged by their assumed motor and cognitive accessibility. Many AAC users were able to physically access the symbols by pointing and relatively little learning was required to use the most iconic symbols. In the past two decades, however, studies have begun to focus on grasping the essence of more of the parameters of graphic symbols that influence accessibility: ambiguity, complexity, figure/ground differential, perceptual distinctiveness and size.

It has become evident that the effects of using graphic symbols extend beyond direct interactive communication to other areas of cognitive, communicative functioning. One such area is literacy acquisition. An obvious question is whether using graphic symbols has a facilitating effect on the acquisition of literacy-related skills. This question has been raised a number of times over the past 15 years. Answers have not been simple. Investigations have, in fact, uncovered more questions. One major question is whether or not the use of graphic symbols facilitates the acquisition of phonologic awareness and other metalinguistic skills deemed essential for reading.

In a series of publications, McNaughton takes the position that the use of graphic symbols can indeed affect the way developing children structure and process orthographic information. She stresses, however, that the effect may be related to the type of graphic symbols to which children are exposed. Picture symbols, which can be processed through recognition, are considerably different from symbols that are not immediately identifiable. Hence, the user of picture symbols processes symbols differently from the user of more abstract symbols. The processes involved in decoding discrete, abstract or semi abstract graphic forms, may more closely resemble those involved in reading.

An intriguing clinical issue relates to how cultural experience may interfere with perception of graphic symbols. Referents can be represented in a wide variety of ways. These representations can be highly culturally specific. Representations for 'woman' and 'teacher', for example, can be very different across cultures. If individuals from one culture are presented with symbols that are not representative of a 'woman' or a 'teacher' from their own culture, but rather from another culture, there may be cognitive dissonance, and they may have difficulty learning them. Providing culturally appropriate symbols is not just a matter of political correctness, it is an issue that must be addressed if clinicians/educators want to facilitate the ability of AAC users to make the connection between graphic symbols and their own internal representational and semantic networks.

Information processing

Which processes are involved when graphic symbols are used in direct interactive communication? It has already been suggested that, depending on the type of symbols, different processes may be activated. If the symbols allow immediate recognition, there may be less need for an intermediate decoding level where symbols are broken down into parts which are assigned individual meaning. If understanding symbols requires analysis at a subsymbolic level, then linguistic or linguistic-like skills must be activated. This is the case for traditional orthography (TO) where sublexical analysis of the parts of the words (graphemes) provide the key for accessing the meaning.

One can gain an understanding of how AAC users access the meanings of graphic symbols by studying existing models of communication. In this section, several communication models that originated from outside the field of AAC are explored in order to generate hypotheses about the nature of the use of graphic symbols.

Forum on graphic symbol relevance

During the summer of 1998, in preparation for the International Society for Augmentative and Alternative Communication (ISAAC) Research Symposium, several scholars exchanged and discussed ideas and theoretical viewpoints related to the use of graphic symbols. They continued their exchange and discussion when they met. The aim of the symposium was to envision and embark on state of the art research and to explore future ways to further understanding of the use of graphic symbols in communication. One of the most striking convictions that became apparent among members of this international group of scholars, clinicians and users is that the importance of this research extends beyond the realm of graphic symbol use itself. The research is expected to contribute to the formation of better and more encompassing linguistic, psychological, and social models of information processing and interaction among people.

Acknowledgement

In the months prior to the symposium, draft manuscripts with useful comments and suggestions were exchanged among researchers and clinicians working around the world in different settings. The authors express gratitude to all who took the time to read early versions of manuscripts and send their reflections. In particular, the authors acknowledge the contributions of Erna Alant (Pretoria, South Africa), Donald Fuller (Little Rock, Arkansas, USA), Manfred Gangkofer (Langwedel, Germany), Mary Blake Huer (Fullerton, California, USA) and Mogens Hygum Jensen (Copenhagen, Denmark).

Chapter 16
Graphic Symbol Use: An Orientation Toward Theoretical Relevance

LYLE L. LLOYD, FILIP T. LONCKE AND
HELEN H. ARVIDSON

This chapter focuses on communication in general, and on the nature of graphic symbols in particular. General communication models are discussed and briefly reviewed in light of how they contribute to the understanding of graphic symbol communication. A number of models concerning internal information processing are also presented as they relate to the use of graphic symbols.

General communication models

Since the middle of the twentieth century, attempts have been made to capture the essence of human communication processing. Shannon and Weaver (1949) proposed a model that describes communication as an exchange of messages between senders and receivers. The process is regulated by feedback mechanisms. Other models provide similar accounts of the nature of communication (Berko, Wolvin and Wolvin, 1977; Fairbanks, 1954).

Communication model applied to AAC: Lloyd, Quist and Windsor (1990)

In the same tradition, Sanders (1976) proposed a communication model that includes the multimodal nature of augmentative and alternative communication (AAC), and that can serve as a basis to understanding graphic symbol use in AAC. The model proposed by Lloyd, Quist and Windsor (1990) can be considered as an elaboration of the Sanders model. Lloyd et al. argued against developing a new AAC model, noting that the Sanders model was robust enough to accommodate the various modalities used in AAC. The strength of the model is that it captures the essential components of message transmission, and the parallel structure of the modes involved. The model does not, however, account for the actual processes that lead to the use of the modes. Some authors (Grove and Smith, 1997) believe the model suggests that communication through non-speech modes is the result of internal transcoding from speech. This interpretation implies that speech representation is essential. As Grove and Smith point out, however, such an interpretation may not account for all observations of language use in different modalities. Rather, it is possible that AAC users go beyond input characteristics.

Although the Lloyd et al. (1990) model does not focus on the way modal information is acquired and processed – possibly, but not necessarily structured around representations of speech – it is not necessarily incompatible with these observations. Lloyd et al. referred to Sanders' brief discussion for insight into the existence of various levels of processing in the encoding and decoding of messages. The model (Figure 16.1) calls attention to the aided–unaided taxonomy for the means to represent, select and transmit. The use of different means to transmit (e.g. devices) may alter the interface of the sender to the transmission environments or signal channels and the receiver. The model illustrates communication interaction between two partners within a communication environment. The illustration is actually a simplification of typical communication showing one dyad in one environment. Communication is typically more complex, often involving multiple partners and/or environments.

The basic elements in the communication process are sender, receiver, message and message transmission. During the process of communication, each sender is at the same time a receiver of his or her own message. Figure 16.2 shows these basic elements.

Feedback and auto-feedback provide a system of fine tuning. In the Relevance Theory, Sperber and Wilson (1986) point out that communication involves much more than the processes of encoding and decoding. Encoding and decoding are guided by implicit considerations about communication partners – inferential processing – the meaning in terms of what is relevant. Relevance is considered to be determined by factors such as communication ease and effect (von Tetzchner et al., 1996).

Clibbens (1997) suggests that the applicability of Relevance Theory to AAC models lies, at a general level, in the relative emphasis it gives to the importance of contextual factors in the interpretation of utterances, and, more specifically, in its explanatory use of the trade-off between effort and effect. The use of AAC techniques may simply often been felt to require too much effort in relation to what the user gets out of it. A typical phenomenon that non-disabled speakers also show when they do not feel like repeating a whole argument, saying 'never mind'.

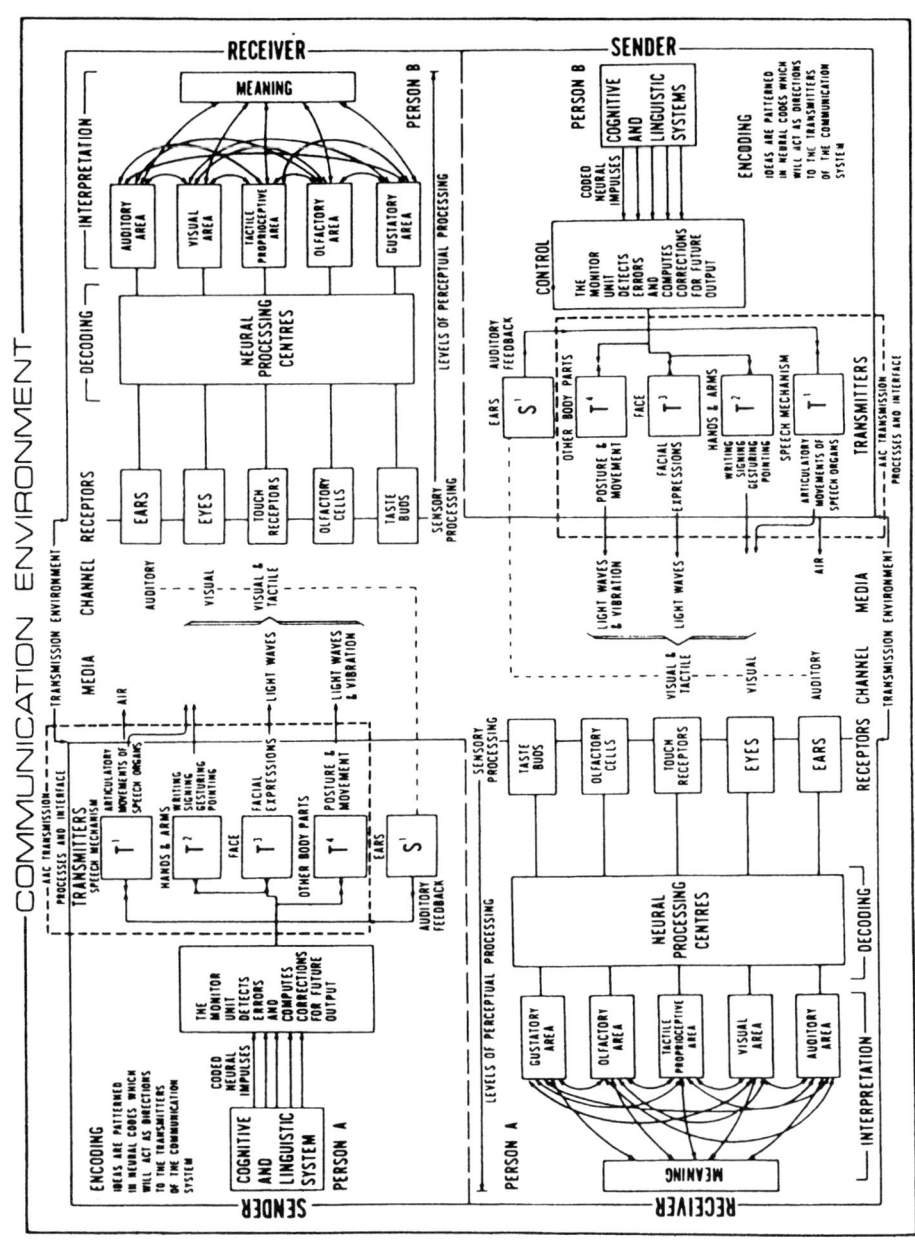

Figure 16.1. AAC communication model (from Lloyd, Quist and Windsor, 1990, pp. 172–180).

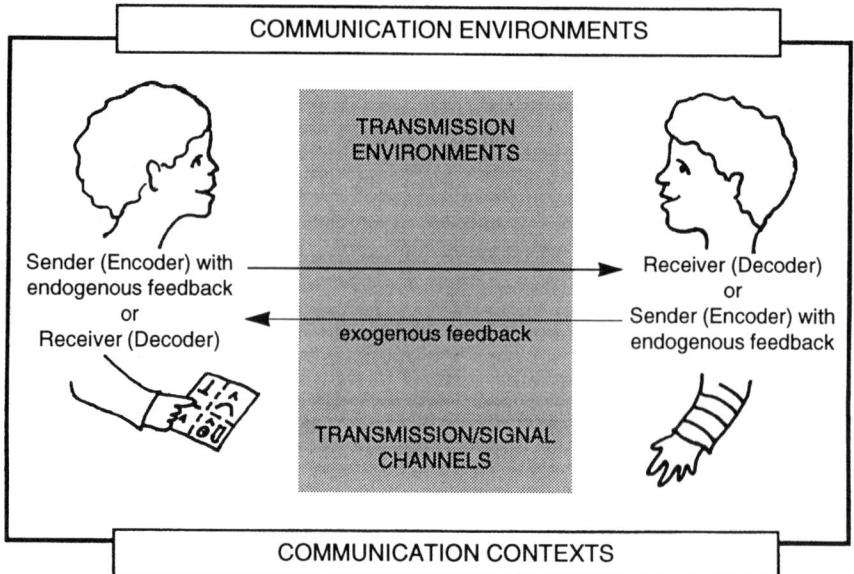

Figure 16.2. Basic elements of the human communication model (from Lloyd, Fuller and Arvidson, 1997b, p. 7).

Terminology

It is important to seek consistency and avoid ambiguity in the use of terms; therefore, we propose the following definitions and discussion of critical terms related to graphic symbols in AAC. Several of the definitions have been proposed earlier (Blischak, Lloyd and Fuller, 1997; Lloyd and Blischak, 1992; Lloyd, Fuller and Arvidson, 1997a); some are new attempts to grasp the essence of the term.

Channel. The term 'channel' refers to the way a message is transmitted. Use of the visual channel implies that the message is received via optic receptors (the eyes), and use of the auditory channel implies reception by auditory receptors (the ears). Communication uses the tactual channel if reception is tactile (e.g. as in Braille reading, spelling in the hand, or the use of tangible/textured symbols as used with individuals with dual sensory impairments).

Language. The general term 'language' has received several definitions, partially depending on the linguistic theory that is adopted. A strong unambiguous definition is needed, especially as the linguistic nature of graphic symbol communication has been the subject of controversy and discussion. Some definitions are not restrictive. All graphic symbol systems with communicative function would qualify as a language according to a definition that defines language as 'A system of symbols (e.g. manual signs, words) and rules for combining them that can be used for a communicative function (e.g. expressing feelings, transferring information)' (Lloyd, Fuller and Arvidson, 1997a: glossary, p. 533).

A more formal definition of language renders the linguistic nature of graphic symbol use less evident. This is illustrated when language is defined as 'A conventional set of arbitrary symbols (spoken or written) and a set of rules for combining them to represent ideas about the world for the purpose of communication' (Blischak, Lloyd and Fuller, 1997, p. 39).

An even stricter definition makes graphic symbol use less qualified for linguistic status in the following definition: 'A natural human language is a conventional system of arbitrary symbols and grammatical rules to combine these symbols into larger units (i.e. phrases, clauses, sentences) in order to convey meaning. A *natural* language is one that has evolved naturally from social interaction between human beings and typically is acquired by children as their first language' (Lloyd, Fuller, Loncke and Bos, 1997, p. 43). While this definition may still leave open the possibility that some graphic symbols do function as a language, the requirement that they need to be acquired as a first language by children may pose an important limitation. This 'first acquisition requirement' is related to the purported inborn nature of linguistic development. Acquiring a system as a first language is considered to be evidence that learning the system is internally motivated by an intrinsic language orientation.

Modality. Modality has been defined as 'The particular channel through which information is transmitted or received' (Lloyd, Fuller and Arvidson, 1997a: glossary, p. 535).

This definition can be further developed when modality is considered to be 'an interaction between using an output form (a mode) and internal organization. The "visual–gestural modality", for example, indicates the specificity of utterance planning, production, reception, and understanding when the message is conveyed through the visual channel.'

Modality form. Once a modality is selected, a communication form can be structured as part of a system. For example, fingerspelling is a gestural communication form transmitted through the visual channel.

Mode. Mode has been defined as 'A particular way of communication (e.g. oral mode, manual-motor mode, ocular-motor mode)' (Lloyd, Fuller and Arvidson, 1997a: glossary, p. 535).

Multimodal approach. A multimodal approach is 'An intervention approach that uses more than one mode of communication (e.g. use of residual speech, gestures, manual signs, graphic symbols)' (Lloyd, Fuller and Arvidson, 1997a: glossary, p. 535). While multimodal communication is more the rule than the exception, multimodal approaches are clinical and educational intervention styles and techniques that seek to capitalize on the natural tendency to express and structure information in more than one parallel, complementary or redundant way.

Multimodal communication. Multimodal communication involves 'The use of more than one mode, channel, or form to communicate (e.g. use of residual speech, gestures, manual signs, graphic symbols)' (Lloyd, Fuller and Arvidson, 1997a: glossary, p. 535). Multimodal communication is more the rule than the exception.

Multimodality. Multimodality refers to the ability and the tendency of human beings to combine and integrate different information sources in message reception and message expression. The term refers to the fact that human beings tend to process information in more than one mode. These information modes refer (1) to the forms of output in communication such as gesture, sign, speech, writing, and (2) to the way information is internally represented: in networks where a word can have a speech representation and a written representation. Both representations are connected with each other. Multimodality is a powerful means to structure linguistic and non-linguistic information.

Symbol. A symbol is '(1) Something used to stand for or represent another thing or concept (e.g. real object, picture, line drawing, word). (2) In communication, it is anything used to represent thought (e.g. acoustic symbols via speech, letters of the alphabet via writing). AAC symbols can be acoustic, graphic, manual, and/or tactile. A symbol may be classified as aided or unaided, static or dynamic, and iconic or opaque. Symbols may also be taxonomically grouped as sets or systems. In some countries (e.g. United Kingdom) the AAC professional jargon limits the use of symbol to refer only to graphic symbols' (Lloyd, Fuller and Arvidson, 1997a: glossary, p. 541).

Symbol types

A symbol may be classified as one of two symbol types according to the processing undertaken (McNaughton, 1998a, p. 66). In *Type One* symbols, each symbol's representation relates to the visual appearance of its referent. It is a picture which is derived from the spatial positioning of the components relative to each other within the whole. A Type One symbol matches its referent's salient visual features. *Type Two* symbols relate to domains other than visual appearance (e.g. phonological or semantic). They portray meaning by the sequencing of their components and the logic or rules by which these components are ordered both on an intra-symbolic level (e.g. components or letters within words) and on an inter-symbolic level (e.g. words within phrases and sentences).

The distinctions made between these two types of symbols were compared by McNaughton and Lindsay (1995) to the differentiation between 'geometric' and 'algebraic' (Jackendoff, 1987), 'analogy' and 'propositional' (Shepard and Cooper, 1986), 'depictive' and 'descriptive' (Kosslyn, 1983), and 'dot matrices, mental models' and 'propositional representations' (Johnson-Laird, 1983) in the cognitive science literature.

Symbol set. A symbol set is '... (a) set of symbols that is closed in nature; it could be clinician-produced or it could consist of purchased symbol books, stamps, and/or cards containing a limited number of symbols. A symbol set can be expanded, but it does not have clearly defined rules for expansion' (Vanderheiden and Lloyd, 1986, p. 71).

Symbol system. A symbol system is '... (a) set of symbols specifically designed to work together to allow for maximum communication. Symbol systems include rules or a logic for the development of symbols not already represented in the system. These rules may be internal to the symbol system ... or may be part of the language coded by the symbol system' (Vanderheiden and Lloyd, 1986, p. 71).

Aided and unaided communication

Lloyd and Fuller (1986) argue that the aided–unaided communication distinction can be used as basis for classification within AAC methods and means. Aided communication is a general term used to indicate a way of communication that implies the use of some external aid or assistive communication device. Unaided communication refers to the production of utterances solely by coordinated use of parts of the body (e.g. natural speech, pointing, manual signing, facial expression).

The aided versus unaided nature of communication affects the way communication is established. For example, the use of an external aid for communicating often diverts the attention of a communication partner away from direct face-to-face contact. Graphic symbol use is a form of aided communication which is typically combined with other communication means. Unaided communication such as natural speech, gestures, and/or manual signing are often included in an individual's communication repertoire. This reflects the multimodal nature of communication. Intervention should be geared at finding the best combination of both aided and unaided communication (Blischak and Lloyd, 1996).

Taxonomy

Taxonomies provide a framework to aid in understanding critical features that distinguish symbol sets and systems. These distinctions aid in the decision-making process involved in selecting the most appropriate symbols for graphic symbol users. Taxonomies suggest important under-lying processes of symbol use. For example, the use of a picture-based graphic symbol system will probably require more global mental opera-tions than the use of traditional orthography or a graphic symbol system in which many of the symbols are combinations of other symbols (e.g. Blissymbolics).

Representational classifications

Graphic symbols may at first glance appear to be nothing more than mere labels for spoken words. This assumption is understandable given the practice of printing or displaying a graphic symbol with a written word, as well as the practice of using a graphic symbol with a spoken or electroni-cally produced word.

Contrary to common belief, the relationship between a graphic symbol and its referent is not necessarily straightforward. Because picture-based graphic symbols are not part of a linguistic system, for example, meanings can be difficult to grasp and are often open to interpretation. Linguistic systems establish a rather strict relationship between referent and meaning, mainly based on a rule-governed system. With picture-based graphic symbols, this strict relationship is, by necessity, overruled by contextual demands (Hjelmquist, 1997). However, graphic symbol sets and systems are often deliberately not meant to be used as strict represen-tations of words. In many cases, graphic symbols represent concepts, or more or less loosely described semantic fields. As is the case in linguistic semantics, semantic fields are not strictly defined but rather subject to individual experience and growth.

Graphic symbols are often combined with spoken or written language. In these cases, it is tempting to assume that graphic symbols are attachments to linguistic units (e.g. words) or vice versa (i.e. linguistic units are attachments to graphic symbols) and/or that graphic symbols fill in 'empty' slots in spoken language. In the first case, graphic symbols may or may not convey redundant information, in the latter case graphic symbols always give complementary information. When used in combination with speech or written language, one possible, but not necessarily true, assumption may be that graphic symbols assume a linguistic role. See, for example, McNeill's 1992 model in which parts of the message are assigned to channels based on the linguistic–non-linguistic dichotomy. This would mean that language assimilates other modes into its system. If that is the case, the question would be at which linguistic level a graphic symbol gets incorporated into language (e.g. lexical, phonological, ...). A tentative answer is that most graphic symbols will be incorporated at the lexical level, sometimes at the grammatical level. If incorporated at the lexical level, a graphic symbol becomes one of the elements that constitutes information stored in the internal lexicon. This lexicon will be multimodal (see, for example, elaboration of Levelt's blueprint for the speaker by Loncke, Vander Beken and Lloyd, 1997).

When a graphic symbol constitutes an action or an extended idea, it may function as a representation at the grammatical level, more or less providing a label for a whole sentence or phrase. For example, a graphic symbol representing a bus may be interpreted as an indication that 'it is time to get dressed and ready to go', regardless of whether one intends to go by bus or by another means of transportation.

Some graphic symbol sets and systems contain information that relates to the sublexical (i.e. phonological or graphemic) level of spoken or written language. This is the case not only for traditional orthography, but also for other phonemic- or phonic-based symbols (e.g. Expanded Complex Rebus, see Fuller, Lloyd and Stratton, 1997). These symbols allow the symbol user to induce strategies based on phonology that can assist in generating and understanding messages.

In order to understand the possibilities and the effects of graphic symbol use, it is important to know which characteristics are relevant in their production and perception. Graphic symbols differ in many respects. Fuller, Lloyd and Schlosser (1992) suggested that AAC systems might be best categorized and compared within a symbol taxonomy that distinguishes between (1) aided and unaided symbols, (2) static and dynamic symbols, (3) iconic and opaque symbols, and (4) whether the symbols are part of a set (i.e. a collection of symbols without combinatorial rules) or system (i.e. a collection of symbols with combinatorial rules for making new symbols or a series of symbols). Graphic symbols fit in one of the categories represented in Figure 16.3.

Lloyd and his colleagues have proposed a number of classifications that may be helpful in understanding the type of system, combined with factors such as mental effort, modality preference and functional similarity (see Tables 16.1–16.3).

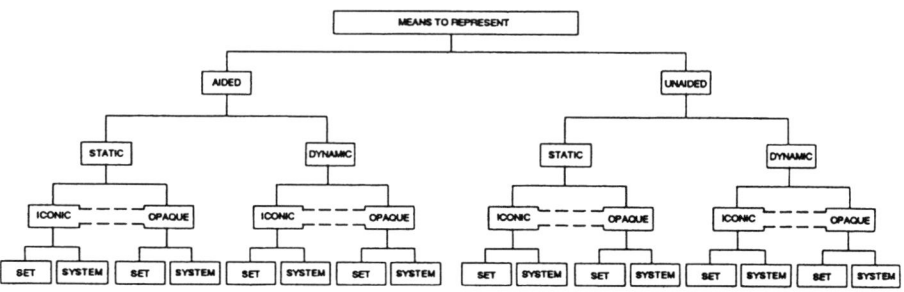

Figure 16.3. AAC symbol taxonomy for the means to represent. The iconic/opaque level is represented as a continuum rather than a dichotomy because of the limited research base (from Fuller and Lloyd, 1997, p. 35).

Table 16.1. Aided and unaided means to represent an idea, means to select the representation of the idea, and means to transmit the representation of the idea (from Lloyd, Fuller and Arvidson, 1997a, p. 34)

Aided	Unaided
Means to represent	
Objects	Gestures (e.g. pointing, yes/no head shakes, mime, Amer-Ind, generally understood gestures, esoteric signs/gestures)
Pictures (e.g. photographs, Picture Communication Symbols or PCS)	Natural sign languages (e.g. ASL, BSL, PSL, SSL; American, British, Portuguese and Swedish Sign Language, respectively)
Pictogram Ideogram Communication (PIC)	Gestuno
PICSYMS	
Blissymbols	Manually coded English (MCE) (e.g. Signed English, Paget-Gorman Sign System or PGSS, Seeing Essential English
Graphic representation of manual signs and/or gestures (e.g. Sigsymbols)	or SEE-I, Signing Exact English or SEE-II, or the manual or gestural coding of other spoken languages)
Synthetic or animated manual signs and/or gestures	Fingerspelling or manual alphabets
Expanded (complex) rebus	Eye blink, gestural and/or vocal alphabet codes (e.g. Morse code)
Other logographs with referent relationships	Eye blink, gestural and/or vocal word and/or message codes
Modified orthography and other symbols	Tadoma and other vibrotactile codes
Arbitrary logographs (e.g. Yerkish lexigrams) and shapes (e.g. Premack symbols)	Hand-cued speech (e.g. Cued Speech and Danish Mouth Hand)
Traditional orthography (TO)	Natural speech
Graphic representations of fingerspelling	
Synthetic fingerspelling	
Braille and other static-tactile codes	
Electronic-cued speech	
Digitized speech	
Synthetic speech	
Electrolarynx-generated speech	

(contd)

Table 16.1. (contd)

Aided	Unaided
Means to select	
Mechanical pointers	Blinking
	Body movements
Switches	Eye gaze
	Gesturing
Other mechanical or electronic indicating	Pointing with a body part
prostheses/devices that may use either	Speech
direct selection or scanning	Vocalization
	Writing
Means to transmit	
Communication boards, charts,	Direct transmission using various body
cards, books	parts (e.g. arms, face, hands, vocal tract)
Microprocessors that can be either adapted	
or dedicated as AAC aids	
Paper and pen	

Table 16.2. Listing of symbol sets and systems according to the AAC symbol taxonomy (from Lloyd, Fuller and Arvidson, 1997a, p. 36)

Aided	Unaided
Aided-static-iconic set	Unaided-static-iconic set
Basic (simple) rebus	(none)
Objects	
PCS	
PIC	
Pictures	
Tangible symbols	
Aided-static-iconic system	Unaided-static-iconic system
Blissymbols	(none)
Expanded (complex) rebus	
Picsyms	
Sigsymbols	
Aided-dynamic-iconic set	Unaided-dynamic-iconic set
Animated gestures	Amer-Ind
Animated manual signs	Gestuno
	Gestures
	Mime
Aided-dynamic-iconic system	Unaided-dynamic-iconic system
(none)	Manually coded languages
	Natural sign languages

(contd)

Table 16.2. (contd)

Aided	Unaided

Aided-static-opaque set
  Premack symbols
  Yerkish lexigrams
	Unaided-static-opaque set
	  (none)

Aided-static-opaque system
  Animated fingerspelling
  Braille
  Graphic Morse code
  Traditional orthography (TO)
	Unaided-static-opaque system
	  Fingerspelling

Aided-dynamic-opaque set
  (none)
	Unaided-dynamic-opaque set
	  (none)

Aided-dynamic-opaque system
  Digitized speech
  Synthesized speech
	Unaided-dynamic-opaque system
	  Cued speech
	  Gestural Morse code
	  Natural speech
	  Tadoma

Table 16.3. Categorization of aided symbols according to their functional similarities (Lloyd, Fuller and Arvidson, 1997a, p. 49)

Object-based symbols

Real objects	Tangible and textured symbols
Miniature objects	

Primarily picture-based symbols without linguistic characteristics

Photographs	Brady-Dobson Alternative Communication (D-DAC)
Simple line drawings (e.g. basic (simple) rebus)	Pictogram Ideogram Communication (PIC)
Core Picture Vocabulary	Mosman Sounds and Symbols
Picture Communication Symbols (PCS)	Other commercially available symbols
Oakland Picture Dictionary	(e.g. Touch'n Talk)

Partially picture-based symbols with linguistic characteristics

PICSYMS	CyberGlyphs (formerly Jet Era Glyphs)
Blissymbolics	Sigsymbols

Primarily picture-based symbols of dedicated VOCAs

DynaSyms	Lingraphica Concept-Images

Aided representations of manual signs and gestures

SIGSYMBOLS (sign-linked symbols)	HANDS
Pictures or illustrations of sign and gestures	Sign Writing
Worldsign	Synthetic or animated manual signs and gestures
Makaton symbols	

(contd)

Table 16.3. (contd)

Alphabet-based symbols	
Traditional orthography (TO)	Morse code
Modified orthography	Aided representations of fingerspelling
Braille	

Phonemic- or phonic-based symbols	
Expanded (complex) rebus	Phonetic alphabets (e.g. IPA, ITA)
Visual phonics	NU-VUE-CUE

Arbitrary logographs and shapes	
Yerkish lexigrams	Premack Symbols

Electronically produced vibratory/acoustic symbols	
Vibrotactile codes	Electronically produced speech
Electronic-cued-speech	

Characteristics

General communication models, clearly defined terminology and taxonomies facilitate understanding of the nature of graphic symbols. It is clear that there is no one typical graphic symbol and that processing depends on multiple variables.

Characteristics of graphic symbols described in this chapter determine how symbols are learned or acquired and how they are processed, but there are additional characteristics. Major factors are related to characteristics of the user's perceptual, cognitive and linguistic strategies and depend on larger schemes of information processing. These factors are discussed in the following chapters.

Chapter 17
Graphic Symbols:
Clinical Issues

HELEN H. ARVIDSON, SHIRLEY MCNAUGHTON,
GILLIAN NELMS, FILIP T. LONCKE AND LYLE L. LLOYD

From a clinical viewpoint, the use of graphic symbols raises a number of interesting issues related to the way in which individual users perceive, understand and produce graphic symbols within the total context of their environment. When selecting and introducing graphic symbols, the clinician/educator must be aware that success or failure is dependent on a number of factors such as the (1) advantages and disadvantages of graphic symbol communication compared with other forms of communication, (2) user's ability to match form and content, (3) user's vision and visual-perceptual system, (4) user's cognitive abilities, (5) interaction between graphic symbol use and language acquisition, (6) impact on literacy, (7) pragmatics of graphic symbol communication, (8) social and cultural status of graphic symbols and graphic symbol communication.

Advantages and disadvantages of graphic symbol communication compared with other forms of communication

When selecting graphic symbols to be used in an augmentative and alter-native communication (AAC) system, it is important to consider their advantages and disadvantages relative to other means of communication (Lloyd and Kiernan, 1984). Table 17.1 summarizes a number of these advantages and disadvantages (Blischak, Loncke and Waller (1997).

In order to capture the essence of graphic symbol communication, one must consider similarities and differences with other forms of AAC. One must also look at graphic symbol features. There are strong indications that a number of characteristic features impact the way graphic symbols are processed and produced. The relationship between these features and processing, however, is dependent on the user's cognitive, perceptual and linguistic experiences.

Table 17.1. Advantages and disadvantages of using graphic symbols (from Blischak, Loncke and Waller, 1997, p. 324, as adapted from Lloyd and Kiernan, 1984)

Advantages	Disadvantages
Are permanent, static	May not be immediately transparent to user
May be accessed by limbs or eyes	and communication partners
Have flexible display options (size,	Require communication partner to be close
spacing, colour, VOCA)	and at an appropriate viewing orientation
May be physically prompted	May discourage face-to-face communication
Have longer duration than speech	Have space and size limitations
May reduce memory demands	Can be damaged physically
Allow for delayed message reception	
May provide a permanent record	

Understanding the distinctive nature of graphic symbol use is critical when making intervention decisions. For example, in deciding whether a graphic symbol approach, a sign approach or a combination of both should be considered for an individual, the clinician/educator must take into account a number of considerations. Jones and Cregan (1986) suggested consideration of indicators, listed in Table 17.2.

Table 17.2. Indicators and contra-indicators for sign and graphic symbol use (from Jones and Cregan, 1986)

Sign use	Graphic symbol use
Indicators	
Client uses meaningful gestures	Responds well to pictures
Can/will imitate	Poor short-term memory
Good recall	Poor recall
Wants to learn (and physically able)	Slow to work things out
Readily interacts	Needs very tight structures
	Severely physically handicapped
Contra-indicators	
Limited motor skills	Poor two-dimensional discrimination
Stereotypic hand movements	Cannot picture-match (but has sign-relevant
Very intermittent attention	abilities)
Frequent changes of caregivers	

User's ability to match form and content

It is important to note that the use of graphic symbols is common in communication and information processing. Information transfer via traditional orthography is essential in contemporary cultural, economic and political organizations. Moreover, graphic symbols outside of traditional orthography have become essential when information needs to be rapidly recognized and processed. A typical example is the use of logos and graphic symbols for marketing and product recognition (e.g. McDonald's arches).

The purpose of graphic symbols can be the same for individuals with disabilities as it is for individuals without disabilities. Cognitive, sensory or social impairments, however, enhance the need for a systematic (literally: belonging to a system) use of graphic symbols. Reliance upon this systematic use of graphic symbols for communication does involve a different purpose and greatly increased exposure than more casual use of graphic symbols. Moreover, individuals who use graphic symbols for communication require appropriate instruction to facilitate the acquisition of literacy. Literacy itself is of critical importance to individuals with little or no functional speech, and any possible support that may be gained from graphic instruction and different types of graphic processing warrants research attention.

For individuals with disabilities who have little or no access to traditional orthography, the use of other graphic symbol sets and systems may provide appropriate alternatives. A number of factors, however, must be considered when determining the appropriateness of sets and systems. One consideration involves the extent to which the introduction of sets will enhance a user's personal development and social participation. If an individual has the cognitive ability to acquire the essence of symbolic communication, the pros and cons of introducing a symbol set versus a symbol system, however, must be considered with care. A symbol set is a relatively closed, restricted collection of symbols that, by its very nature, does not offer combinatorial ways to go beyond the set. Using a set instead of a system may hinder maximal development by creating a ceiling effect in learning. A set does not provide for progress once all the symbols are learned. However, observations show that some individuals may not allow themselves to be limited by the restrictions of a set, and may find ways to expand it. For example, the user may suggest combinations of existing graphic symbols to represent new referents (Blischak and Lloyd, 1996). It is important that clinicians and educators recognize such communicative creativity. This creativity may, however, be a good reason to consider the use of graphic symbol systems rather than sets. Graphic symbol systems are, by their nature, more open than graphic symbol sets, and provide more possibilities to explore and create new combinations. In other words, graphic symbol systems are more language-like, and may indirectly stimulate a user's linguistic potential.

The question of whether or not the use of graphic symbols facilitates linguistic communication is important. The issue has particularly high relevance because of its role in the debate as to whether graphic symbols may or may not have a direct or an indirect effect on the acquisition of literacy (see McNaughton and Lindsay, 1995).

User's vision and visual–perceptual system

One has only to observe individuals engaged in conversation to realize the importance of good senses of hearing and sight. For speaking individuals, hearing is key. For individuals who use aided or unaided AAC, sight may be more critical. Individuals with hearing and visual impairments often wear hearing aids and corrective lenses to improve their abilities to engage in a wide variety of routine activities, not the least of which is communication. Individuals with hearing and visual impairments who have additional disabilities can also benefit from these aids, but there are barriers. The underdetection and undermanagement of hearing and visual impairments in individuals with severe disabilities are two of them (Blischak and Wasson, 1997).

The precise prevalence of visual impairments in AAC users is difficult to determine; however, the rate of visual impairments among individuals with multiple impairments and disabilities is much higher than in the general population (Batshaw and Perret, 1992; Brett, 1983; Schorr, 1983), and the impact can be complex (Bailey and Downing, 1994). Because multiple, overlapping disabilities can cause a concomitant effect, careful assessment of vision to determine optimums for even the most basic characteristics of graphic symbols becomes critical.

Visual assessment must certainly provide information related to visual acuity, the clearness or sharpness of vision, but it should also provide information related to a number of other optical-motor skills and abilities such as accommodation, attention, binocularity, convergence, eye–hand coordination, localization, scanning, tracking and tracing. Perceptual skills and abilities involving colour, cortical functioning, closure, figure–ground discrimination, inner–outer detail, integration, laterality and direction-ality, light and contrast sensitivity, parts-to-whole and spatial relationships, three-to-two dimensional representations, visual memory and visual sequencing should also be considered (Steciw, 1995).

At a conference to discuss research needs for the 1990s, Lloyd (1990) expressed concern about the paucity of information about the critical characteristics of graphic symbols to guide the use of graphic symbols with AAC users. He noted that we 'lack the basic information to ask the serious questions about: (1) what helps and what hurts in our attempts to use symbol enhancement or elaboration; (2) what can we trade in the symbol to increase rate and at what costs; (3) what about graphic (and other) symbols can be exploited in clinical, educational, and communicative activities' (p. 67).

While there has been some research related to these issues since that conference, more is needed to determine the benefit of manipulating symbol characteristics to capitalize on the visual strengths of the individuals who use them. Information is needed to guide not only the initial selection of appropriate symbols, but also the subsequent manipulation of symbol characteristics so they can be optimally matched to the skills and abilities of individual AAC users.

Mollica (1997) pointed out that intuitions about perceptual and cognitive accessibility of graphic symbols may be misleading. For example, the recognition of a photograph as a symbol referring to an object or another external referent may not be as straightforward as it seems. In order to be able to recognize and interpret a photograph, a number of perceptual and cognitive operations must be activated. The study of visual perception (especially visual perception prerequisites) must necessarily be relied upon in order to better understand symbol recognition and interpreting processes (see, for example, the work of Gibson, 1969). Gangkofer (1990, referred to in Schlosser, Lloyd and McNaughton, 1997) noted that the understanding of pictographic representations is dependent on several preconditions: (a) daily exposure to and experience with pictographs in a given society, (b) learning of codes that have been agreed upon in a given society, (c) differentiating design of the symbols to avoid confusing symbols, (d) rule-governed development of pictographs, and (e) the cognitive construction of meaning (requiring the 'symbolic function').

Which characteristics of symbols have an influence on the way they are perceived and how they are processed is dependent on the perceptual strategy. Perception of symbols will be different depending on the level of perception. For example, if a person has been using the symbols for some time, he or she may need to focus on only a limited number of critical features to allow recognition.

User's cognitive abilities

One of the most critical questions relates to which characteristics of graphic symbols render them more or less accessible. This issue is important because it touches upon one of the essential elements of the philosophy of AAC: the selection of communication means that are maximally accessible for the cognitive abilities and style of a user.

The following characteristics of graphic symbols have been suggested as characteristics that play a role in the way symbols are processed by AAC users: ambiguity, complexity, figure–ground differential, iconicity, perceptual distinctness and size. They are listed in Table 17.3.

As stated before, the impact of graphic symbol characteristics is not unambiguous; it is largely dependent on the cognitive and perceptual strategies of the graphic symbol user. If symbols are approached and decoded from an internalized linguistic system, the user is more likely to scan symbols for features relevant within the system. In traditional orthography, for example, the user may try to find phonemes, phoneme combinations, or morphosyntactic cues and overlook other characteristics, such as iconicity. In general, it is expected that the better the user internalizes a rule system, the less relevant other characteristics may become.

Table 17.3. Characteristics of graphic AAC symbols

Characteristic	References
Ambiguity	Fuller, Lloyd and Stratton, 1997; Silverman, 1995
Complexity	Fuller and Lloyd, 1987; Fuller, Lloyd and Stratton, 1997; Hayes, 1996; Hern, Lammers and Fuller, 1996; Luftig and Bersani, 1985a,b; Nail-Chiwetalu, 1991/ 1992
Figure/ground differential	Cooper and Fuller, 1996; Fuller, Lloyd and Stratton, 1997; Silverman, 1995
Iconicity	Bloomberg, Karlan and Lloyd, 1990; Clark, 1984; Fuller, 1987/1988; Fuller, Lloyd and Stratton, 1997; Goossens, 1983/1984; Hayes, 1996; Hern, Lammers and Fuller, 1996; Koul, 1994/1995; Lloyd and Fuller, 1990; Luftig and Bersani, 1985a,b; Mizuko, 1985/ 1986; Mizuko and Reichle, 1989; Musselwhite, 1982; Musselwhite and Ruscello, 1984; Nail-Chiwetalu, 1991/1992; Yovetich and Paivio, 1980
Perceptual distinctness	Fuller, Lloyd and Stratton, 1997; Lloyd and Karlan, 1983, 1984; Lloyd and Kiernan, 1984; Silverman, 1995
Size	Fuller, Lloyd and Stratton, 1997; Silverman, 1995

For example, a Blissymbol user may primarily pay attention to the combination of elements that make up the symbols and decode them as bundles of features rather than concentrate on their image-like qualities. Such an approach is similar to the psycholinguistic behaviour of language users. One of the major assumptions of present-day psycholinguistics is that this abstract type of information coding and decoding allows fast processing (Pinker, 1994). This may explain the finding that deaf sign language users tend to ignore the obvious iconic qualities in signs during real-time, on-line communication. This has been noted not only with experienced deaf signers, but also with deaf children acquiring a sign language (Pettito, 1988).

However, if the user cannot rely on an internalized rule and combination system, other characteristics will become more relevant in allowing understanding and producing the symbol. Direct visual recognition (possible with photographs) will facilitate access if no linguistic-like rules are available to the user. However, as Mollica (1997) pointed out, even 'direct visual recognition' may not be as direct as one might think. The recognition of a two-dimensional drawing or a photograph probably requires cultural familiarity with this type of representation, as well as the use of perceptual strategies.

Clearly, cognition and perception impact an individual's use of graphic symbols, but there are converse considerations. For example, does the use of graphic symbol communication affect cognitive growth? It is most likely that the introduction of the use of graphic symbols has an impact on direct communication (with partners present in the user's direct physical environment). Any increase in the scope of communication induces an increase in potential social interaction, social recognition and information exchange.

Moreover, the use of graphic symbols may lead to other interesting effects. Graphic symbols may offer a means to visualize concepts and relationships. The use of graphic symbols may also help to visualize structural aspects of language. For example, two graphic symbols in juxtaposition may help the user understand the nature of compound words. Also, the visual nature of graphic symbols can be used as a scaffolding for memory. Visual symbols may be cognitively easier to access.

Finally, the use of graphic symbols can have a growth effect through increasing experience that feeds into itself. An expanded vocabulary and success experience is likely to lead to more communicative initiatives. For example, when two graphic symbols in juxtaposition help the user understand the nature of compound words and Blissymbolic indicators serve as linguistic markers, there may be increased opportunities for novel communication and language development. Additionally, knowledge of the structural aspects of language has been found to be associated with literacy acquisition (Gottardo, 1995).

Interaction between graphic symbol use and language acquisition

An intriguing question about graphic symbol use is how it may affect language acquisition. Is the use of graphic symbols similar to the use of linguistic symbols? Are the same or similar linguistic skills emerging through graphic symbol use as through typical language acquisition? This matter has been the issue of important studies and considerations (for example, see the section on language development in this book).

One major distinction to be made here is between structure and use. Symbols may or may not originate from a linguistic system; i.e. they may share structural characteristics with other symbols of the system that give them linguistic status. In general, a system can be considered to be linguistic if it (1) has developed through direct communication within a community of humans, (2) has a lexicon of elements that are formed on the basis of sublexical formational rules (phonology and phonotactics), (3) has a set of rules about how lexical elements are combined and modified in combination (syntax and morphosyntax), and (4) has duality of patterning.

The communities in which many languages have developed and are functioning can be very large and can exist over a long period of time. Spoken languages can have billions of users and exist over many centuries. Changes over time are generally very gradual. On the other hand, languages may emerge in a very short time and in very limited groups of users. The study of pidgin and creole languages demonstrates the flexibility of individuals to create a linguistic system if the circumstances require it. In general, new languages emerge when one critical factor exists, such as the lack of access to a common language with other humans. Linguistic creativity is strong enough to stimulate individuals to invest in modes other than speech if access to spoken forms is limited. The study of sign languages in deaf communities has shown that lack of access to speech is not an obstacle for creating a language. The human system simply switches to a different and more accessible mode and establishes a communication system that shares the same principles as spoken languages: lexicon, sublexical combinatorial rules and morphosyntactic rules. Observations of deaf children show that the circumstances of having no or only limited access to sign language allow for the creation of a multi-level communication system that is structurally similar to languages (e.g. Goldin-Meadow et al., 1994).

In his analysis of language, Lindblom (1990) discusses both the phonological level of letter component combinations in words as well as the syntactical level of word combinations in phrases of sentences. In his description of the difference between human language and animal communication, he presents examples of Type Two structure (human language) and Type One structure (animal communication):

> ... human language makes combinatorial use of discrete units at two levels of structure1. At the phonological level they combine vowels and consonants to form words and other forms. And at the level of syntax they use rules for combining words into phrases and sentences. This combinatorial method is so powerful that, for practical purposes, it sets no upper limit on the number of messages that languages can convey. It is the key to their expressive power. Since it operates both on the units of phonology and on the units of syntax, it has dual structure. In the terminology of the linguist, human languages are said to exhibit duality (Hockett, 1958).... Animal communication systems do not have this dual structure. Their signals are Gestalts. They do not make combinatorial use of signal elements. They communicate by means of holistic patterns .... As a result, the number of messages that they can transmit must necessarily be limited. (Lindblom, 1990, p. 227)

The developmental model of reading, with its four phases of development in learning to read words, offers an explicit description of orthographic symbols being processed first as Type One symbols and then as Type Two symbols (McNaughton, 1998a). In the logographic phase, words are processed holistically, similar to the processing of pictures. As the child progresses through the transitional and alphabetic phases, the processing becomes increasingly analytical. Individual letters (typically at the beginning of words) begin to be associated with their corresponding sounds and eventually the grapheme–phoneme correspondences are processed for all the letters. The work of Byrne and his associates (Byrne, 1992; Byrne and

Carroll, 1989; Byrne and Fielding-Barnsley, 1989) has shown that 'breaking free of the logographic stage depends on achieving phonemic awareness' (Byrne, 1992, p. 6). In exploring the possible relationship between the processing of multicomponent (Type Two) symbols and the processing of words, it should be remembered that phonemic awareness in beginning reading requires the visual analysis of words into their letter components as well as the phonological analysis of speech sounds.

Impact on literacy

Two speculative positions have been proposed regarding a possible relationship between graphic symbols and literacy acquisition. Bishop, Rankin and Mirenda (1994), in a paper entitled 'Impact of graphic symbol use on reading acquisition', argue that the use of graphic symbols may facilitate specific components of print and word awareness, but that the overall impact of these symbol sets/systems on beginning reading may be minimal' (p. 113). Their argument is based primarily on reading research that confirms the central role played by phonological recoding on reading acquisition, and they reference eminent researchers in the reading acquisition literature such as Rayner and Pollatsek (1989), Share et al. (1984) and Stanovich (1986, 1988). As they point out, little is learned through most AAC graphics regarding the phonological processing required for reading print. They do not consider, however, the visual processing component within phonological recoding. They acknowledge that a contribution may be made by graphic symbols through their power to enhance an AAC user's language through increased communication with others and through their facilitation of such emergent literacy skills as awareness of directionality of print, that print conveys meaning, and the concepts of sounds, letters and words. Bishop et al. (1994) do not distinguish between different types of symbol processing, however, discussing all graphics as if they were picture based or logographs.

McNaughton and Lindsay (1995) take a counter position to that of Bishop et al. (1994), first arguing that two types of symbols must be considered: those that are processed holistically (Type One, picture-type symbols) and those that can be analysed into their component parts (Type Two symbols such as Blissymbols). Their argument as to the potential importance of graphic symbol usage rests upon the need to consider the orthographic processing within reading acquisition. Stanovich (1992), supported by the findings of Barron (1986), Ehri (1987), Juel, Griffith and Gough (1986), Patterson, Marshall and Coltheart (1985), Tunmer and Nesdale (1985), and his own work with associates (Cunningham and Stanovich, 1990; Stanovich and West, 1989), cautioned that phonological processing is not necessarily 'the end of the story' (p. 318). Further, he suggested that there might be individual differences in the ability 'to form accurate orthographic representations, to access orthographic representations, or both' (p. 319). In a comprehensive review of the reading acquisition literature, Share (1995) recognized the secondary, but necessary ability of storing and retrieving word-specific orthographic information. He stated that differences in this ability 'will determine how quickly and accurately orthographic representations are acquired' (p. 156). The question must be asked, 'Can graphics play a role in preparing the learner to form accurate visual representations and/or access them, and to process visual information quickly and accurately?'

Given (a) the reliance of the AAC user upon graphic symbols (and the optional processing capabilities depending on symbol type and method of instruction), (b) the growing capabilities within technology to enable the AAC user to read and write graphic symbols (e.g. BlissInternet, Writing with Symbols), and (c) the recognized limited literacy competencies of many AAC users, there is ample justification for research to move the debate beyond speculation.

In examining the possible relationships between graphic symbol use and literacy acquisition, two domains of knowledge can serve as resources for AAC researchers. The first comes from the language acquisition literature and requires viewing both graphic symbol usage and literacy acquisition within the language learning continuum. The second is derived from the mainstream reading acquisition literature.

McNaughton and Lindsay (1995), through adapting Snow's (1991) language proficiency model to depict the language pathway to literacy for AAC users, identified five strands within the pathway: visual, auditory, motor, social and symbolic. The learning that occurs in each of these strands, through the use of AAC graphics can be considered as developmental steps toward literacy. As recognized by both Bishop et al. (1994) and McNaughton and Lindsay (1995), the language experience gained by the aided AAC user who relies on a visual medium to gain access to expressive communication warrants attention in the study of literacy acquisition. This experience begins with the first attempt at aided communication whether it be through controlling a voice-output device by selecting visually labelled keys, or by indicating symbols sequentially to produce a message to be interpreted by a communication partner. A view of the language continuum that relates specifically to literacy acquisition and provides skill areas to be examined has been proposed by Miller (1990). She suggests that there are two levels of language processes that contribute to literacy acquisition: Level 1 processes comprise phonology, morphology, syntax, semantics and basic pragmatics; Level II processes comprise metalinguistic awareness, discourse knowledge and higher level pragmatics.

Findings in the mainstream reading acquisition literature provide support for a developmental approach (Ehri, 1992; Frith, 1985; Share, 1995; Vandervelden and Siegel, 1995) and the need to study such language related factors as semantics, syntax, working memory, metalinguistic knowledge, etc. (Daneman, 1991; Siegel, 1993). Stanovich (1986) provides insight with his description of reciprocal relationships, situations where the causal connection between reading ability and the efficiency of a cognitive process is bidirectional. Another important aspect of Stanovich's approach is the Interactive Compensatory Model (Stanovich, 1980) in which skills at one processing level can help compensate for deficiencies at another level.

In a developmental approach to reading, stages are identified as learners move from processing words holistically as sight words or as paired associates, through analysing components of words to the eventual stage of becoming skilled readers who use their extensive knowledge of spelling–sound relationships to identify unfamiliar words. One may consider the possibility of similar phases occurring during the learning of a symbol system such as Blissymbolics. Equally, there may be processing levels attained in using AAC graphics having some influence upon the visual processing involved in print acquisition. The findings of an empirical pilot study undertaken by McNaughton (1998b) suggest that future research would need to use a methodology that can accommodate developmentally limited relationships as described by Stanovich (1986). A developmentally limited relationship is one in which 'the individual differences in a particular cognitive process may be a causal determinant of variation in reading achievement early in development, but at some point have no further effects on the level of reading efficiency' (p. 362). The methodology recommended by McNaughton is that of a longitudinal study designed to permit cohort group comparisons of AAC users. Collaborative international projects would be needed in order to obtain the number of subjects required for reliable statistical analyses. Much could be learned through documenting and studying the development of AAC users from their introduction to AAC graphics through the 'reading to learn' level of literacy acquisition.

In order to portray the complexity of the issues involved, Hetzroni and McNaughton developed a model, Figure 17.1, at the ISAAC 1998 research symposium.

In considering Communication, Graphics and Literacy, they used the premise underlying the Interactive Compensatory Model proposed by Stanovich (1980) (i.e. skills at one processing level are capable of compensating for deficiencies at another level). In Figure 17.1, the levels comprise (1) Learning to Use an AAC Graphic Symbol Set/System and Print, (2) Building a Language, World Knowledge and Cognitive Base, and (3) Using both Graphics and Print to Learn. The double arrows at the top depict interactive relationships. The factors that influence the entire learning process are shown by the arrows pointing toward the box. They include culture, life situation, degree of disability, symbol type, extent and quality of instruction, family and school expectations and feedback, opportunity to use a voice output communication aid (VOCA), and broader environmental support.

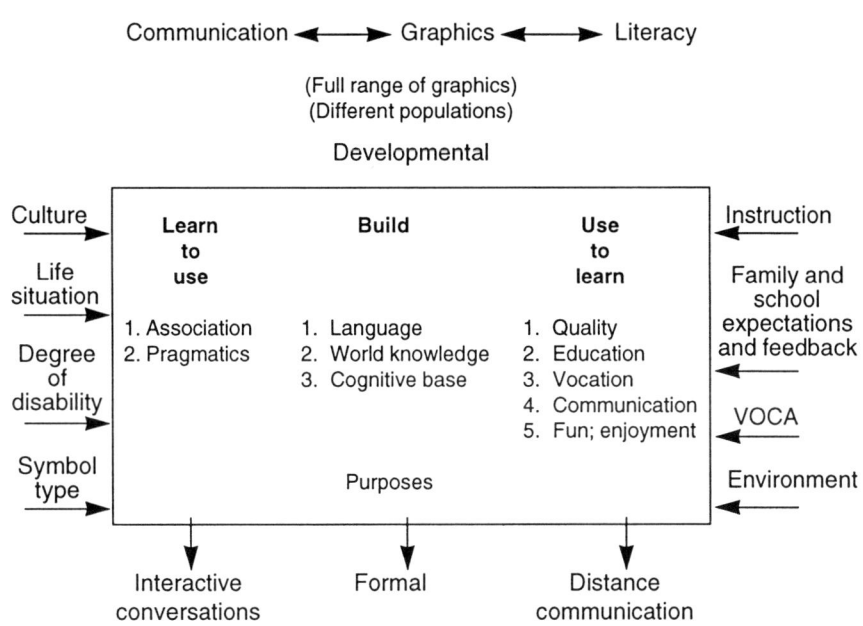

Figure 17.1. Proposed model of communication, graphics and literacy based upon Interactive Compensatory Model.

It is important to consider different purposes of communication and literacy including (a) interactive (direct, face-to-face) communication and literacy; (b) formal (presentations, reports, business letters) communication and literacy; and (c) distance (telecommunications, computer mediated) communication and literacy. Additionally, it is critical to remember the developmental continuum of different types of symbols (and the processing they required) and the different factors affecting different populations.

A distinction should be made between the early stage of Learning to Use Graphics/Print, and the later stage of Using Graphics/Print to Learn. At the early stage, one must consider the learning factors that might be developmentally limited. The type of instruction and family expectations also warrant attention at this stage. At the later stage of using print to learn, consideration must be given to the language, world knowledge and cognitive base attained through using graphics prior to reading print. An assessment of reading proficiency at least at a grade six level seems essential in any evaluation of the relationship between graphic usage and literacy acquisition. Rankin, Harwood and Mirenda (1994) wrote a discussion paper relating to this topic. In the Building component, which involves many factors that are difficult to assess, attention must be directed to variables that have been identified within the mainstream literacy acquisition literature, but which have received little attention in the AAC literature. The multifaceted nature of the relationships between communication, graphics, and literacy must not be overlooked. All forms of symbols, whether they be pictures, Blissymbols or traditional orthography, must be studied within the domain of literacy. Graphics should be considered as being on a continuum extending from pictorial illustrative graphics, through a rule-governed generative graphic system to traditional orthography.

Pragmatics of graphic symbol communication

Graphic symbols can only be used as aided communication. This affects the nature of exchange of information in several ways. One major characteristic in aided communication is that face-to-face contact must be interrupted to access the symbols, both by the sender and by the receiver if there is no VOCA. In typical communication, eye contact functions as a regulator that helps to indicate times for changes such as when to take turns and when to maintain or yield the floor. In other words, eye contact is important in the fine tuning of the interaction. The use of graphic symbols may make this more difficult. For example, it has been observed that communication partners who are not familiar with graphic symbol users sometimes tend to focus on the device or on the communication board and ignore the graphic symbol user.

The use of graphic symbols may also affect the content of the messages. In typical face-to-face communication, crucial information is not only conveyed through speech, but also through gestures and prosody. Very often, these means provide a back-up and redundant channel for the spoken information. Graphic symbol users can rely on these means to build a message to a much lesser degree, putting a heavier burden on how graphic symbols must be used in order to make sure messages will be understood.

Finally, it may be that the nature of graphic symbol communication leads to a different pattern of metalinguistic awareness. In typical speech communication, metaphors and puns are often nothing other than a play with sounds and word formation. In visual-linguistic communications, puns often reflect an awareness of how visual forms can be put in contrast (Klima and Bellugi, 1979). It is not clear if users of graphic symbols spontaneously find original and new effects in symbol selection that reflect a 'visual form' play similar or equivalent to puns in spoken language.

Social and cultural status of graphic symbols and graphic symbol communication

The status of AAC generally is extremely poor, not only in the wider population, but also is many environments which should provide greater emphasis and status for all AAC users and particularly graphic symbol users. To date, the lack of awareness given to multilinguistic issues in the field of graphic symbols is a matter for great concern. Two particularly relevant areas of sociolinguistic research should be applied: bi/multilingualism which refers to the language patterns of the community, and bi/multilinguality which refers to the language patterns of the individual.

The areas of multilingualism and multilinguality interact with each other, as the language patterns of the individuals are affected by the community of graphic symbol users. The community of graphic symbol users and the relative status of graphic symbol use are key elements in a discussion of multilingualism. AAC in general, and the use of graphic symbols in particular, are generally seen as being a 'lower status' form of communication which could be compared with the use of minority languages the world over. High status languages such as English are spoken by large communities, but graphic symbols fall into a category similar to that of a minority language, not only in the world at large, but also often within the very communities which purport to help develop language skills. Therefore, an asymmetric relation arises between the spoken language of the majority and the expressive language of the graphic symbol user. Even within school environments, for example, graphic symbol users rarely see staff members using graphic symbols to communicate. Users are typically spoken to but expected to reply using graphic symbols. They do not have the advantage of seeing these higher level spoken utterances communicated through graphic symbols. Even when a high level of graphic symbol use has been achieved, without a suitable community of users, graphic symbol users are likely to lose skills over time (Barnett and Bax, 1996).

Within the issue of relative status, graphic symbols are not only perceived as having lower status than speech or signing when used on a communication board, but also than when used on a voice output communication aid (VOCA). Barnett and Woll (1998) discuss the relationship between social purposes of interaction and communication usage. Commonly, within a multilingual community, different languages may have different spheres of use (i.e. formal, vernacular, colloquial). Graphic symbols on VOCAs may have different spheres of use than graphic symbols on communication boards. For example, a VOCA may be used in class with a group of listeners, but a graphic symbol communication book may be used at home with family.

Within AAC, a profound asymmetry between reception and production is common. A person may receive input in the form of spoken English while producing output using Blissymbols (Barnett and Woll, 1998). This asymmetry emphasizes the lack of a multilingual community of users, which graphic symbol users need. A considerable amount of research is required in this area, but changes can be made now within schools and establishments where there are graphic symbol users.

AAC in general and teachers of graphic symbols can create a truly multi-lingual community for their users by becoming users of AAC systems with graphic symbols themselves. This not only teaches through use and demonstration, but raises the status of the AAC system. For example, in one small school in London, children with communication books were in the majority, but speaking children asked for communication books as these were seen as having considerable status within that environment. This example should provide us with the conviction that multilingualism is an achievable aim.

The perception of graphic symbols is closely linked to world view and everyday life experience; that is, the interpretation of graphic symbols is dependent upon one's culture and life experiences. This can be observed from emergent literacy: a child who experiences that marks on a paper mean certain things may start making marks on paper and give it meaning. Through socialization, interaction and acquisition of language and literacy, meanings that are assigned to symbols become restricted and often specific. This explains the surprise and the amusement individuals experience when they find out that a specific symbol used within one language context refers to a totally different meaning in another language context. For example, hot water taps in bathrooms are often labelled with the letter 'H' and cold water taps with 'C'. However, in countries where a Roman language is used, the hot water tap is often labelled 'C', referring to the word 'caldo' (Italian) or 'chaud' (French).

Once used to a meaning, individuals may find it hard to realize that meanings are based upon convention, and may not be universal or strict. Within American cultures, a capital letter 'H' refers to 'hospital'. However, as demonstrated in Lloyd's Initial Symbol Test (Lloyd, 1994), 'H' can have other meanings, in various cultures and contexts (e.g. 'hydrant', 'hotel'). Some cultures readily recognize that a red cross means medical help services, while other cultures (e.g. Arabic) recognize and use a totally different symbol, a crescent, and find it just as obvious .

The meaning which is attached to any given symbol is often dependent on the culture of the individual looking at the symbol. Huer (1998) examined perceptions of graphic symbols across four different cultural groups: African-American, Chinese, European-American and Mexican. Results indicated that individuals from four ethnic groups perceived graphic symbols differently within symbols sets/systems (Blissymbols, DynaSyms and PCS), as well as within parts of speech (verbs and modifiers).

Individuals from different cultures attend to different features of symbols when initially viewing symbols (Huer, personal communication, August 1998). The colours within symbols represent different meanings. Colours are culturally linked, and, therefore, may please some consumers while offending others. An example of the different messages conveyed by the perception of colour is found in DynaSyms. Carlson reported that she selected black for the action characters because it seemed to be an appropriate background colour, yet black for action was perceived as stereotypical by African-American individuals when first viewing the dynamic screen on the DynaVox. The selection of this colour caused African-American persons to reject the symbol set upon initial examination (Huer, personal communication, August 1998). The thickness of the lines, as well as the colour of the lines, also communicates different messages to individuals across cultures.

Translucency has been identified as one of the important features influencing the learning of graphic symbols. Several researchers (Fuller, 1997; Hooper and Lloyd, 1988; Koul and Lloyd, 1998; Schlosser, 1995) have used the adult translucency ratings of the 910 Blissymbol study by Lloyd, Karlan and Nail-Chiwetalu (1994) designed to investigate differences in learning Blissymbols by children and adults. Possible criticisms for using these translucency values, however, are that (1) children who typically use Blissymbolics as a transition to reading are usually 6–7 years of age and may perceive Blissymbols differently from adults, (2) cultural differences may influence perceived translucency, and (3) individuals with disabilities who use Blissymbols may perceive them differently from individuals who are not disabled.

In order to answer these questions, Quist et al. (1998) obtained translucency ratings from 161 elementary school students (pre-readers, 6–7 years) in the Netherlands and the United States. In addition, translucency data were obtained on 22 deaf children in Belgium and 16 children with severe disabilities in the Netherlands. Children evaluated the translucency of 100 Blissymbols spoken by a teacher by indicating one of three smiley faces (representing high, mid, or low translucency) in prepared booklets.

The findings of this study indicate that children, although more variable in their ratings, generally rate the translucency of Blissymbols similarly to adults. Those Blissymbols rated high in translucency by adults were, for the most part, rated high by children. On the low and mid-translucency Blissymbols, however, children rated about 50% in the same category as adults, suggesting, in this case, that the children may have been using more of a dichotomous scale. The translucency ratings of children in the Netherlands and in the United States were similar. An interesting finding in this study was the similarity in the ratings provided by children with disabilities. The samples were very small; however, the significance of these correlations is high. There may be a number of reasons for these differences (e.g. creativity, experiential differences, teacher influence); however, the data indicate overall high correlation with the adult ratings and argue for their use in training and research.

Chapter 18
Graphic Symbols and Information Processing

FILIP T. LONCKE, LYLE L. LLOYD, HANS VAN BALKOM
AND HELEN H. ARVIDSON

In typical communication, information is processed at different levels at the same time. For example, in a largely parallel process, a listener makes phonological discriminations and lexical decisions, and decodes the syntactic form of a speaker's utterance. Communication using graphic symbols also appears to involve parallel processing but with the co-occurrence of more analytic and more global perception.

Numerous models have been proposed to account for the way specific information is processed (e.g. accessed, recognized, retrieved) and for the various aspects involved (e.g. visual perception, speech production, language understanding, reading, writing). This chapter reviews a number of models that shed light on the way graphic symbols may be understood and produced in interactive communication.

Paivio's dual processing model

One of the first models of processes applied to augmentative and alternative communication (AAC) was based on Paivio's model of dual processing (Paivio, 1971, 1986). Paivio's central thesis is that performance in memory and other cognitive tasks is mediated not only by linguistic processes but also by distinct non-verbal imagery of thought.

From this perspective, graphic symbols are interesting because they offer the user the opportunity to process information on the basis of representativeness. Representativeness is the degree to which a naive subject perceives a symbol as representing the word label of the referents. Yovetich and Paivio (1980) conducted a series of studies on the learning of Blissymbols, and concluded that the learnability of Blissymbols increased as representativeness increased (Yovetich and Young, 1988). The concept is that representativeness comes close to most operational definitions of translucency (Fuller and Lloyd, 1991).

The importance of this approach for the use of graphic symbols is obvious: the higher the translucency value of the graphic symbols, the more likely it will be that the user will access the symbol by focusing on its imagistic characteristics. The model of dual processing may be visualized as in Figure 18.1.

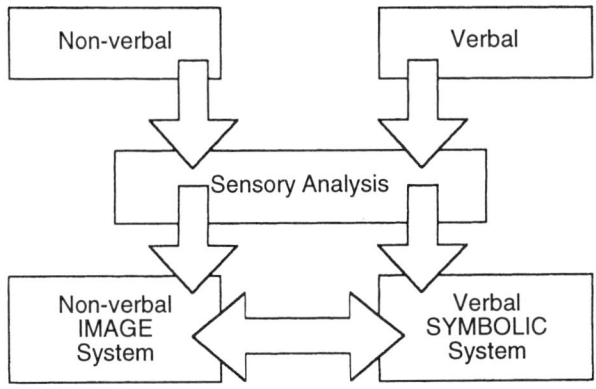

Figure 18.1. A visualization of Paivio's dual processing model.

McNeill's gestural model

McNeill (1985, 1992) has proposed a dynamic approach in understanding how a speaker generates an utterance. McNeill focuses on the fact that natural gestures occur simultaneously with speech, and seem to have a common underlying computational stage. Gestures and speech constitute an intrinsic whole in which each mode expresses part of the message – sometimes in a redundant way, sometimes in a complementary way. Each mode takes on a part of the message for which it is best equipped. That is, in typical communication, speech carries linguistic–analytic information while gestures carry more imagistic–global information (Goldin-Meadow and McNeill, in press). Loncke, Blischak, McNeill, Vander Beken and Verbanck (1997) have suggested that this distribution of functions is relative and subject to change. There is a balance in the distribution of functions. The type of information that will be assigned to each channel depends upon (1) the characteristics of the channels, (2) the accessibility of the channels, and (3) the potential sharing of code by communication partners. Figure 18.2 shows an attempt to visualize McNeill's model.

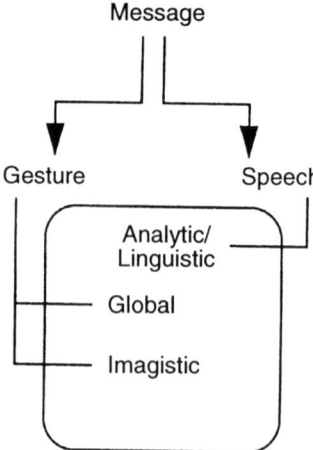

Figure 18.2. A visualization of McNeill's model of relationship between gesture and speech.

Levelt's blueprint of the speaker

Levelt (1993) proposed a blueprint that illustrates critical processes involved in speaking. This model (Figure 18.3) deals primarily with the psycholinguistic aspects, and ignores other communicative modes (the non-verbal part of messages) that are concurrent with speech. Essential elements in Levelt's blueprint are (1) the central position of the lexicon, and (2) the production and understanding of speech as linear processes in which grammar, morphosyntax and phonology play successive roles.

Elaboration of Levelt's blueprint

Just as the term multimodal describes the communication of individuals with natural speech, it also describes the communication of individuals who use augmentative and alternative communication (AAC). Speaking individuals naturally incorporate a variety of modes such as facial expression, gestures and writing as substitutes or supplements to spoken words. Individuals who use graphic symbols are also multimodal communicators (Beukelman and Mirenda, 1992; Kangas and Lloyd, 1998; Lloyd, Fuller and Arvidson, 1997; Millikin, 1997; Vanderheiden and Yoder, 1986). While it is generally agreed that multimodal communication is preferred to unimodal communication (Blischak and Lloyd, 1996; Vanderheiden and Lloyd, 1986; Vanderheiden and Yoder, 1986), it is often more easily achieved by speaking individuals than by AAC users, who must rely on others to provide multiple modes.

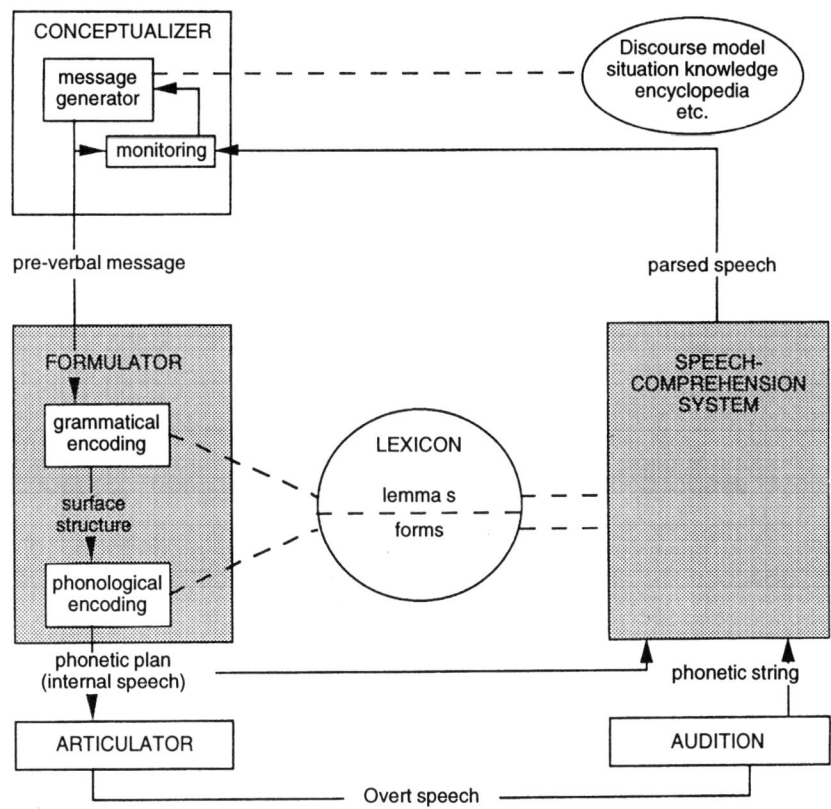

Figure 18.3. Levelt's blueprint of the speaker (from Levelt, 1993, p. 9).

Blischak and Lloyd (1996) described the multimodal communication system developed for Cathy, a young woman with severe-profound bilateral, sensorineural hearing loss, quadriplegic athetoid cerebral palsy, and estimated mild-moderate cognitive disability. Over the course of 25 years, Cathy used facial expressions and body movement, manual signs, graphic symbols and a voice output communication aid (VOCA). Analysis of conversational samples at Cathy's group home revealed that Cathy used the following modes during interactions with her supervisor: gestures and manual signs (64%), VOCA (21%), communication book and traditional orthography (8%) and vocalization (7%). Each of these modes contributed in different ways to Cathy's ability to communicate. They also provided different opportunities for cognitive, linguistic and pragmatic skill development.

Iacono, Mirenda and Beukelman (1993) compared the use of multimodal and unimodal AAC approaches with two young children with intellectual disabilities. Benefits from the use of multimodal communication may relate to intellectual abilities; however, there is evidence to suggest that multimodal AAC can have a facilitating effect on language development. While neither the multimodal nor the unimodal treatment emerged as being more effective than the other for one of the children, the multimodal treatment was found to be more effective than the unimodal treatment for the other.

In a paper discussing research needs for the 1990s, McNaughton (1990) expressed the need to examine 'various approaches and development of technology and software to allow AAC users to select their own vocabularies and AAC systems' (p. 9). Individuals who use graphic symbols as their main mode of communication should have the opportunity to choose additional modes to incorporate into their systems. More research, however, is needed to investigate just which modes are the best complements to graphic symbols across contexts, partners and time. Research should focus on the advantages and extent to which specific modes can improve communication for individuals with different abilities. The effects that different modes have on increasing frequency of initiations, improving quality of interactions, and enhancing efficiency in sending messages should be investigated for AAC users in a variety of communication contexts with different partners over time. The development of an effective multimodal system demands it.

Loncke, Vander Beken and Lloyd (1997) departed from Levelt's blueprint of the speaker (Levelt, 1993) and proposed a number of adaptations to grasp the essence of multimodal communication, as illustrated in Figure 18.4.

In order to understand this adapted model, a number of terminological specifications must be made:

- Instead of 'speech comprehension system' the term 'message comprehension system' is used. It is obvious that the term 'speech' is not appropriate here, because of the multimodal nature of what is expressed and what needs to be processed by an understanding system. The term 'message' may not be the best choice, but other options like 'surface expression' might be unclear.
- Phonological encoding is to be understood as the process in which the constituent elements of the message are identified and assembled. In speaking, these elements are the phonemes of the spoken language. For manual signing, they include such elements as hand configuration, movement, place where a sign is performed (Loncke and Bos, 1997).
- Instead of 'audition', the term 'reception' seems to be more appropriate to account for multimodal communication.

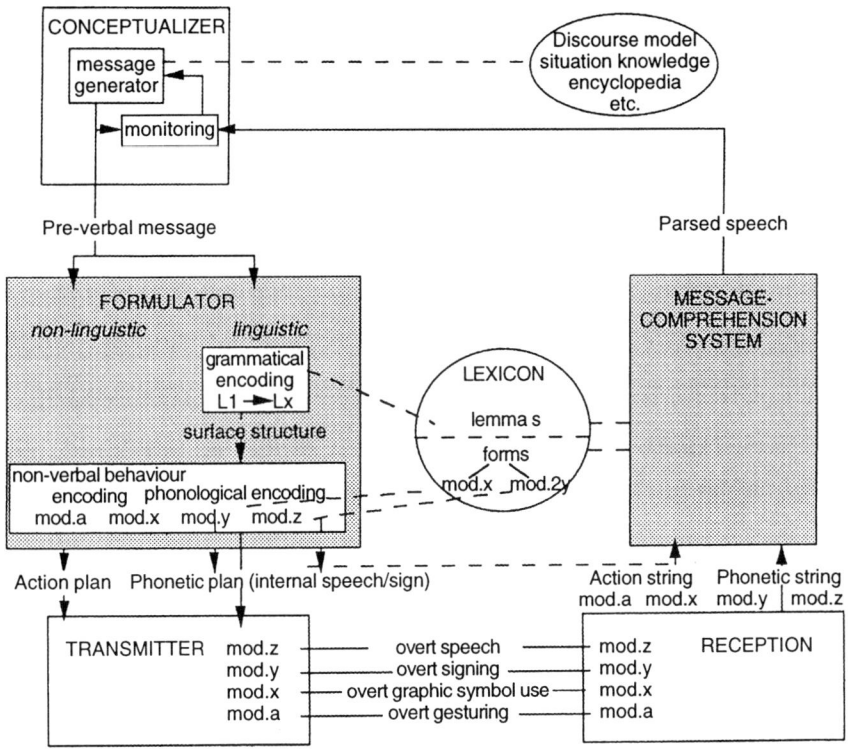

Figure 18.4. Elaboration of Levelt's blueprint of the speaker to include the multimodal aspects of communication (adapted from Loncke, Vander Beken and Lloyd, 1997, p. 106.).

The adapted model has three assumptions:

- There is only one internal lexicon, in which several types of forms are stored. These forms may belong to different modalities. They are organized in the mental lexicon in relation to each other, influenced by the way an individual – especially an individual acquiring language and communication skills – is exposed to language and communication. The practice of using a graphic symbol together with speech may help an AAC user make an internal association between the two forms.
- Different modalities are generated at a stage just prior to phonological encoding (i.e. when the system begins to prepare for actual expression). This means that generating speech or manual signs and selecting graphic symbols are the results of a chain of processes that is linked to a

modality only in the last stages. Production of communicative utterances is therefore considered to be the result of a process that begins largely modality-free. Evidence for this hypothesis comes from studies in gesture and sign language. For example, McNeill (1985) proposed that both gesturing and speech share the same underlying basis. Similarly, the comparison between the acquisition of sign language and spoken language as first languages suggests that they are both driven by modality-free structuring strategies.

- Parallel to the linguistic formulator, is a non-linguistic formulator which generates actions such as pantomiming, pointing, gesturing.

The model accounts for the use of different modalities:

- Manual signing will most likely follow a similar path as speaking. A lexical decision in the mental lexicon will activate phonological encoding which leads to a phonetic plan in which the execution of the sign is prepared.
- Pointing to a graphic symbol may result from processes within the non-linguistic formulator.
- Simultaneous use of modalities will most likely be reflected in parallel processing.

Reading acquisition models

The use of graphic symbols appears, in many ways, to be similar to typical reading and writing processes. It is natural that researchers have been trying to compare graphic symbol use with reading. Access to the meaning of the symbol in recognition or expression may or may not be similar to accessing the lexicon in reading and writing. Just as in reading and writing, the use of graphic symbol communication requires some combination of analytic and global processing.

Berninger (1987) undertook a study to examine different types of processing of printed words in beginning reading. She drew on the work of Rayner (1976), who suggested that the relative importance of different kinds of visual information (individual letters or overall word shape) may change at various stages of reading acquisition. Berninger was interested in both 'developmental changes in attention to different sources of information in a stimulus word' and 'the kind of linguistic representations accessed in memory during the reading act' (p. 388). She relied partially on the work of Kolers and Roediger (1984), who argued for a process-oriented view of information processing in which both stimulus information and 'procedures of mind' for manipulating symbols are represented in memory. Their model assumes that different units of visual information can be extracted from the same stimulus and predicts that competence in applying the different procedures will change as an individual learns to read. It also predicts that the unit of visual information extracted from the word will affect the process by which visual codes are translated into linguistic codes during word decoding. Berninger found that non-readers remembered a whole word more accurately than a letter in a word or a letter sequence in a word. Beginning readers remembered a whole word more accurately than a letter sequence in a word, but not more accurately than a letter in a word.

In summarizing results Berninger reported that '(a) visual perceptual structures imposed on printed words are affected by the unit of stimulus information available for differentiating among similar stimulus words; and (b) visual procedures for remembering whole-word patterns, component letters, and serial multiletter units are not acquired simultaneously, are not perfectly correlated, and have different relationships with criterion measures of word decoding' (p. 415).

Berninger (1987) considers that global, component and serial procedures for single words (different levels of visual processing) may all contribute to the decoding process. Global procedures may anchor attention to the visual configuration of a written word in a running line of text and may facilitate a preliminary search of potential matches with representations of words in memory. Component procedures may facilitate attention to individual letters and thus application of phonic rules of letter–phoneme correspondence and discrimination among alternative matches with representations in memory. Serial procedures may facilitate attention to letter sequences '... and thus abstraction and application of the orthographic code as well as discrimination among alternative matches with representations in memory' (p. 414).

Berninger's work (1987) is of interest, as she adds the theory and findings of a visual-perception study to the developmental studies in the beginning reading literature. Her approach offers a view of various types of visual processing working in harmony, yet changing their roles as the individual develops and gains increasing experience with print. Her conclusions appear to complement those of many researchers within the area of reading acquisition (e.g. Bryant et al., 1990; Byrne, 1992; Byrne and Carroll, 1989; Byrne and Fielding-Barnsley, 1989; Cunningham, 1990; Lundberg, Frost and Petersen, 1988; Tunmer and Hoover, 1993).

The findings of the researchers cited above provide interesting empirical results to consider along with the theoretical proposal offered by Olson (1997). In seeking congruities between the work of Smith (1971, 1973, 1979) and Adams (1990), Olson has offered an interpretation of the relationship between phoneme awareness and exposure to print which helps unify the findings of a reciprocal relationship from many empirical investigations (Ehri and Wilce, 1980; Foorman, Jenkins and Francis, 1993;

Mann, 1986; Morais, Alegria and Content, 1987; Stanovich, 1986; Vandervelden and Siegel, 1995). Olson theorizes that reading requires the analysis of speech into a novel set of categories, which are arbitrary and determined by the model of the writing system. He suggests that the processing of written material be conceived as a model by which one discovers knowledge of one's own speech, previously undetected (i.e. the discovery of the phonemic level of speech, not recognized prior to processing print), is derived from experiences with print. If the work of Berninger (1987) along with that of the reading researchers who advocate phonological instruction is considered within the context of Olson's theory, the case can be made for explicit instruction directing attention to both visual and phonological analytic processing.

It is of special interest that both visual and phonemic analytic processing be considered as factors influencing movement from a dependency on holistic processing to the analytic process required in reading. The possible relationship to reading acquisition of explicit instruction relating the visual analytic processing of Type Two AAC symbols prior to the processing of print cannot be addressed directly in this chapter. It is hoped, however, that the findings regarding performance on the visual tests using AAC symbols (picture identification, visual matching and visual analysis retrieval) will stimulate future study. There is a need to explore possible relationships between the type of graphic representation system used for communication, explicit instruction and reading acquisition.

Adams's model of reading acquisition

Graphic symbol use and reading/writing have a striking similarity: the graphic nature of the symbols and the fact that they are transmitted visually. This has led researchers to wonder if and how much the underlying processes of graphic symbol use and reading/writing are alike or different. In particular, the effect of graphic symbol use on the acquisition of literacy has become a central topic within AAC (McNaughton and Lindsay, 1995; Smith and Blischak, 1997).

Adams's (1990) model of reading acquisition has been used by AAC researchers, because it indicates which components appear to be most critical in the acquisition process: a context processor, a meaning processor, an orthographic processor and a phonological processor.

McNaughton and Lindsay's model of acquisition of graphic symbols and literacy

McNaughton and Lindsay (1995; see also McNaughton, 1998a) present a model (Figure 18.5) that illustrates how the use of graphic symbols in

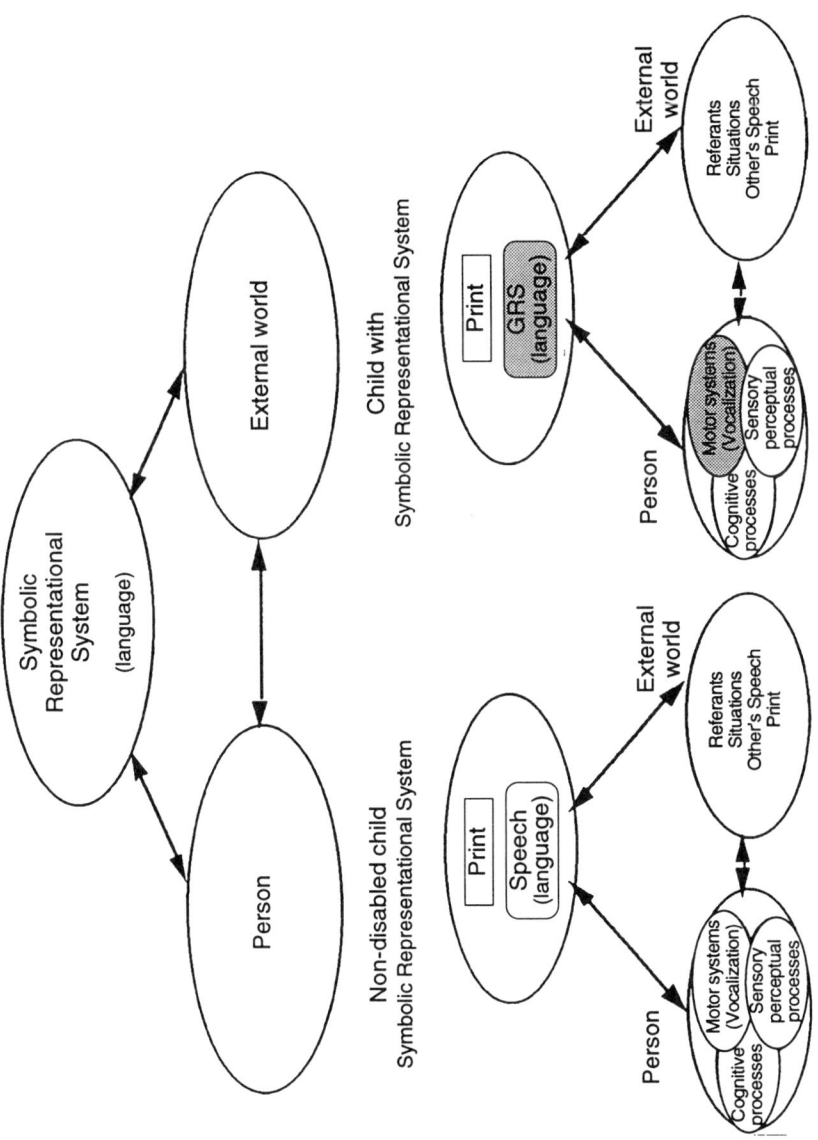

Figure 18.5. McNaughton and Lindsay's model of symbolic representational system learning (from McNaughton and Lindsay, 1995, p. 214). GRS – graphic representation symbol.

children is interconnected with cognitive development, motor systems, sensory perceptual processes and the external world. It focuses on the question of whether or not the use of graphic symbols may have a facilitating effect on the acquisition of literacy.

Conclusion

Several models have been designed to reflect underlying processes in the treatment of information through perception, direct communication by linguistic and non-linguistic means, and reading and writing. These models offer interesting aspects that inspire understanding of graphic symbol use, which may serve as a basis for generating hypotheses and testable predictions about how graphic symbols are recognized, learned and produced. There is still, however, a need for an empirically-based, comprehensive model that captures the essence of graphic symbol use. Development of the model is worthwhile work for the years to come.

Chapter 19
Research Issues and Graphic Symbol Use

Lyle L. Lloyd and Filip T. Loncke

Research in the use of graphic symbols within augmentative and alternative communication (AAC) is important from at least two perspectives. First, graphic symbol research enhances understanding about which intervention techniques are most effective. Second, it yields data and information on topics such as human information processing, symbol acquisition, the potential of visual symbols to carry linguistic information, and emergent literacy.

Researchers and practitioners are encouraged to focus on a broad scope of issues and implications relevant to the study of graphic symbols. Because AAC is a transdisciplinary field, it engages the interest of researchers and practitioners with a wide range of expertise who can seize the opportunity to address the following questions and considerations.

- How does one decide what graphic system to use from a research point of view?
- Is there any inherent linguistic structure to symbol use when the grammar of the native (spoken) language is imposed upon a symbol user? With virtually all the graphic symbol sets/systems, there is no way to mark all the refinements of grammar. Rebus may be the exception, because traditional orthography is used as part of the graphic representation to support symbols where necessary.
- What are the implications for literacy with graphic symbol use, and does one set/system offer more opportunity for developing literacy skills than another? Teachers frequently ask how to introduce reading and writing (particularly) to children with little or no functional speech.
- What is the role of voice output and graphic displays on literacy learning?
- Which characteristics of graphic symbols (e.g. iconicity, complexity) are

most critical? Is there a hierarchy among these characteristics?
- Do iconicity and complexity point to relevant distinctions according to symbol type?
- How do characteristics of graphic symbols interact with characteristics of manual sign when a multimodal approach transcending the aided and unaided domains is used?
- How do other characteristics (e.g. memory, motivation) interact with graphic symbol characteristics in the learning process?
- Even with all the scepticism toward prerequisites, it appears that vision, generally, and visual perception, specifically, are essential for graphic symbol use. The problem is that very few children have actually had their vision investigated in depth, and it is not known what their vision is like. Although this may be specifically related to graphic symbols, it impacts whatever AAC system is selected for the user.
- More attention should be focused on the most basic issue of perception of graphic symbols. This would include investigating a variety of visual abilities in addition to simple acuity so that the presentation of symbols is tailored to the abilities of the user. Studies could be planned around manipulating variables (e.g. size, location, contrast) to determine the impact that they have on learning different types of symbols and on using them effectively for communication.
- Ways of improving the effectiveness and efficiency of communication by capitalizing on opportunities for using multiple modes should be investigated. While graphic symbols may be central to an AAC system, the use of other modes (both aided and unaided) should be systematically investigated to determine how they can be incorporated to improve general parameters of efficiency and effectiveness as well as specific skill areas related to initiating and interacting.
- The role of culture in the perception of AAC symbols should be investigated as the understanding of pictographic representations is probably related to 'world view' and culture.
- The impact of the purpose for which graphic symbols are taught and the way in which symbols are learned or acquired should be studied. Increasingly, Blissymbols have been used to facilitate the development of language and literacy skills in children with limited speech, who are expected to speak in the future (e.g. supported use of AAC in children with Down syndrome; von Tetzchner, 1996). It seems that these children learn symbols differently. Because the intensity with which these children learn symbols differs from the intensity with which other children with little or no speech learn symbols (they are able to express themselves) they tend to pay less attention to detail, depending more on iconicity.
- Alant (personal communication, 28 August 1998) has expressed concern about the use of graphic symbol sets/systems (e.g. PCS, Blissymbols) as a means to facilitate the development of language and

literacy. Research has shown that teachers tend to use symbols at what they expect the expressive language level of the child to be (e.g. five-word sentences) without facilitating the receptive language level of the child (which may be a seven-word sentence). They pitch the receptive level on the child's expressive level (i.e. how many symbols the child will recognize).

- Some work has been done bridging the gap between concept symbols (e.g. PCS, Blissymbols) and letters (traditional orthography), but the process of moving from concept to word to letters is not clearly understood. Perhaps there should be a transitional phase/system between, for example, the use of Blissymbols (concept) and traditional orthography (letters) by creating a word-based system (e.g. adapting Blissymbols to become more specific) to facilitate transfer to word and phonemic recognition?
- The types of graphic symbols used and types of instruction prior to and during acquisition of reading/writing skills should be documented.
- The relationship between type of instruction and type of graphic processing should be examined.

It is critical that, in addition to describing types of instruction implemented to facilitate literacy, future research should elaborate on outcomes. The advantages and disadvantages of each graphic symbol type used in AAC should be examined. Attention should also be directed toward procedures that support transition between different graphic symbols and to how different symbol vocabularies relate to each other.

As new software makes it possible to mix symbols from different sets/systems, there is a need for increased understanding of the issues involved. The new technological capabilities raise new questions and enable researchers to study problems they would have been unable to address previously.

In summary, a number of research issues in the area of graphic symbol use and literacy within the AAC field require attention: clarification of terminology, longitudinal documentation of graphic symbol use and literacy performance of AAC users, sharing clinical learning, and identifying and documenting successful practices.

Section IV
Outcomes Measurement in AAC

Chapter 20
Outcomes Measurement in AAC

Mats Granlund and Sarah Blackstone

Life can only be understood backwards
But must be lived forward.
Kierkegaard

What is outcomes measurement?

Outcomes research is meant to increase our understanding of what has already happened so that positive changes can be made along the way. The measurement of outcomes is common practice across disciplines and within healthcare and educational systems. Outcomes research is designed to 'measure and establish a baseline of what works; how well something works; for which clients it works; and, at what level of economic efficiency it works' in a clinical service delivery system (DeRuyter, 1997, p. 95).

In the area of practice known as augmentative and alternative communication (AAC), a multitude of outcomes occur as a result of various interventions. While it is clear that AAC has a large number of remarkable outcomes to report, it is also true that relatively few are measured and not many outcomes studies are published. Instead, we have a proliferation of anecdotal accounts in the form of stories, case reports and biographies. We also have a growing number of efficacy studies that focus on the effectiveness of intervention processes (see *Augmentative and Alternative Communication*, March 1999) conducted by researchers under controlled conditions. In these studies the desired outcome of intervention is defined by the researcher in relation to a specific research question or theory rather than by a specific stakeholder (e.g. user, family member or clinician). In contrast, outcomes research focuses on the evaluation of everyday AAC interventions and their results in relation to the outcomes desired by different stakeholder groups.

The AAC community is not excluded from having to participate in the accountability and performance monitoring agendas of public policy makers, nor is it exempt from the challenge of having to evaluate the worthiness of its services, devices, providers and various delivery systems (DeRuyter, 1997, p. 95). This chapter strives to raise some issues about the complexity of the task we confront in measuring outcomes in AAC.

To understand the effects of AAC services and devices and to improve the quality, efficiency and effectiveness of AAC interventions, more information is needed about (a) the outcomes of specific AAC interventions with different populations; (b) the circumstances that have an impact on the effectiveness of AAC strategies and devices used with different populations; (c) the types of services and devices consumers find most satisfactory and why; (d) the cost effectiveness of AAC interventions; and (e) how consumers (and others) perceive the costs of AAC services and devices relative to their benefits.

Studying the outcomes of AAC interventions is not simple. It means confronting issues related to the evaluation of a complex, comprehensive and collaborative area of service delivery that is designed to address the communication needs of both children and adults with a variety of disabilities and conditions. Solutions are necessarily diverse because of the nature of the communication problems to be solved. In addition, AAC interventions involve a number of stakeholder groups who have different perspectives. While it is reasonable to assume that all stakeholders desire a successful outcome, it is unreasonable to assume that each group desires the same outcome. Thus, outcomes research necessitates determining the information needs, expectations and perspectives of the important stakeholders in the intervention. These and other characteristics inherent to the field of AAC have an impact on how research questions are framed and design methodologies are carried out.

AAC researchers who become familiar with measurement models and theoretical constructs that address similarly complex areas of service delivery are far more likely to conduct research that leads the field of AAC toward better practices. One paradigm that can be used is systems theory (Bateson, 1972). According to systems theory, a system emerges from the interaction of its parts. Thus, when the relationship among parts becomes known, the system may be better understood. Systems theory also suggests that all systems strive toward an endpoint or final state (von Bertalanffy, 1968). There are two kinds of final states: (1) static finality and (2) dynamic finality. Static finality means that the relationships among the parts are always the same. This is observed in the relationship between letters and words, because letters make up words. Dynamic finality means the relationship among the parts change so that the final state (or desired outcome) can be reached from different initial conditions and in different ways. Communication and interaction are obvious examples of systems with dynamic finality. For example, an individual using AAC techniques may, with varying degrees of success and independence, successfully communicate his menu preferences to a waiter in a restaurant using speech, gestures, a voice output device, or an interpreter.

Domains of outcomes measurement

Traditionally, outcomes research can be carried out across five separate, but related domains of intervention. Each domain addresses a pivotal aspect associated with judging the merits and best practices of goods and services, programmes and practitioners. Researchers can collect qualitative and quantitative data on the effectiveness, comprehensiveness, and efficacy of what was delivered across domains (DeRuyter, 1997, p. 99). The domains of outcomes measurement are briefly described below.

Clinical status

Outcomes measurement of clinical status/results reflects changes in an individual's level of impairment, e.g. dysarthria, dyspraxia, language disorder/delay. Because AAC interventions do not typically purport to address clinical status (i.e. the underlying impairment), changes across this domain are rarely considered a major part of outcomes research in AAC. However, clinical changes do occur; and speech-language pathologists, occupational therapists, psychologists and others involved with AAC intervention do measure these behaviours. Clinicians who feel that AAC approaches are having a facilitative effect on speech (e.g. improved intelligibility), language (e.g. increased skills in syntax) and motor skills development (e.g. enhanced fine motor skills) may decide to measure this domain more closely. However, changes in clinical status are also a reflection of developmental factors in children and the natural recovery process in adults with acquired disabilities, rather than a particular AAC intervention.

Functional status

The primary focus of AAC interventions is to improve functional communication. By definition, AAC devices are communication prostheses. They replace a function that is less available, e.g. expressive communication using speech and/or writing. Measurement of functional status, together with consumer satisfaction, accounts for most of the focus on outcomes in AAC. Measurement of functional status focuses on the development of specific communication skills or device use in daily life. Currently, anecdotal reports, testimonials, case studies and efficacy studies show, for example, that AAC interventions result in an increase in the use of symbols and devices at school, with families, in the community, and increased use of requestion and commenting behaviours using AAC techniques. Few AAC studies report changes in the interaction patterns of AAC users across the day or with multiple communication partners. Interestingly, in a recent review of intervention studies, McCollum and Hemmeter (1997) did not find the interactional patterns between child and parent to be more balanced after communication intervention.

Functional status measurement tools currently used in rehabilitation settings focus on a variety of functions (mobility, activities of daily living, communication). They are, therefore, not very sensitive to demonstrating change or improvement in communication skills. More recently, an emphasis on the development of discipline specific measures of functional status have resulted in the increased use of the Canadian Occupational Performance Measure (COPM) (Law et al., 1994) and the Functional Assessment of Communication Skills for Adults (FACS-A) (Frattali et al., 1995). However, even these measures do not take into account the unique nature or complexities associated with assistive technology and augmentative communication (DeRuyter, 1997, p. 94).

Quality of life

This domain measures changes in opportunities and the ability of individuals to participate in social, educational, community, vocational and family activities. AAC interventions that target changes in a person's quality of life tend to reflect a participation model of service delivery. By definition, quality of life is a subjective construct, so it is important to make clear whose perceptions of change are being measured (Beukelman and Mirenda, 1998).

Satisfaction

This domain addresses the level of satisfaction with AAC services and devices. Typically, researchers measure the opinions of consumers. However, other stakeholders may also be more or less satisfied with AAC interventions. Their satisfaction levels may also be measured.

Cost

The area of cost seeks to determine and analyse the costs associated with AAC intervention and may include an analysis of cost benefit, cost utility, and cost effectiveness (Persson and Brodin, 1996).

Level of outcomes measurement

There are three levels of outcomes measurement: individual level, programme level and system level.

Individual level (immediate setting)

Most clinical evaluation data are collected at the level of the individual. Desired outcomes (goals) are defined and data collected to reflect changes in an individual's communication skills within the immediate environment (often limited to a clinical setting). Measurement at this level typically is of most interest to the clinicians/teachers who provide services, as well as to AAC users and their caregivers. Other stakeholders (manufacturers, researchers, policy makers), while interested in outcomes at this level, want and need information about the impact of intervention on a larger number of individuals. Because clinicians and consumers are most interested in outcomes at this level, the focus of measurement is often on clinical and functional status, as well as satisfaction and quality of life.

Programme level

Outcomes research at the programme level involves aggregating data collected at the individual level. This requires that the type and manner of measurement and the data collection procedures are consistent. Research at this level addresses questions about clinical and functional status, cost, quality of life and satisfaction for particular AAC services/devices with different groups of individuals. Because programme managers, funders, AAC 'specialists', and manufacturers are particularly interested in outcomes at the programme level, the focus is often on functional status, satisfaction and cost.

System level

At the system level, programme data are further aggregated to provide information about AAC interventions across centres, agencies, assistive technology teams and programmes. These data may be used to set or change practice guidelines and policy. Administrators, policy makers, heads of agencies/programmes and third-party payers are seeking information about costs and the relationships between cost and functional status, clinical status, quality of life and satisfaction data.

In order for outcomes management systems to be effective and meaningful, linkages, both vertically and horizontally, between stakeholder groups, dimensions and levels are needed. Without these linkages, the relationships among the components of the system and their impact on AAC service delivery will remain forever unclear (DeRuyter, 1997).

Granlund and Steénson (1998) completed a study that included all three levels of outcomes measurement. They followed five professional teams of special education consultants over a five-year period. Each team consisted of four members. Members were specialized either in autism, visual disability, motor disability or hearing disability and provided services for school-aged children with profound and multiple disabilities. At the individual level, researchers collected data in five areas for each student who received services. This was an effort to measure individual outcomes of functional status and satisfaction as well as the quality of the intervention process. The five areas measured were: (a) changes in functional status as the result of specified interventions which were measured with goal attainment scales; (b) the quality of the intervention process as measured with the help of ratings of logical coherence in the intervention programme (i.e. criteria related ratings of the extent to which problems and goals are related and problem explanations and intervention methods are related); (c) the quality of the intervention process as measured with the help of ratings of the functionality in goals and methods (i.e. criteria related ratings of the degree to which goal attainment will increase the autonomy and self-determination of the person receiving services); (d) teacher satisfaction with services, and (e) the quality of collaboration in the intervention process as measured with teachers' perceived involvement in the intervention process.

At the programme level, each team's data were aggregated according to two categories: qualitative efficacy and quantitative efficacy each year, over the five-year period. Qualitative efficacy included both outcome measures and process measures: (a) proportion of goals with expected level of goal attainment, (b) mean rating of logical coherence, (c) mean rating of functionality of goals and methods, (d) teachers' mean satisfaction with the services received, and (e) teachers' mean ratings of their involvement in the intervention process. Quantitative efficacy included measures of the amount of services provided; these were process measures in relation to client outcomes and as an outcomes measure for the programme: (a) number of students given services; (b) number of individual education plans (IEPs) written; (c) number of Goal Attainment Scales (GAS) constructed; and (d) number of GAS evaluated.

At the system level, the mean score for each variable in each efficacy dimension was calculated for each year. This enabled the researchers to compare functional outcomes of the students, satisfaction of teachers, and intervention process measures across teams. Teams that scored below the average in at least three out of the five years on a majority of the variables in an efficacy dimension were classified as low in quantity or quality. Teams classified as low or high in the dimensions were compared regarding team characteristics such as type of leadership, team culture, communication between team members, resources and staff turnover. This allowed the researchers to identify factors related to positive outcomes of intervention both within individual team members and within teams as systems. For example, at the system level, the results revealed that team characteristics relating to high quantitative efficacy (e.g. clear and distinct routines for service coordination) had a minimal overlap with the team characteristics that related to high qualitative efficacy (e.g. consensus among team members regarding what constitutes good outcomes of services). As a result of this study, in-service training activities of team members were coordinated to enhance consensus regarding 'good' outcomes of services. Another result was that documentation of services was refined to correspond with the desired outcomes of services to a larger extent (i.e. the qualitative efficacy measures became a part of monthly team reports).

In addition to measuring the outcomes across the domains and levels, it is important to know the interrelationships among the domains and levels of measurement and to relate the various dimensions with the needs of various stakeholder groups. Realistically, the costs associated with carrying out such a comprehensive outcomes study agenda in AAC at the system level currently would preclude it from happening.

One might expect that positive outcomes in consumer satisfaction would correlate with positive outcomes in functional status, quality of life and cost. However, this is not necessarily the case. The interrelationship between satisfaction measures and other outcome domains is commonly low (McNaughton, 1994). When one considers that satisfaction measures tend to focus on the way services are given rather than on the outcomes of services, this is not surprising. Satisfaction measures focus on the processes rather than the outcomes of AAC interventions.

Status of outcomes measurement in AAC

Ten years ago, it was sufficient to demonstrate that persons with severe speech impairments could communicate effectively when they used AAC strategies, techniques and devices. Today, the testimonials of practitioners, AAC users, manufacturers and family members are no longer sufficient. According to Guralnick (1997), the field of AAC has already answered the first-generation outcomes research question: 'Do AAC interventions have positive outcomes?' The answer is 'Yes.' Outcomes measurement in AAC must now begin to address the second generation of outcomes research questions: 'For whom?', 'Under which circumstances?', 'With what treatments?', 'For how long?', 'At what cost?'

Research studies in AAC are typically designed and implemented by highly trained specialists under rather ideal conditions rather than in natural clinical contexts (Blockberger, 1994). While these studies may demonstrate the efficacy of an intervention approach, they are not outcomes research. For starters, they produce results that are not easy to generalize.

A quick review of outcomes research in AAC reveals a paucity of published studies. For example, the journal *Augmentative and Alternative Communication* has fewer than five articles that purport to be AAC outcomes research.

Four examples of outcomes studies reported by AAC researchers follow:

1. In an unpublished study, Mathy (1998) investigated the outcomes (functional status, satisfaction) of AAC intervention in 24 adults with amyotrophic lateral sclerosis (ALS). Two groups participated: those with bulbar presentations and those with a spinal presentation. Each client had access to and used many AAC methods. Data showed that

both groups of individuals used multiple approaches. They relied on no-tech or low-tech strategies for conversations and used high-tech devices to tell stories, convey detailed information, talk on the telephone and write. They reported being 'generally' or 'very' satisfied with AAC intervention. The one area of dissatisfaction was their ability to carry on a conversation. In a second study of six patients, Mathy reported they used no-tech communication across all settings and were more likely to use high-tech devices primarily at home. Factors influencing choice of AAC methods included speed, simplicity of use, ability to use in multiple positions and partner acceptance. On the basis of these studies, Mathy concluded that when individuals with ALS are provided with a range of AAC options and taught to use them effectively, they strategically use what they feel is most effective. Their choices are likely to depend not only on their motor abilities, but also on their communication partners, the setting and the demands of the communication activity.

2. DeRuyter (1994, 1999) followed 122 subjects (55% male; 45% female), ages 2 years 11 months to 21 years 8 months (mean age 13 years 7 months). He collected data across all five measurement domains on each person to determine changes in the user's environment, use of assistive technology (AT), perceived value of the technology relative to cost, clinical status, frequency of assistive technology breakdowns, functionality of equipment and satisfaction with services. Follow-up data were collected for each person at 6 months, 1 year and 2 years after their equipment was delivered. Results suggested that the families and children and youth who had AAC devices (60%), computers (25%), environmental control technology (14%) and other technology (5%), perceived the value of AT relative to costs as good or fair and were satisfied with the services they received. Cognitive/clinical changes occurred in at least half of the children over this period while environmental changes were minimal. Regarding their use of the prescribed equipment, the researcher found that after six months 66% were using their devices as designed and after two years, 45% used their devices as prescribed. Fifteen per cent had discarded the equipment after two years. It was interesting to note that the reasons for discarding equipment were related mostly to equipment breakdowns. Nearly half reported occasional or frequent breakdowns during the first year, while 60% reported occasional and frequent breakdowns within two years. These data suggest that although the everyday use of AT was likely to decrease over time, it remained relatively consistent over the two-year period.

3. In a longitudinal study of AAC intervention following traumatic brain injury and stroke, DeRuyter and colleagues developed a database of 500 non-speaking individuals seen at Rancho Los Amigos Rehabilitation Center. Thirty-eight per cent were non-speaking as the

result of traumatic brain injury (TBI); 18% had suffered a cortical/subcortical stroke; and 3% had a brainstem stroke (personal communication, December, 1998). DeRuyter, Doyle and Kennedy (1990) followed 72 TBI adults who were non-speaking at the time of discharge from the inpatient acute rehabilitation programme for two years. Sixty-five per cent had regained speech to a functional level within that period of time. Of the 35% (n = 25) who did not regain speech, more than half (56%) were using their AAC devices in the manner for which they were designed. Twenty-four per cent had totally discarded their systems and 20% were using their systems in certain environments. The researchers point out that while on the surface, these usage data may not appear to reflect a positive outcome, closer examination of these data show a number of positive outcomes. For example, two-thirds of the individuals discarding their systems had recovered speech and the remaining third had upgraded their original ACS. Thus, functional communication abilities of most individuals with TBI had improved. Most (83%) also had improved cognitively. The researchers found that the provision of an AAC device during initial stages of recovery had enabled rehabilitation staff to conduct cognitive–linguistic assessments. This allowed many of the non-speakers to participate in multidisciplinary rehabilitation programmes, which facilitated their recovery by ensuring appropriate treatment programming and placement. Thus, as a result of the functional usage of an AAC device by TBI non-speakers, determining rehabilitation potential earlier and providing appropriate programming controlled costs. Both factors decreased length of stay in hospital.

4. DeRuyter, Kennedy and Doyle (1990) examined the appropriateness of AAC device selection and AAC device usage in 23 non-speaking patients who had suffered a left cerebral vascular accident. An independent panel determined the appropriateness of the AAC device selected. They concluded that all devices chosen at the time of hospitalization discharge were appropriate and that six months post discharge, 83% were still appropriate. However, while 87% of these adults were using their systems as designed at discharge, only 43% were using their devices six months post discharge and 39% had abandoned their devices. Underlying variables such as changes in lifestyle and interactive needs following a cerebrovascular accident seemed to underlie the poor outcome in usage noted.

In summary, outcomes can be measured across five different domains and three levels. Data collected will reflect the views of the stakeholders involved with the design and implementation of research. Given the complexity of the area, researchers need to clarify their outcome perspective (e.g. user, administrator). From their chosen perspective they need to select the most important outcomes to measure and then use stringent designs and methodologies to conduct their research. These data and their subsequent analysis will help to determine the ecological validity of the complex interventions studied in AAC outcomes research.

Steps toward determining what to measure

It is clear that to measure the outcomes of AAC interventions effectively, researchers must first clearly define both the desired outcomes of intervention (i.e. the dependent variables) and what the intervention consists of (i.e. the independent variable). Goals lead to actions (or intervention approaches); and outcomes are the effects of those actions (Granlund, Blackstone and Norris, 1998). A major step in conducting outcomes research, therefore, is to define clearly the goals or desired outcomes of the intervention. It is important to note that the desired outcomes of intervention are never the only outcomes; however, they are the outcomes that should be measured. Defining the desired outcomes is a key to good outcomes research (and good AAC intervention). In traditional intervention research the desired outcomes are equal to the dependent variables. They are defined by the researcher in relation to the research questions of the study. However, in investigating the outcomes of clinical intervention there are several different stakeholders who might favour different outcomes. Therefore, in defining the desired outcome, it is important to ask, 'Whose outcome is it?'

At Alliance '95, an international conference on AAC outcomes evaluation (Blackstone and Pressman, 1995), participants developed the following consensus statement about outcomes measurement in AAC.

> Outcomes measurement should be consumer driven, flexible and enduring.
> The result of AAC interventions should be an improved quality of life for people who use AAC.
> The results of outcomes measurement also should be used to improve cost-effectiveness and to improve the quality of equipment and services.

We know that goals are value-laden. Goals always reflect the values of the stakeholder(s) who set them. This means that the desired outcomes of different stakeholder groups will differ. For example, in a survey completed in 1995, various AAC 'experts' were asked how they would rate the importance of different domains of outcomes research for different stakeholder groups. Results demonstrated that these experts thought that AAC consumers consider quality of life issues the most important outcomes, service providers focus on functional communication, and administrators are concerned mostly about consumer satisfaction and costs (Blackstone, 1995).

Unlike AAC intervention research where goals reflect the professionals' values, outcomes research is meant to measure the impact of AAC intervention on the lives of AAC users and their primary partners. AAC users and their caregivers should actively participate in selecting the goals and, therefore, the intervention approaches. For example, a speech-language pathologist and teacher might write an IEP objective as follows: 'The child will *answer* questions in class using pre-programmed and spontaneous phrases on an AAC device.' A parent, on the other hand, might prefer the objective written as, 'The child will use the AAC device to *ask* questions in school, at home and in an after-school programme.' While such differences are subtle, the impact on intervention and outcomes can be significant. Collaboration and consultation are necessary before making decisions about the desired outcomes of AAC intervention approaches.

A second important step in defining what to measure is considering how to relate desired outcomes measured in one domain to the intended or desired outcomes in another domain or across levels of measurement. For example, Dunst (in Bruder, 1997) evaluated the effectiveness of a curriculum for young children with profound disabilities. He asked questions such as: 'Do the outcomes of this particular child-focused AAC intervention have positive effects on the feelings, attitudes and behaviour of the adults who interact with the child?' The curriculum consisted of learning games to enhance a child's interactive competence and contingency awareness. Dunst collected data on 42 children and 66 caregivers at four levels of measurement. First-level effects were defined as behaviours displayed during intervention sessions such as children exhibiting attention, excitement, vocalization and caregivers exhibiting verbal, non-verbal and affective behaviour. Second-level effects were defined as behaviours demonstrated as a result of, or in response to, the contingency behaviour of the children. These included the recognition behaviour of children and behaviours exhibited by caregivers in response to contingency behaviours of the children. Third-level effects were changes in behavioural repertoires following increased skills in children, including changes in the cognitive styles of children and increased enjoyment of children in the caregivers. Fourth-level effects were defined as behaviours that resulted from the increased learning capacity of children that were spatially and temporally removed from the learning situation. These included the (a) health status of the children, and (b) increased availability of caregiver's time. Results suggested positive outcomes at each level, as well as interaction effects between levels.

A third important step in selecting the outcomes to measure is to consider the relationships among intended and unintended outcomes, within and between outcome domains and levels. Relevant questions could be: 'Is parent satisfaction with AAC services related to the perception of decreased family needs?' and 'Is parent satisfaction with services or decreased family needs related to the goal-attainment of children?' These questions were asked by Granlund and Björck-Åkesson (1996a) in a study of the processes and outcomes of training pre-school consultants in family-centred habilitation interventions. They found no statistically significant relationships between the outcomes 'satisfaction', 'decreased family needs', and 'goal-attainment for child-focused interventions'. The authors explain the result as follows: *Satisfaction* is a measure of the way in which services were given. Therefore, it is not related to outcome measures such as decreased family needs or goal attainment for child-focused goals. *Decreased family needs* is a generic measure covering several areas of family needs (e.g. needs for information, support, receiving help with family relations). It is not necessarily related to specific intervention goals and outcomes for the children, which may only affect a restricted part of family needs.

The Granlund and Björck-Åkesson (1996a) study illustrates the importance of analysing the theoretical and logical relationships among different measures by asking (1) whether there is a logical reason to believe that different outcomes are related, and (2) what relationships can be expected between outcome domains and between outcome measures within the same domain in AAC outcomes research. It is important to measure several outcomes and also to investigate their interrelationship. Such investigations must be based on a sound theoretical model for plausible outcomes and their interrelationships (see Dunst, in Bruder, 1997).

To summarize, researchers face a formidable task in accounting for the diverse and dynamic nature of AAC interventions. It is necessary to clearly state the value-base for decisions made in measuring the outcomes of AAC intervention. In addition, defining the desired outcomes and taking into account measurement across various domains and levels of measurement are crucial to this area of research.

Characterizing the independent variable

The independent variable may be defined as the actions taken to reach the desired outcome. In clinical AAC interventions, independent variables rarely consist of a single intervention or a fixed treatment. Instead, AAC interventions are better defined as 'a menu of possibilities accompanied by a series of supports that facilitate consumer's interaction with these possibilities' (Knapp, 1995, p. 7). A major challenge for outcomes research in AAC is to provide a comprehensive description of these possibilities, the series of supports that facilitate the interactions among the possibilities, and their interrelationships. The possibilities may consist of the typical characteristics of an intervention, e.g. a symbol set, a speech output system and a specific training programme to be used. Such specific AAC intervention characteristics will not be further discussed in this chapter. They are the focus of most efficacy research efforts.

A second set of intervention components or possibilities is generic to all interventions but is not always included in AAC outcomes research. These involve characteristics of (a) the professionals and the programme,

(b) the milieu surrounding the intervention being carried out, and (c) the AAC user who is receiving services as well as those in their immediate context.

(a) Characteristics of the professional and the programme

The professionals involved and types of intervention programmes affect outcomes in AAC because they determine who delivers the services, how services are provided and the way in which services are evaluated. In a review of the effectiveness of early intervention on deaf children and children with hearing loss, for example, Calderon and Greenberg (1997) argue that the variables with the greatest effect on client outcomes reflect factors related to personality, training, philosophy and generic communication skills of the professional who delivered the services. Several other studies in human services (e.g. Orlinsky and Howard, 1986) have also demonstrated that factors related to characteristics of professionals providing intervention have an important impact on client outcomes. To date, the influence of professional characteristics are seldom mentioned or described in AAC outcomes research. It would be interesting to investigate the interrelationship between the interventionist's ability to improve the disabled person's sense of efficacy in relating to others and the measured outcomes of AAC intervention.

In defining variables related to characteristics of the programme, AAC researchers can consider the programme's 'theory of action' (Patton, 1978). Theory of action refers to the assumptions upon which the interventionists rest their actions. Assumptions include official policies as well as traditional beliefs and cultural values. An example is the practice of simultaneously introducing an AAC device to a user and training the user's parents/spouse/caregiver to facilitate the use of the device. This approach reflects a belief on the part of professionals and programme administrators that communication partner training increases the probability that assistive technology (and AAC intervention) will be successful. By spelling out the logic behind such an approach and by specifying the underlying hypothesis/theory/belief, AAC researchers are more likely to collect data that test the assumptions by asking questions like, 'Does partner training increase the use of the device during interactions? Under what circumstances and in which settings?'

To investigate theories of action, a qualitative approach is necessary because factors underlying clinical practices are not always explicitly stated or documented. Therefore, a document analysis would have to be supplemented with interviews of professionals and administrators.

(b) Characteristics of the intervention milieu

Variables, such as where services are delivered, how intense the training is, and the nature of the intervention decision-making process, also affect the outcomes of AAC interventions. A good example of how to investigate these characteristics is the ongoing Castle project (McConachie, Clarke, Wood, Price and Grove, work in progress). The project aims to document the amount and type of speech and language therapy intervention during one school year for up to 30 children with motor disabilities. It also aims to make an analysis of the relationship between parameters of the interventions and their outcomes by measuring the children's use of aids and their progress in communication skills. Researchers are documenting the independent variables by measuring:

- The structure and type of delivery of speech and language therapy (hours of therapy, place of delivery, communication modes encouraged, objectives for each session, etc.).
- The child's attendance in school during the year.
- Vocabulary available to each child.
- Periodic audit of the availability of the AAC system.
- Interviews with AAC users, speaking children in the classrooms, teachers and parents.

Data collected for each intervention factor are subsequently related to specific AAC-focused outcomes using measures such as Goal Attainment Scaling and the amount of AAC system use in school when the child was observed.

(c) Characteristics of persons who use AAC and their immediate setting

Personal characteristics strongly influence the outcome of an intervention. Bronfenbrenner (in Sontag, 1996) identifies three types of personal attributes: (a) physical attributes; (b) personal stimulus qualities; and (c) developmentally structuring attributes. In addition, Bronfenbrenner suggests that personal stimulus qualities and developmentally structuring attributes, because of their tendency to affect the emotional content of the interaction with the environment, may have a stronger impact on a person's function and development than physical attributes.

- *Physical attributes* include factors such as bodily characteristics, type of disability (e.g. visual disability, cognitive disability and physical disability), age, sex and gender. Physical attributes are often well described in AAC research. However, several studies have shown that physical attributes have only a weak to moderate relationship with the outcome of AAC interventions (e.g. Romski and Sevcik, 1992).
- *Personal stimulus qualities* (e.g. bio-behavioural state, temperament/behavioural style and affective expressions) invite or discourage reactions from the environment. For example, a number of recent studies have shown that the frequency of communication interactions, as well as the type of communication interactions, are related to

personal stimulus qualities in persons with profound multiple disabilities. Guess and his colleagues (1993) studied the relationship between bio-behavioural states (e.g. degree of alertness) and communication interaction. They found that persons with profound multiple disabilities spend only brief periods of time in the alert bio-behavioural states necessary for mutually rewarding communicative turn-taking to occur. The authors noted that because bio-behavioural states seem to be intrinsically controlled, they are difficult to relate to environmental events. However, they also noted that communicative behaviours within the environment often came before periods of alert bio-behavioural states and that these behaviours seemed to prolong the periods of time spent in alert bio-behavioural states.

• Developmentally structuring attributes refer to a person's 'active orientation toward and interaction with the environment' (e.g. intellectual curiosity, exploration) (Bronfenbrenner, 1992, p. 219). In working on early communication and microtechnology with children who have profound multiple disabilities, Schweigert and Rowland (1992) reported using different intervention strategies for training 'contingency awareness' based on the type of stimulation (e.g. social stimulation) the child found reinforcing.

Characteristics of the immediate setting also influence the outcomes of communication intervention. Affleck et al. (1989) evaluated the outcomes of interventions designed to assist the families of premature infants in their transition from neonatal intensive care programmes to the home environment. The intervention, which included information regarding child development, resources and input on child activities, consisted of weekly home visits for 15 weeks. Results revealed that while the severity of the infant's medical condition was unrelated to the mother's perceived need for support, the mother's need for support moderated the effects of intervention. Thus, when mothers felt a strong need for support, the intervention approach seemed to increase their sense of control and responsiveness. In contrast, when mothers perceived less of a need for support, intervention did not increase their sense of control or their responsiveness.

To summarize, several aspects of the independent variable (i.e. the actions taken to reach the desired outcome) affect the outcomes of AAC interventions. Outcomes researchers need to describe and document components that are specific to a single intervention as well as those that are generic to all interventions. The generic components may include characteristics of (a) the interventionist and/or change agents, (b) the intervention milieu and way it is implemented, and (c) the user who is obtaining services and the immediate context (partners, locations, tasks, etc.). The multiple dimensions and components of the independent variable in AAC reflect the complexity of the field. Therefore, in conducting research on heterogeneous groups, such as persons in need of AAC, paradigms that require group assignment, experimental control and rigorous measurement procedures are generally not applicable.

Attributing results to influences

To document the relationships between interventions and outcomes, one has to analyse carefully the quality of evidence associating the intervention and observed changes (Simeonsson, 1995). Simeonsson (1995) proposes a framework for evaluation that is built on a legal paradigm and focuses on three levels of 'certainty of evidence for change': suggestive, preponderant and conclusive. (1) Suggestive evidence indicates that there is a possible relationship between the intervention and the outcomes. (2) Preponderant evidence shows proof that there is a probable relationship between intervention and outcome. (3) Conclusive evidence proves that the relationship of an intervention to subsequent outcomes exists. In this framework, the levels of certainty of change relate to available information about five different aspects of the intervention cycle. The first four levels pertain to a thorough description of the independent variable: (1) the purpose and nature of intervention; (2) how ecologically valid the intervention is; (3) the fidelity of the implementation and maintenance of prescribed intervention methods, i.e. how the intervention is implemented in comparison to what was planned; and (4) how anticipated outcomes, as well as unexpected effects, are documented. The fifth aspect pertains to whether the association between the intervention and the outcomes are investigated. Simeonsson (1995) suggests the use of two alternative approaches to traditional group designs: single subject designs and the case studies.

- *Single subject designs* are frequently used in AAC efficacy research when the focus of intervention is on changing the clinical or functional status of a person with disabilities through a specific intervention. However, when patterns of interaction or comprehensive effects of several interventions are the focus of evaluation (as they are in outcomes research), it becomes difficult to use single subject research designs.
- *Case studies* range from subjective narratives to analytic reports (Simeonsson, 1995). The adequacy and rigour of the case study approach is dependent on central features such as (1) a theoretically derived framework; (2) detailed documentation; (3) use of multiple sources and methods in data collection; and (4) explicit criteria (preferably set beforehand) for evaluating outcomes. In addition, replication is important as it offers the possibility of generalizing the findings.

Multiple case studies, in which the same set of measurements make it possible to aggregate data on programme or system level, can be useful in outcomes research. Detailed documentation over extended time-periods makes it possible to identify comprehensive outcomes for several consecutive and/or parallel interventions. At present, case studies are primarily used to evaluate the impact of communication interventions in realms of social interaction and communication rather than in the area of symbol acquisition or specific use of communicative functions. An example is Goldbart's (1994) detailed case reports on assessment and intervention data, which is included in a communication curriculum for students with profound, multiple disabilities.

To analyse data from multiple case studies, researchers can use a cluster analysis strategy (Youngman, 1979). In AAC outcomes research, the focus can be on different subject characteristics or characteristics of the intervention in relation to the relative strength of the effects across different outcome measures. Instead of factor analysis of test-items, however, this approach enables researchers to analyse groups of individuals, i.e. 'case-clusters' who represent persons in need of AAC and who respond in similar ways to AAC interventions.

It is also possible to combine case studies with more traditional group designs using a three-tired model of data analysis (Light, 1999). In this model, the first level of analysis uses traditional statistical methods based on group data and focuses on variables of interest in relation to the outcome(s) of intervention. The second level of analysis consists of finding and describing groups of individuals who are representative (or not representative) of the pattern in the group data on outcomes. The third level of analysis uses a case study approach to further describe the individuals representing the different patterns found at the second level analysis. Thus, group results can be reconciled with individual performance data.

In summary, the heterogeneity of the target group for AAC intervention, as well as the diversity in the way interventions are actually implemented, make it necessary to find alternatives to traditional group designs in order to investigate the association among factors related to interventions and their outcomes. Such alternatives can combine the results of individual case studies with the possibilities of finding ways that enable researchers to generalize results that are available using group designs.

The intrusiveness of the design

Outcomes research is commonly not a part of everyday intervention and can therefore be intrusive. It may change the way that an intervention is implemented (i.e. threaten the ecological validity of the outcomes evaluation) and/or may be ethically unsound (i.e. threaten the personal integrity of the person in need of AAC or others involved in the intervention).

Ideally, evaluation tools and activities used to conduct outcomes research should not affect the way in which services are provided. In reality, this is more or less impossible. By applying chaos theory-based research approaches to organizations providing services to persons with disabilities, Granlund and Steénson (1998) and Schalock et al. (1994) showed that by simply documenting aspects of services, outcomes measurement and other data collection processes act as a strong force in 'pulling' those services in ways indicated as desirable by the documentation instruments. One way to decrease these forces is to base the evaluation on existing documentation methods and observe service settings as they exist. However, in quality assurance activities and outcomes research, there is a deliberate use of documentation measures and activities to change the services provided in the desired direction. According to several authors (e.g. Nelson, 1977; Bailey, Buysse and Palsha, 1990), this type of reactivity and reliability are compatible. People can (and do) give reliable ratings of their behaviour even as they react to the measurement by changing their behaviour in the desired direction.

If the aim of outcomes measurement is to affect the way interventions are implemented, then the evaluation tools used should be: (1) reactive in the desired direction of change; (2) reliable; and (3) possible to integrate into the current practices and routines for providing services. This means that the professionals and persons in need of AAC must consider the measurement tools useful. This requires collaboration. An example is the earlier mentioned longitudinal evaluation of team functioning reported by Granlund and Steénson (1998). Evaluation data were based on existing documents such as (a) written educational plans, (b) existing statistics of frequency of services, (c) reactive measures of the functionality of goals, (d) logical coherence of educational plans, and (e) classroom teachers' ratings of involvement in the decision-making process. Researchers used both existing measures and those developed by team supervisors to give feedback on team performance. The data collected on the implementation of intervention were compared with goal attainment for student-focused interventions with the help of Goal Attainment Scaling (GAS) (Kiersuk, Smith and Cardillo, 1994) and a satisfaction measure. The combination of data collection methods enabled the researchers to demonstrate both the ecological validity and the reactivity of their outcomes evaluation.

Outcome research activities also have to be analysed with regard to: (1) the personal integrity of the person in need of AAC and others in their immediate setting; (2) the advantages that follow from participation in the outcome evaluation activities for the person in need of AAC and his/her immediate setting; and (3) the integrity and availability of the results of outcome evaluation in the dissemination of evaluation data. The *personal integrity* and privacy of the person in need of AAC and others in his/her immediate setting are threatened to a lesser degree if participation is anonymous. However, anonymous participation makes it impossible to change practices in individual cases as a consequence of evaluation. The *advantages of participating* in the outcomes evaluation activities become less obvious to the person in need of AAC and others involved in their lives. In relation to *dissemination of outcomes* data, two factors are important to consider. First, the *personal integrity* of participants must be protected when data are presented. Second, data should be presented in a way that is *readily understood by the participants*. One way to handle these issues is to use an aggregation approach with coded data, as described in Table 20.1.

Table 20.1. Outcomes research and personal integrity

Level of outcomes	Integrity in data collection	Advantages from participation	Dissemination of evaluation results
Person in need of AAC and others in the immediate setting	Clinicians collect data from users and others in the immediate settings and apply codes to the data of individual users	Clinicians discuss evaluation results with each user and make adjustments to the interventions implemented	Evaluation data and conclusions are presented in oral and written form for users and others involved before official release. Users judge integrity and validity of results.
Clinician	Person responsible for evaluation at programme level assigns codes to individual clinicians. Data are aggregated for each clinician	Person responsible for evaluation at programme level provides each clinician with summarized data and gives feedback on important issues	Evaluation data and conclusions are presented in oral and written form to clinician before official release. Clinician judges integrity and validity of results
Programme	Data are aggregated at the programme level	Data aggregated on programme level are presented to programme participants	Evaluation data and conclusions are presented in oral and written form to programme participants before official release
Organization	Data are aggregated across programmes	Data are aggregated on organization level and may be available to participants	Evaluation data are officially released

As can be seen in the table, data are not collected anonymously at the user or clinician levels. This might lead to users, their caregivers and clinicians being less honest in responding to questionnaires to measure satisfaction, for example. However, 'open' ratings are necessary if clinicians are to follow up on the ratings with their clients and if supervisors are to support the professional growth of clinicians. Open ratings enable clinicians/supervisors to look at the 'profile of ratings' and ask follow-up questions on items that deviate from the most common responses. AAC users and others in their immediate settings often give valuable information during meetings that address follow-up questions.

Regarding dissemination of evaluation results, Miles and Huberman (1994) give recommendations for developing an 'integrity check-list' so users and others can judge the integrity and availability of the results disseminated. Items to consider are: 'Are descriptions of interventions and services meaningful?' i.e. do they 'ring true?', 'Does the description match my standards for personal integrity?', 'Is the report written in an understandable and available manner?', 'Is the knowledge offered usable?', and 'Have users of the findings experienced any sense of empowerment, or increased control over their lives/professional behaviour?'

In summary, questions about the intrusiveness of a research design are interrelated: 'Is the design a threat to the ecological validity?', and 'Does it protect the personal integrity of the participants?' Ecological validity is higher if evaluation activities do not affect service participants and are not a part of the services. Generally, however, the collection of data is a component of the services delivered. Personal integrity is related to the advantages that users and others involved directly in the intervention gain from participating in the evaluation. When outcomes research is a part of continuous quality improvement activities, then 'open' ratings from users and others in their immediate settings are recommended so that the quality of intervention can be improved for individual users. However, when aggregating data at the programme and system levels, coding data is recommended to protect personal integrity. If possible, those involved in the intervention should be involved in preparing the dissemination of evaluation results.

Conclusions

Outcomes measurement in AAC is a relatively young phenomenon that has recently entered the second generation of outcomes research. Questions now must address important professional and public policy issues such as: 'For whom?', 'Under which circumstances?', 'With what treatments?', 'For how long?', 'With what outcomes?' The divergent questions asked and the divergent outcomes that occur necessitate that AAC researchers become familiar with a wide range of research designs, multiple research methods and theoretical models and paradigms that address other complex areas of service delivery. Not only do desired outcomes of AAC intervention need to be described and specified, but also components in the communicative system involved (the person in need of AAC and others in the immediate setting, the context milieu for intervention, and characteristics of the intervention itself) need to be defined. Important issues to address include:

- The interrelationship between the domains and levels of outcomes.
- The perspective and needs of various stakeholder groups (e.g. whose outcome is it anyway?).
- Characteristics of the interventionists (e.g. superexpert or typical clinician?).
- Specific and generic characteristics of the intervention (e.g. ecological validity? client centred?).
- Characteristics of users/immediate setting (e.g. life style and temperament?).
- Personal integrity (e.g. do users feel dependent or threatened?) and advantages for users and others in their lives that result from participating in the outcomes evaluation (Does participating make any difference?).

Section V
Family Issues and AAC

Chapter 21
Moving Forward with Families: Perspectives on AAC Research and Practice

Lynn A. Sweeney

Introduction

Research on family issues in augmentative and alternative communication (AAC) is growing but still limited in comparison with other focus areas in the field of AAC (Angelo, Kokoska and Jones, 1996; Blackstone, 1994; Blackstone and Williams, 1994). The goal of this chapter is to present an overview of what we believe is known now and help to organize these perspectives and findings into a practical menu of considerations to guide future steps in research and programme development. Inclusion of a family member who uses AAC impacts on family dynamics, child-rearing practices and the development of relationships. Fostering independence, healthy interdependence, self-determination and the development of relationships with family, friends and community members are crucial components for successful and meaningful AAC outcomes. Findings from several countries suggest that the ways in which families are involved in decision-making, planning and instruction contribute significantly to long-term success with AAC (Sweeney et al., 1998). Current theories and models from a variety of fields as well as the vitally important information beginning to be collected from family members and people who use AAC themselves point us toward a new and fruitful journey in partnership with families.

Defining 'family' for AAC purposes

What is and who is a family? It was a question asked by Blackstone (1994) and raised again at the 1998 ISAAC Research Symposium on Augmentative and Alternative Communication (AAC) in Dublin, Ireland. The fact that the community of AAC families, researchers and service providers continue to struggle with this primary question suggests at least three points of importance to family-related AAC research and practice at this time:

231

1. Families are dynamic and ever-changing systems with compositions that are culturally, circumstantially, individually and at times even legally determined.
2. People who use AAC often experience literal or figurative departures from traditional family structures such that their close and significant supports in situations may or may not involve biological relatives.
3. Despite the overwhelming importance of family, research on family issues in AAC is in a first tier level of development (Björck-Åkesson in Sweeney, Björck-Åkesson and Granlund, 1998).

In order to move forward with the study of family issues in AAC an operational definition of family is needed. This definition must be both broad enough to encompass a range of family compositions and flexible enough to be applied in unique as well as more traditional and frequently occurring family situations.

Blackstone (1994) cited the following description (Winton et al., 1990) as capturing the 'essence of family'.

> Families are big, small, extended, nuclear, multi-generational, with one parent, two parents, and grandparents. We live under one roof or many. A family can be as temporary as a few weeks, as permanent as forever. We become part of a family by birth, adoption, marriage, or from a desire for mutual support. A family is a culture unto itself, with different values and unique ways of realizing its dreams. Together, our families become the source of our rich cultural heritage and spiritual diversity. Our families create neighbourhoods, communities, states, and nations. (Blackstone, 1994, p. 1)

Considering the complexity and diversity of family compositions and the concurrent need for a research friendly reference point, Sweeney (in Sweeney, Björck-Åkesson and Granlund, 1998) offered this family definition for research discussion purposes: 'Family is: a system of significant others who provide various forms of care, guidance and support.' The range of potential emotional connections and interdependency are implied underpinnings of the key words (i.e. care, guidance, support) in this definition.

Carpenter (1998) has suggested that as a result of multiple social changes and influences '... our traditional role definitions of the family are no longer valid and could in fact hinder professional interactions with families if professionals adhere to them' (p. 181). Given the decreasing number of families reflecting the traditionally stereotyped member and role features (e.g. two married parents with father as provider, etc.), Carpenter has recommended a move to 'self-defined family' (1998, p. 181) as a reality-based reflection of meaningful support. 'Not all relatives, but nevertheless forming a closely knit social network, with a focus upon mutual support and interest in each other' (Carpenter, 1998, p. 181). Although the family 'members' may not all be blood-related they do

'... carry out the functions traditionally associated with the patriarchal, blood-related family' (Carpenter, 1998, p. 181).

Perhaps equally perplexing as it is at times necessary is the tendency to broadly connote family in terms of characteristics rather than members. After all, it is the forms rather than the functions of family that have principally changed over time (Dahlstrom, 1989). For each person the classic roles of the nuclear family members such as parents, spouses and siblings may be enhanced or replaced by a variety of individuals who touch and support a life in significant ways at different points in development. Departures from more traditional ideas of caregiving and support become more likely when the life in question is influenced by the presence of one or more significant challenges. The need for functional and supportive family social structure is heightened when disability of a family member is present (Carpenter, 1998). Commensurate with this need there may be an increased probability of including supportive others, beyond blood relatives, who function as part of a self-defined family.

Researchers and those who use AAC appear to agree that the definition of family and distinction of family members must be determined by each person individually. This suggests that in order to identify, match or compare participants for family-related studies of AAC the person who uses AAC should (whenever possible) be consulted regarding who they consider to be a member of their family. Regardless of the operational obstacles research must overcome, families are the experts when it comes to identifying 'who' and 'what' they are. Investigators should accordingly avoid uninformed assumptions regarding family membership.

The task of family definition would be made much simpler if researchers could assume reciprocity on the part of all those identified as family 'members'. However, reciprocity in the perception of 'belonging' to a family group cannot be assumed, particularly in situations where the person with a disability has experienced impoverished support systems and contacts. In some situations the only regular contacts available for the person who uses AAC may be paid care providers. It has been suggested that paid and non-paid participants in the person's life be viewed differently when family and supports are defined. Some believe this distinction should be maintained regardless of the degree or quality of contact the employed person may have. It seems reasonable to assume that motivational factors would play a role in this concern. Certain motivations for involvement in the life of another, such as financial gain, duty or emotional connection, can be considered distinctively different from one another. However, in terms of relationships, human beings are rarely singularly motivated over time. Some individuals do form bonds above and beyond those expected between recipient and paid provider of service. Providers of care may leave their paid positions but continue supportive, connected relationships with the person who uses AAC. Some consumers of care provision ultimately marry a care provider. On the other hand, (for various reasons) blood-relatives and spouses may become paid service providers or care aides for family members with disabilities. It may therefore be premature to categorically exclude paid providers of service from a potential pool of defined family members. Role multiplicity among immediate and extended family members and paid providers of service offers an intriguing arena for study relative to people who rely on AAC. It suggests the need for further situational examination, review of additional research outside of the field of AAC and perhaps design of more role-sensitive data collection tools. Reciprocity in the concept of 'belonging' to a family may consequently prove to be an important aspect of defining family.

Research efforts must anticipate and include consideration of the range of family compositions before family issues may be studied in comprehensive ways. Attention to family composition will be particularly needed in studies requiring group assignments. On a micro level researchers must attend to family forms and functions when selecting or attempting to match participants/groups. On a macro level similar care must be exercised when comparing groups on the basis of family involvement.

How are families viewed?

In certain areas of family research, particularly those involving the process and effects of intervention, definition of and rationale for the family view/approach taken are important. Potential variables affecting the appropriateness and effectiveness of intervention may be more or less highlighted by the family view/approach from which the study has been designed and carried out. Equally important in understanding the relationship of the independent and dependent variables of the study would be the control of factors affecting the proposed approach (e.g. philosophy, practices and interaction styles of the implementers). Assuring that the research methodology and procedures are consistent with the family approach selected would assist other researchers in replicating a study so that objective comparisons of results may be made.

Since working with families attempting to integrate the use of AAC into daily life involves unique adaptations relative to the communicative histories of the interactive partners, the approach taken by a researcher or clinician could have significant influence on the findings obtained or adaptations made. Granlund, Björck-Åkesson and Carlhed (1999) have proposed distinctions of professional views and approaches to working with families and the related roles and tasks families are assigned accordingly (Table 21.1).

When families are viewed as decision-makers and service coordinators their roles and needs become central to team functions and programme development. Family-centred approaches are generally considered the most viable for working with families of children with disabilities (Angelo,

Table 21.1. Early intervention and the family system

Focus	Goal/objective	Intervention	Role assigned to family	Family task
The family as developmental/functional environment for the child with disabilities	The child with disabilities interacts optimally with persons within the immediate setting and has a 'rich environment'. Family has desired lifestyle	Stimulation outside home is provided, e.g. activity centre Parents are give advice, adapted toys etc. Supervision and interaction coaching	Providers of 'rich environments' Interaction partners	Stimulate child with disabilities Adapt environment to needs of child with disabilities
Family in crisis	Family has a normal family life cycle and 'accept' actual child, e.g. cope with grief reactions	Crisis therapy Respite care Redefine behaviour of child with disabilities	Patient Client	Solve/cope with emotional reactions 'Work on' perceptions of child with disabilities
Family as trainers	Optimal child development within specific area	Teach training programme Supervise parents	Student Trainer	Implement programme designed by professionals
Family as a needs entity	Decrease in perceived family needs	Assess needs Fulfil needs	Recipient of services	Identify needs Use available services
Family as decision-makers and/or service coordinators	Family is actively involved in and perceives control over the intervention process	Provide opportunities for involvement and control Teach problem-solving strategies	Decision-maker Service coordinator	Express needs Design goals and methods Select from service options Evaluate

From Granlund, Björck-Åkesson and Carlhed (1999).

Kokoska and Jones, 1996; Begun, 1996; Sweeney et al., 1998, Zuckerman and Brazelton, 1994). Educational guidelines in the United States attest to this 'best practice' conviction. Family-centred practices are closely aligned with the principles of empowerment and informed choice-making. Under different circumstances the roles of family members and service providers may necessarily change. However, preservation of family self-sufficiency and proactive planning by the family members may be plausibly linked to the family's decision-making capabilities and perspective of situational control. The positive effects of preserving the sense of control among family members using AAC has been demonstrated even in circumstances requiring short-term use of AAC (Costello, 1998).

In situations where service providers have exercised long-term authority and control of goal-setting and programme design, family members may feel anxious or disconnected. As the family's well-being is diminished other team members may judge the family to be passive and complacent or reactive and aggressive. Both are predictable responses to the loss of control. Once an unbalanced pattern of power has been established and practised team interactions become increasingly ineffective and/or strained (Dunst, Trivette and Deal, 1988; Trivette, Dunst and Deal, 1997). Ultimately, the person who uses AAC will lose opportunities and the potential for powerful support through the combined energies of family and providers of service. In order to effect transition smoothly from family-centred to person-centred planning the family and the family member who relies on AAC will need to become self-determined and empowered in an atmosphere of objectively offered options and informed choice-making (Bersani et al., 1998; Sweeney and Van Tatenhove, 1998; Wehmeyer, 1999).

Developing a framework for family research

In addition to attending to the definition of family and family-related approaches, a review of theoretical models of family functioning and involvement may assist investigators in research efforts. Non-linear and more dynamic-based theories of human development, interactions and system functioning (including family systems) have gained growing attention in the past decade (Fogel and Thelen, 1987; Smith and Thelen, 1993; Vasta, 1992). Theories of ecology (Brofenbrenner, 1979, 1992) and chaos (Gleick, 1987; Guess and Sailor, 1993) are of particular interest in the study of families that include a person with disabilities.

For studies of family involvement in AAC, Björck-Åkesson (in Sweeney, Björck-Åkesson and Granlund, 1998) pointed out that there is a need for a theoretical framework that 'encompasses different aspects of family involvement' and that this framework should 'deal with the complexity and dynamics' of AAC use and family functions. Because such a framework has not been comprehensively established or agreed upon in relation to investigation of family issues in AAC, one might consider work in this area to be in the 'first tier' stage of development (Sweeney, Björck-Åkesson and Granlund, 1998). Björck-Åkesson (Sweeney, Björck-Åkesson and Granlund, 1998) with additions from Sweeney (present text) proposed a set of theoretical frameworks and models which may be useful in describing aspects of family involvement in AAC (Table 21.2).

Table 21.2. Applying theoretical frameworks to encompass aspects of family involvement in AAC

Model	Authors
Systems theoretical model	Bertalanffy (1968), Fogel and Thelen (1987), Smith and Thelen (1993)
Ecological systems theory	Bronfenbrenner (1992),
Transactional theory	Sameroff and Fiese (1990)
Philosophy of intervention Perspective of intervention	Dunst (1990), Bailey and Simeonsson (1984, 1988)
Social cognitive theory	Bandura (1992)
Ethological and relationships approaches Helplessness theory	Hinde (1992) Seligman (1992)
Behavioural theory	Bijou (1992)
Model of human occupations (MOHO)	Kielhofner (1995)
Empowerment	Rappaport (1987), Dunst et al. (1988)
Theory of communication action	Habermas (1984)
Ecocultural theory	Tharp and Gallimore (1989), Bernstein (1971, 1973)
Self-determination	Wehmeyer et al. (1998)
Chaos theory	Gleick (1987), Guess and Sailor (1993)

Theoretical frameworks encompassing different aspects of family involvement, complexity and dynamics (adapted from Björck-Åkesson, 1998 with additions by Sweeney, 1998).

Several of these theories share common properties of focus, with discrete differences. Each provides the researcher of family issues in AAC with different degrees of dynamic perspective from which to develop research questions and select variables for investigation. Much of research and practice in AAC up to this point has focused upon dyadic relationships and individual perspectives. Cochran and Woolever (1983) noted that family research has also tended to be focused at the micro-level. Evolving applications of systems and transactional theories place greater emphasis upon multilevel interactions and the dynamic dimensions of family and individual development. When addressing family issues in AAC it no longer seems sufficient solely to study discrete interactions, individual opinions or unilateral effects. Rather, the concept of the family as a 'system' invites investigators to address the multilevel, multidirectional and interrelated nature of family perspectives and functions. In doing so consideration should be afforded to the effects of the person who uses AAC on the family system as well as the effects the family and societal systems have on the AAC user.

In the ecological view Bronfenbrenner (1979) described an interconnected layering of environmental systems which operate at four levels of proximal to distal relationship to an individual (e.g. micro-, meso-, exo- and macro-systems). These systems might be viewed as concentric circles (e.g. Berger and Thompson, 1996, p. 5) with the individual and micro-system (e.g. activities and relationships at home, school, etc.) at the centre and the macro-system (e.g. characteristics of a society, culture, etc.) in a more distal but over-arching relationship to all other systems. The meso- and exo-systems described components and connections within and between the other systems that could affect the developing person. Bronfenbrenner's conceptualization has served as both a model for human development and a framework from which to study human dynamics. In a more recent chapter Bronfenbrenner (1992) took himself to task for overlooking certain important individual variables and characteristics (e.g. temperament, beliefs, life course options, etc.) in his original model. In revising the original system definitions, and his own view, Bronfenbrenner advised future researchers '.... apply the mighty process-person-context model – perhaps even with a timely chronosystem component – and a rich research reward is sure to come' (p. 241). Such advice seems particularly wise in relation to family-based AAC research. The researcher has only to consider the multitude of typically benign environmental variables, such as the weather (e.g. bright sunlight on a dynamic display), that might affect AAC interactions in order to understand the importance of examining interactions within and between environmental systems as well as individuals and contexts.

Further insights are sure to be gained from integration of empowerment and self-determination perspectives in the construction of programme and research design (Bryen, Slesaransky and Baker, 1995; Schlosser, 1996; Sweeney, 1993; Wehmeyer, 1999). The importance of both theories is echoed in the comments of people who use AAC and their families, and in other portions of the present text.

The confines of this particular chapter do not allow for individual review of each of the models and theories represented (Table 21.2). The reader is directed to the references provided above for further exploration of these perspectives and related applications. Perhaps future studies with families who use AAC will lead to the development of new theoretical models or special adaptations to existing ones in order to depict the AAC experience more comprehensively.

Core learnings: establishing lessons from the field

'Core learnings' are statements that are used to encompass a current and global knowledge base in a specific area/field of study. They are in essence 'lessons from the field'. The 'learnings' are taken from both research-based and practical wisdom in an effort to improve understanding and bring organization and priority to empirical study and practice-based goal setting. Following a review of current information, including extensive input from families and those who use AAC, these core learnings are offered for consideration. There are several additional points for inclusion, review, and further study related to each core learning. Some related points of interest are summarized in the core learnings introduced in the following text. It is hoped that by illuminating the wisdom of the present, the direction and priorities for architecture of future family research in AAC will be made more clear.

Proposed core learnings

1. Families want their members to communicate effectively

Regardless of their current level of family involvement in AAC development/application, the majority of families repeatedly indicate their desire for a family member to be an independent communicator. Research and practice have shown that some of the care and helping routines of significant others may enhance communication development while others may inadvertently thwart the development of more independent communication and/or acceptance of AAC (Basil, 1992; Hjelmquist and Sandberg, 1996; Sweeney, 1989 ; Sweeney et al., 1998; von Tetzchner and Martinsen, 1996). In the busy schedule of the day families often report that it is simply easier to communicate for their family member or make use of their special skills in interpreting less symbolic message forms rather than arrange or wait for the use of an augmentative system. As use of highly individualized interpretive strategies continues, it becomes increasingly apparent to family members that the person attempting to use AAC may have a very limited number of regular communication partners or have difficulty generalizing skills outside of the family setting (Sweeney, 1992, 1996). Families need acceptable alternatives for fostering communication independence that they may choose from as routines, time and lifestyles allow (Björck-Åkesson, Granlund and Olsson, 1996; Granlund and Björck-Åkesson, 1996). It is only in a relatively small number of cases (typically abusive situations) that barriers are purposefully used among family members to limit communication in significant ways. In the majority of families there is not only the goal of effective communication but a sincere willingness to take steps to achieve this goal if those steps are family sensitive, practical and meaningful.

The incorporation of AAC involves changes in the family's interaction patterns (Hjelmquist and Sandberg, 1996; Light, Collier and Parnes,

1995a,b; Parette, 1994). If these changes cannot be readily accommodated complications may arise. For example, in the absence of more symbolic forms, an individual may begin to use challenging behaviours as a communication form. Others may redirect the positive communication functions of intent and initiation because the message form itself is unacceptable. Helping families to uncover and address the links between communication and behaviour represents a necessary step in establishing more effective interaction. Mirenda (1997) and others have indicated that an AAC system needs to be more effective in obtaining communicative outcomes than challenging behaviour in order for the communication system to be embraced.

> If desire, usefulness and need are not apparent or if the chosen AAC method is not considered at least as effective as already established forms of communicating, the likelihood of acceptance is decreased (Sweeney, 1998, p. 222).

The author (Sweeney, 1996) established a proportional relationship whereby as 'surrogate communicating' (Sweeney, 1989) and message formulation/initiation by others increased, apparent interest in and use of AAC by the individual decreased. A resulting assumption by onlookers in such situations may be that the potential AAC user is unable or unwilling to communicate differently. Patterns of helplessness may ultimately develop (Basil, 1992; Sweeney, 1989, 1992).

Future research must strive to identify programme approaches and strategies that help families to realize the goal of effective communication with those who use AAC. Sensitivity to family needs and priorities, establishing partnerships and the timing of information gathering and instruction figure prominently into a formula for success. Compilation of the range of approaches and strategies already naturally developed and effectively used by families may represent a logical first step.

2. Families function better under conditions of mutual understanding and positive interdependency

There is abundant literature from the fields of psychology, counselling, social work, human development, and communication to substantiate the role of mutual understanding in dyadic and group functioning (Berger and Thompson, 1996). Mutual understanding and good communication among family members may seem like an idealistic expectation. Some current self-help literature disputes the existence of 'functional' or truly 'healthy' families altogether. The dynamic and ever-changing nature of families makes it difficult to measure or even define their functionality. Families regularly strive to accommodate new members and situations and all of the joys and crises that go along with them. In the process of change and the presence of stressors family member roles fluctuate and reorganize in order to attempt to re-establish the sense of 'homeostasis' no matter how fleeting or atypical that status may seem to an outside observer. The family that appears chaotic today may transform to stability tomorrow.

Despite their ever-changing nature, it is difficult to dispute the positive impact of respect, understanding, good listening behaviour, appropriate discipline and healthy boundaries within family units (Berger and Thompson, 1996). Although culturally, generationally and individually influenced, these characteristics within and between family members contribute significantly to stability and positive interactions of the family as a whole.

Many successful adults who use AAC reflect on the most valuable lessons and opportunities from their childhood years. Stories repeatedly note the importance of 'being allowed to make mistakes', 'learn consequences for actions', 'being allowed to make choices', 'having independence valued', 'being included as others are', and 'finding communication forms early in life', etc. Early identification and provision of acceptable communication modes and opportunities for participation and decision-making are frequently cited as personal growth factors (Millen, 1996). The retrospective voices of long-term users of AAC have revealed that often one family member (most frequently the mother) is identified as the principal teacher/provider of opportunities. At times opportunities are missed because all of the family members do not fully perceive the abilities and interests of the family member who uses AAC. It is not uncommon for individual family members (and service providers) to have different perceptions, fears and aspirations for the person who uses AAC. Future goal setting and life planning practices provided for non-disabled family members may be delayed or overlooked for the person who uses AAC if more immediate barriers and crises are not resolved. Through the myriad of scenarios, the greater the individual's ability to be interactive with all family members the greater the likelihood of mutual understanding and complementary goal setting.

Angelo, Jones and Kokoska (1995) and Angelo, Kokoska and Jones (1996) have identified some of the AAC-related priorities of mothers and fathers. Their study of families of adolescent and adult users of AAC (Angelo, Kokoska and Jones, 1996) showed that the fathers surveyed placed a focus on the technical aspects of device operation and maintenance. Mothers on the other hand ranked needs for social and community integration as higher priorities. Both mothers and fathers placed emphasis on 'planning for future communication needs' (p. 18). It is interesting to note that integrating the use of assistive devices at home was a high ranking priority for fathers but did not appear among the most significant needs of mothers.

Given more typical caregiver roles, it is not surprising that the majority of literature on families that include a member with disabilities has focused on the role, perspective and actions of the mother. In most societies and culture groups it is the mother who will assume primary responsibility for care provision and teaching. Research regarding the different communication patterns of mothers, fathers and siblings relative to the person who uses AAC is extremely limited. While it is clearly important to maintain a holistic view of the family system, many valuable lessons stand to be gained from information gathering relative to the other family members, in addition to the mother.

McConkey (1994) has identified the father as the hard-to-reach member of the family. Carpenter and Herbert (1994) concluded that fathers sometimes viewed themselves as the 'peripheral parent' and provided insights to encourage future work with fathers (Carpenter and Herbert, 1997). In clinical situations fathers frequently lament over their limited ability to communicate with their child who is experiencing communication challenges. In one review of communication experiences of fathers over 60% of those interviewed indicated that they had poor to no communication with the child who used AAC (Sweeney, 1998). These same fathers rated communication between the mother and child as 'good'.

Among siblings there is often a reported pattern of the oldest child or the one closest in age to the child who uses AAC acting as a mentor or interpreter for their sibling in much the same way as interpreting is accomplished with a primary caregiver (typically a mother). Studies with families that include both deaf and hearing children of deaf parents reveal similar patterns of interpreting and more adult responsibilities on the part of the oldest hearing sibling who also knows sign language. Padden (1983) noted that the patterns of interpreting and establishing contacts on behalf of other family members may place hearing children of deaf parents in demanding roles and that these children may continue in such roles once they are adults. Similar studies of the varied roles and related expectations of siblings of those who use AAC do not currently exist. Review of the literature regarding sign language use and interpretation within families with deaf and hearing members may yield a situationally analogous backdrop for framing similar work in AAC.

Grandparents may function as supports or sources of stress for the parents of a child with special challenges (Seligman, 1991; Mirfin-Veitch, Bray and Watson, 1996; Mirfin-Veitch and Bray, 1997, pp. 76–77). Whether or not a grandparent is able to come to terms of acceptance of a child's disability seems to be a critical factor related to these potential and dichotomous roles. Since in many sociocultural groups grandparents are becoming more vital and regular child-rearing and family supports, increased attention to the role/s of grandparents in AAC development and use is warranted. Mirfin-Veitch and Bray (1997, p. 78) note that comprehensive identification of positive support attributes and parent-accepted support practices among grandparents has not yet been accomplished.

When all family members are able to communicate with each other, mutual understanding is possible and the person who uses AAC will have enhanced opportunities for learning and personal growth. By sharing communication responsibility each family member has a greater chance for positive experiences using AAC. Supporting families in this process and determining which types of support are needed/available requires that the clinician or researcher remain aware and sensitive to the roles various family members assume in relation to the family member who uses AAC and the level of understanding present (cf. Hjelmquist and Sandberg, 1996).

3. Each family has unique circumstances, perceptions, stressors and supports that impact communication development/recovery

Genograms and in particular ecograms or maps are helpful tools for identifying family stressors and supports. Ecograms completed for families of AAC users frequently show that one or more family members are so overwhelmed by the agency, financial and therapeutic demands related to the communicatively challenged family member that the entire family is ultimately challenged. Though all ecograms/maps are highly individual, a reasonable example was previously described by the author (see Sweeney, 1997) and is depicted in Figure 21.1.

The mother who completed this ecomap identified only one constant support in her life, the maternal grandmother. Although others were concerned, their own stressors, obligations and needs kept them from offering reliable support. The father's work schedule and income were also irregular and this further jeopardized the parental relationship. A range of unhealthy family secrets (including blaming the mother for her child's birth-related disability) on the husband's side of the family kept relationships with them strained. The mother had given up her part-time job and all other contacts that offered an outlet from her stress.

> .... the mother routinely made at least 12 agency contacts per week in order to secure funds, therapy, and other services for her child who needed AAC. Her time spent filling out forms, making phone calls, transporting her disabled child to school and services and meeting with doctors and professionals meant that she had little time or energy left to address the needs of her other children, have a relationship with her husband or any type of personal life ... Her other children were having problems in school ... Despite her heroic efforts she perceived herself as a 'bad mother'... (Sweeney, 1996, p. 227).

It is not surprising that under such circumstances families lack the time and energy to provide AAC experiences in the home and community. When AAC presents a burden to the family it will be viewed as a burden by the person who is expected to use it (Sweeney, 1996, 1998). Angelo (in Scott, 1998) indicated that approximately 50% of the families in a statewide survey reported that use of AAC did not fit well into their family

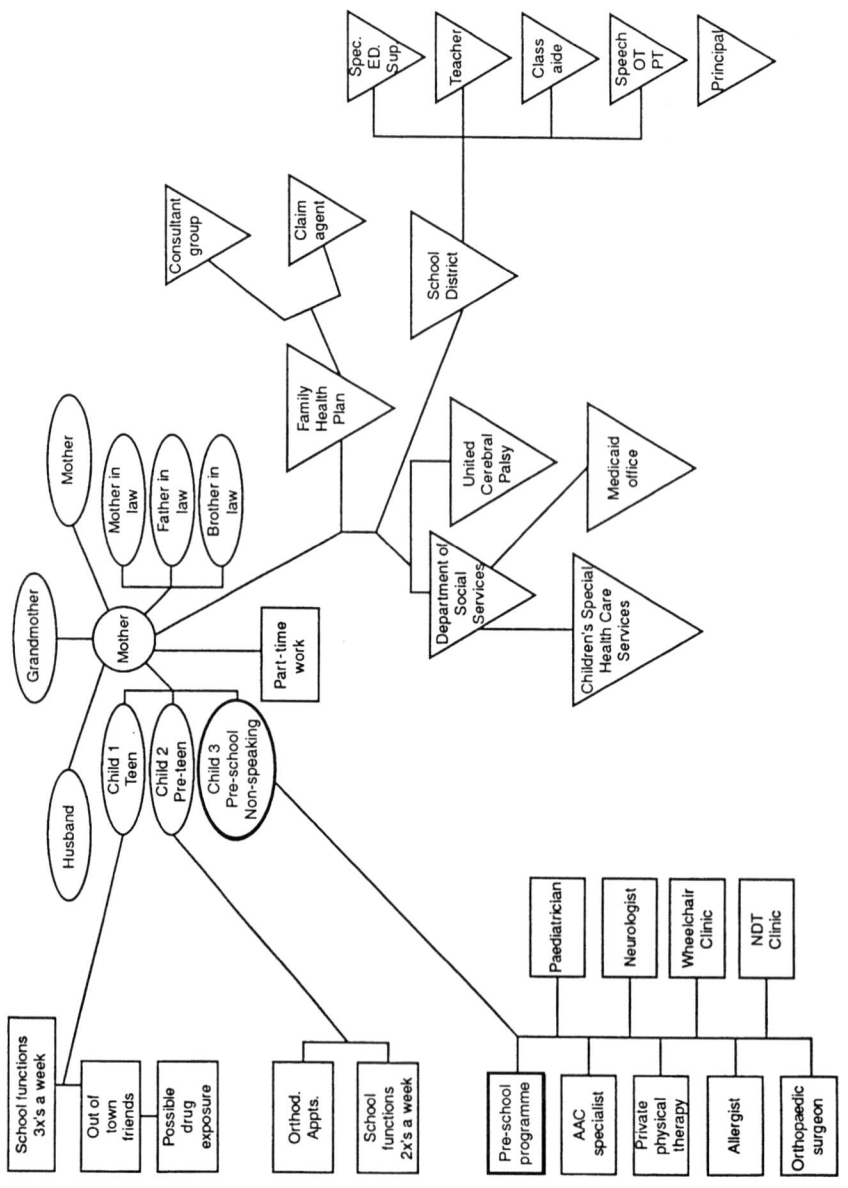

Figure 21.1. Practical ecomap for mother of a child who could potentially use AAC.

lifestyle (p. 8). At various points in time families may have medical and emotional concerns that outweigh or even contraindicate the importance of applying new communication strategies. Equally important, and as previously noted, each family will have different support composition and intensity both in terms of the number of family members who provide support as well as the roles they can and do fulfil. Whether or not families choose to explore and/or share the details of their stressors and supports, service providers must approach family members with the understanding that only they know what is possible and reasonable in their family life. More studies are needed in order to identify common stressors, supports and system effects in families where an adult or child uses AAC. Working in partnership, researchers need to examine what works for families under different circumstances and how stressors may be reduced through use of supports and service integration (Dunst, 1997).

If the family does not perceive a need, a programme cannot be fully effective. Sweeney and Engwis (1996) found that perceptions of skills and needs varied significantly between family members and professionals in AAC assessments. Clinical and research reports suggest that family members may actually feel more satisfied/less stress (at least for defined periods of time) when they are more passive in their approach to communication change (Granlund, 1998, personal communication). When family members use all of their skills to adapt to (rather than change the course of) a communication problem on a regular basis they may lose sight of how dependent the family member is for help with communication/interpretation.

4. Each family has unique cultural, inherited and developed beliefs and practices that should not be imposed upon in the intervention process

The beliefs and practices of families will determine which types of communication tools or strategies will be acceptable (Angelo, 1998; Parette, VanBiervliet and Huer, 1998). To truly be a part of cultural and familial rituals and routines one's assistive technology and strategies must fit into those rituals and routines. If the family interacts sitting on the floor, an AAC strategy must be available and accessible in this situation. If a prayer is to be sung in a native language, the voice output system should accommodate this. If the family's religious beliefs reject the use of technology, a non-tech system should be explored. It is a matter of listening to and learning from families. Families do not need to explain or justify their beliefs and practices. Support persons just need to understand what is important to families and assist them in finding ways to meet their needs.

Zuckerman and Brazelton (1994) provide several examples of how understanding of a cultural viewpoint or parental interpretation could impact on a professional's information sharing and recommendation development with families. The authors give examples of Hispanic,

African-American and Haitian parental interpretations of child behaviour/motivations and their related approaches to problem solving which appeared culturally specific. In each situation the failure or success of the service providers involved could be viewed as largely dependent upon their ability to relate to these culture-based beliefs.

Comparative language studies show that communication content and styles that may be admired in one culture/language are less valued or considered inappropriate in another. For example, in working with various Native People of North America the author has learned that some forms of eye contact are not considered acceptable. While considered inappropriate by the Native cultural group these same behaviours would be considered appropriate evidence of good listening and interest among the caucasian, non-native members of the same geographic area. The length and frequency of expected comments, types of information sharing and other communication related factors also vary greatly across different groups and individual families. Understanding all of these factors within a particular culture group is important for conducting appropriate assessments and building partnerships with families. Equally important is the avoidance of over-generalization and stereotyping of members within a cultural group. Garcia (1994) has suggested a helpful distinction between a 'culture group' (p. 254) and an 'individual-oriented culture' (p. 254). He described the latter as:

> ... the person's own participation in and practice and understanding of the traits of the culture. As an individual, the person can follow, reinvent, or ignore practices passed along by other members (p. 254).

Matching the needs of the person and their sociocultural group with the appropriate AAC forms, devices and strategies is a complicated and delicate task. Arnott (1990, 1997) proposed a device design that is sensitive to and adaptable for particular individual *and family* needs.

5. The development of independence potential, autonomy and relationships are of critical importance in the life of a person who uses AAC

Deci (1975) identified competence and self-determination (i.e. autonomy) as principal psychological needs that relate to 'intrinsically motivated' activity. Goal oriented actions that are achieved principally through the directives of others are not likely to share the same properties or levels of personal motivation and satisfaction as actions that are self-determined. In psychological terms, 'relatedness' with others provides an additional intrinsic motivator that is not only crucial for optimal development (Bowlby, 1988) but for energizing '... interpersonal explorations and interactions ...' (Ryan, Deci and Grolnick, 1995, p. 620). Accordingly, people who use AAC must experience competence in the use of their communication systems, opportunities for autonomous actions and independent access to avenues for building relationships with others. These important components of psychological development and self-directed behaviour are viewed as relevant across the life-span transitions of AAC users (Bersani et al., 1998; Sweeney and Van Tatenhove, 1998; Wehmeyer and Schwartz, 1997).

Interviews with successful adult AAC users are helpful in realizing the importance of independence, autonomy and the development of relationships. When asked to rank the importance of various abilities/life factors such as mobility, ambulation, vocation, communication, etc., relationships and communication are often at the top of the list of adults who use AAC. Of course, several of the stated factors are interrelated but the perceived importance of relationships is undeniable. Engwis and Sweeney (1997) found that despite considerable life-long medical needs and severely restricted mobility and communication, one middle-aged adult awaiting provision of augmentative communication in a skilled nursing facility ranked having relationships with others above all else (including AAC) in importance.

In another example, a non-speaking man who had been on life-support equipment for over a decade promptly and inexplicably (from the medical perspective) died when the only person he had a relationship with, his long-term roommate who regularly talked to him, was transferred from the health care facility where they both resided. Countless other examples of the effects of transfer trauma and loss of relationships demonstrate the ultimate life-enhancing and indeed potentially life-sustaining importance of relationships. Providing the life opportunities and communication skills for developing and nurturing relationships can open the potential for leading a self-determined and rich life. A desirable outcome for anyone.

6. The use of AAC does not exclude use of more traditional or uniquely individualized communication forms

At the 1996 ISAAC Research Symposium on AAC a key topic of discussion among family researchers (Sweeney, 1997) was related to the information families receive from professionals and the impact this information has on the family. Those present provided evidence that many service providers give false prognostic messages or appear to delay provision of communication alternatives. Many families are left to believe that if they just wait long enough their child or adult family member will talk. Some are also told that if they use an augmentative communication system it will negate the potential for speech development. It is difficult to believe that after two decades of advancements in the field of AAC the service network still struggles with a misinformation problem of this significance. Representing AAC as a 'last resort' is surely a disservice to a child or adult attempting to develop or regain communication and their family members who wish to make appropriate intervention choices.

People who use AAC and their family members have the right to make informed choices based upon objective input from service providers. They have the right to continue to work on oral speech development, whether or not they use a voice output communication device, and they have the right to literacy education and access. To truly *serve* individual and family consumers, professionals need to objectively present available intervention alternatives, provide well-founded prognostic information and temper their own convictions regarding an advised course of action with respect for the choices of those who will ultimately be most affected by the outcomes related to the choices made.

Family members also need to have their unique forms of communicating respected. The addition of symbolic and/or technology-based communication forms does not require the family to abandon attention to other (often more efficient) forms they have grown accustomed to using. Rather, an emphasis should be placed upon providing the person with a range of communication tools and strategies that will allow them to interact effectively with a range of partners in different ways. As long as idiosyncratic forms of communicating are not the sole methods attended to, they are not likely to preclude communication growth (Sweeney, 1996). Many of the message intentions underlying idiosyncratic communication forms may become the inspiration for future transfer to more symbolic/technology supported modes. The current knowledge base on working with families indicates that suggestions for altering family patterns of communicating are best accomplished in a family-centred process where the family members help to identify the problems and possible solutions and feel in control of the decision-making (Björck-Åkesson, Granlund and Olsson, 1996; Sweeney, 1996; Sweeney and Van Tatenhove, 1998).

7. Families are more engaged and effective in supporting communication efforts when their knowledge is valued and they are included in programme development

The relevance of including families and other communication partners in the programme planning and intervention process has been established by many researchers and service providers (Angeloa, Kokoska and Jones, 1996; Basil, 1994; Björck-Åkesson, Granlund and Olsson, 1996; Dunst, 1990; Dunst et al., 1991, 1997; Heim and Jonker, 1996; Johansson, 1988; Jonker and Heim, 1994; Light, Collier and Parnes, 1985a,b; Paget, 1992; Sweeney, 1992, 1996). Goals that are unilaterally designed by professional members of an intervention team may not prove to be meaningful or productive for the person using AAC and their significant others. Björck-Åkesson, Granlund and Olsson (1996) point out that despite the importance of including the person with disability and their significant others in development of a functional intervention plan, most are not given this opportunity (p. 326). It is more typical for professionals to provide a plan and ask for agreement/compliance.

Björck-Åkesson, Granlund and Olsson (1996) describe an intervention model based on empowerment, collaborative problem solving and real-life desired outcomes which makes use of individual and family knowledge and goals. Principles from this type family-centred model and additional methods designed by the author (Sweeney, 1992, 1996) were applied with 10 families struggling to achieve communication change over a significant period of time. Following application of family-centred problem-solving with the family, the individual using AAC and other team members, each family reported at least one significant change within less than a two month period of time. Eight of the 10 families reported multiple significant and positive changes in communication/related areas within two weeks to one month. Some of these changes were dramatic. Family members expressed amazement and relief in discovering that communication goals could be met so easily. Where multiple other approaches had been limited in producing change, an approach focused upon family priorities and lifestyle considerations produced immediate, positive results.

8. Communication needs and forms may differ within and outside of the family, under various conditions, with different partners and across stages of life development

Alm and Newell (1996) note that 'A person's very concept of self is bound up with their social persona which is projected out to the world through each day, through interacting with a wide variety of people' (p. 174). They stressed the importance of the AAC user learning to manage everyday interactions outside of the security and patience of family and close friends. Community-based assistive device use is a frequently reported problem and need (Allaire et al., 1991; Culp et al., 1986; Scherer, 1993). While those most familiar with and invested in the life of the person who uses AAC may have developed extensive partner skills, the majority of people in the community at large have not. The same techniques that work beautifully at home may fail miserably with less familiar or less invested communication partners.

Instructional programmes for AAC development are often written from the perspective of a single service provider, based on a limited number of environments or partners. This may prove effective early in the development of AAC. However, unilateral or environmentally sparse forms of assessment and intervention may fail to incorporate important information for understanding and expanding existing skills. Several members of the service community are expanding use of environmentally sensitive data collection instruments that strive to identify tangible supports for augmentative communication use (e.g. Sweeney, 1988; Gamradt, 1998).

The author has observed several situations where school- and home-based team members were not aware of various message forms or modes used in the different environments. For example, in one assessment interview where school-based team members were identifying communication barriers they explained a situation in the lunchroom where the non-speaking child was responded to with time-out or redirective intervention for 'self-stimulatory behaviours' that were interfering with mealtime choices and the feeding routine. The extended finger hand-waving of the child was viewed as an 'undesirable' departure from the tasks at hand and 'autistic-like' in nature. The child's mother quickly pointed out that the hand motions in question had been used mutually by herself and her child for years as an indication for eating pudding. This unique gesture arose partly out of the mother's perception of her child's motor capabilities and partly from the fact that the pudding cups she used contained 10 spoonfuls, one for each finger of the waving hands. Had a more careful inventory of communicative modes, messages and functions been taken across environments and partners this child's persistent communicative attempt might well have been expanded upon and successfully integrated rather than redirected and discouraged. The well-intentioned and highly invested service team had regretfully missed an important opportunity to reinforce and refine communication skill due to their more contained focus in relation to communication contexts, modes and behaviours.

In early intervention, interviews with significant others and attention to unique or partner-specific communication forms are important for both economy and degree of success in programme development. The importance of identifying, preserving and refining existing communication skills has been emphasized (Sweeney, 1992, 1996; Sweeney and Van Tatenhove, 1998; Granlund and Björck-Åkesson, 1996). As the communication situations, partners and demands of life increase, the person who uses AAC and family members need to develop additional strategies. The sooner the person who uses AAC is supported in the development of a menu of workable interaction strategies and equipped with the knowledge of when and with whom to use them, the less likely there will be motivational drain in different communication situations or reluctance to engage new partners.

A review of interview information from hundreds of families seeking AAC assistance for a developmentally disabled child shows that there are trends in perceived needs or in some cases a sense of communication crisis as the potential AAC user approximates the ages of 4, 8, 16 and 21 years of age (Sweeney, 1998). Is this trend coincidental, or can it be substantiated by the experiences of other families, researchers and clinicians? It is interesting to note that within the range of a year or so, these ages represent turning points in the development of all children, youth and young adults. When faced with these stages of development, do families more keenly sense the differences and impending loss of opportunities for their children who communicate in unique ways? It has been suggested that departures from expected developmental milestones may reignite the sense of grief among family members (Birenbaum, 1971). In their review of the Model of Human Occupation, Henry and Coster (1997) make reference to several studies highlighting the changing influences on and perceptions of competency from childhood to adulthood. Review of the available information from both individual and family system perspectives may be helpful in identifying critical junctures for developing supports with families.

9. Development of AAC is a multilayered and ongoing process affected by significant others. Family, friends and neighbours are the most constant significant others

For many people who use AAC their most frequent and competent communication partners are one or more of their therapists or teachers. Therapists and teachers will come and go from the individual AAC user's life and therefore do not represent the most constant/available partners across the life span. Rather, family, friends and neighbours represent the most available and potentially long-lasting communication contacts.

Children between the ages of 8 and 12 years who used AAC or communicated primarily with severely dysarthric speech were interviewed regarding available communication partners. In the majority of cases they identified less than seven people who 'understood' them (Sweeney, 1992, 1997). These people were typically one or both parents, a grandparent or aunt, teachers and therapists at school or a clinic, and sometimes a sibling or friend. The children demonstrated a significant partner deprivation compared with other children their age, who typically had 40 or more regular communication partners and no trouble gaining new ones. None of the children indicated that all family members understood their communication attempts. Few of them indicated more than one neighbour or peer who regularly and successfully interacted with them.

Fostering peer relationships is a current area of interest in the field of AAC. There is a growing recognition that modelling and having role models may be of significant importance for the developing person using AAC. There is a definite need for more research to delineate the important factors in the social layer of the multilayered process of AAC development.

10. The most meaningful outcomes for the individual who uses AAC and his or her family members are those that transfer to home and community and last beyond individual instruction

Because life circumstances and the availability of communication partners are always in flux, people who use AAC need communication tools and strategies that will empower them beyond the classroom, clinic, day programme and individual service providers (Bryen, Slezaransky and Baker, 1995; Sweeney and Van Tatenhove, 1998). A focus on additional research to identify meaningful outcomes from the perspective of long-term AAC users, how families contribute to self-determination, and how service providers can support skills that have life-long value, will have tremendous impact on the development and success of AAC practices (Granlund, Blackstone, and Norris, 1997; Schlosser, 1996).

Identification of desirable outcomes for people who use AAC and their families can help direct the development of future research questions and studies which will have the most practical applications in daily life. A set of individual and family oriented outcomes have been suggested based on input from people who use AAC, their families and those contributing to family research and practice (Sweeney, Björck-Åkesson and Granlund, 1998; Sweeney and Van Tatenhove, 1998). Each of the following may be associated with one or more of the ecosystem designations from Bronfenbrenner's model (1992). Of the outcomes listed, 'life planning' and 'enhanced/supported family accommodations' appear to involve all levels of the ecosystem. Perhaps for this reason they should be afforded increased attention in future research and practice.

Desirable outcomes for individuals who use AAC

1. Empowerment
2. Development of relationships
3. Language-based AAC systems and literacy
4. Use of AAC to participate: school, employment, advocacy, life plan, etc.
5. Self-advocacy/determination
6. Life planning

Desirable outcomes for families of AAC users

1. Enhanced/supported family accommodations
2. Maintenance of self-esteem
3. Respected priorities and decisions (support what is needed)
4. Meaningful/functional interactions among family members

Members at the 1998 ISAAC Research Symposium, many of them family members of people who use AAC, indicated that a crucial question is 'How does AAC affect families and what are the costs?' Partnership with families in the process of designing programmes and research offers the best opportunities for answering this and related questions.

Core learnings provide a palate for both reflection and projection of research and practical needs based upon an existing focus and knowledge base. As a first attempt to identify the family-related lessons from the field the aforementioned points are sure to undergo revisions in time. However, even in this developing form they may facilitate directions for research and practice that ultimately link with desired outcomes for people who use AAC and their families.

Summary

Human service fields are moving from single cause/source perspectives to dynamic system perspectives, from clinically controlled to family and individual-centred models of service and from discrete skills-based to outcome-based design and measurement of programme effectiveness. These paradigm shifts hold great promise for people who use AAC and their families. As families and individual AAC users become more active in defining their services and planning their futures, many changes in prevalent modes of service study and practice will be required. Assuring that research and programme development in AAC follows these trends will require much of those who study and work with families. Researchers must draw insight from the extensive base of current information on human development theory, family function and family service models in light of the significance of rearing a child or living with an adult who has unique communicative modes and experiences. They must be ever vigilant regarding definition of the family itself as well as the theoretical, philosophical and service models which have direct and dynamic influence on research design and findings. Merging these perspectives and guidelines with core learnings and desired outcomes from AAC will serve to strengthen future project design. Ideally, future researchers will propose questions resulting in answers that will provide the most valuable information for serving people who use AAC and their family members.

Service providers will benefit from careful review of the philosophy and approach of their current service systems. Many administratively stated service philosophies and proposed practices are inconsistent with what truly occurs in day-to-day service delivery. When the structure and operation of a service system does not support its philosophical model the chances for effective outcomes are radically diminished. Similarly, when the philosophical model is outdated or incompatible with knowledge of 'best practice', team members will be unable to fully invest their knowledge and efforts. Models of operation that emphasize single causal agents, singular sources of support or disintegrated resources cannot effectively address the multiplicity of needs of a person who uses AAC or their family. The result of such approaches may be a significant drain on all of the people and other resources (material, financial, community, etc.) involved for little meaningful communicative or life change. Situational changes in circumstances for a family may suggest at least temporary shifts in approaches. In family- and person-centred approaches service providers (and the systems they function in) must be willing and able to share and/or 'give up' power and control of many facets of programming to the consumers of service. Empowerment for people who use AAC and their family members does not necessarily equate to an easier service process but it does bring hope for a more effective one with life-long and self-determined results.

Acknowledgement

The author wishes to recognize, with gratitude, the contributions of Eva Björck-Åkesson and Mats Granlund.

Section VI
Consumer Issues and AAC

Chapter 22
An Introduction to Consumer Perspectives in AAC Research: Approaches, Techniques and their Theoretical Underpinnings

RALF W. SCHLOSSER

Consumer perspectives in research have only recently entered the methodological debate in augmentative and alternative communication (AAC). In fact, the 1998 ISAAC Research Symposium held in Dublin represented only the second Research Symposium with a strand on this issue, entitled 'Methods and strategies for assessing the perspectives of consumers in AAC research'. To introduce the three papers that emerged from the 1998 strand, this chapter aims (a) to present the theoretical underpinnings of various approaches to the study/involvement of consumer perspectives, and (b) to discuss how these theoretical underpinnings may inform some of the methodological debates raised in these and earlier papers.

Researchers' theoretical orientations have implications for every decision made in the research process, including the choice of method and techniques (Mertens, 1998). To date, the following *approaches* for assessing consumer perspectives and/or involving consumers throughout the research process in AAC have been discussed at the Symposia: (a) social validation (Schlosser, 1997b; in press), (b) participatory action research (PAR) (Balandin and Raghavendra, Chapter 23, this volume; Bersani, Chapter 24, this volume; Krogh, 1997), and (c) emancipatory research (Balandin and Raghavendra, this volume). In addition, focus groups (Huer and Parette, Chapter 25, this volume) and questionnaires (O'Keefe et al., 1997) have been discussed as two specific *techniques*.

Theoretical paradigms

These approaches and techniques are associated with different theoretical paradigms (see below). In order to understand a specific paradigm and discuss its implications for assessing consumer perspectives or including consumers in the research process it is helpful to ask three paradigm-defining questions phrased by Guba and Lincoln (1994) as adapted by Mertens (1998). The ontological question asks, 'what is the nature of reality?' The epistemological question asks, 'what is the nature of knowledge and the relationship between the knower and the would-be-known?' And, the methodological question asks, 'how can the knower go about obtaining the desired knowledge and understandings?'

The *positivist/postpositivist paradigm* accepts that there is one reality, which is knowable within probability in the case of group studies, or knowable through observable and reliable differences between baseline and intervention in the case of single-subject experiments. Objectivity is important – the researcher manipulates and observes in a dispassionate, objective manner. The methodology is primarily quantitative, interventionist, and decontextualized.

The *interpretive/constructivist paradigm* is situated within multiple, socially constructed realities. There is an interactive link between researchers and participants; the values are made explicit and the findings are thought of as created by an interaction between researchers and participants. The methodology is primarily qualitative; hermeneutical or dialectical; contextual factors are described.

The *emancipatory paradigm* acknowledges multiple realities shaped by social, political, cultural, economic, ethnic, gender and disability values. There is an interactive link between researchers and participants; and, knowledge is socially and historically situated. In the following section, each of these approaches along with the focus group technique shall be examined as to their best fit with these three theoretical underpinnings.

Approaches, techniques and their theoretical underpinnings

Social validation

Social validation, the process of assessing the social significance of the goals, methods and outcomes of interventions (Wolf, 1978), is most closely associated with postpositivism as it is manifested in applied behaviour analysis. Single-subject experimental designs are used to gather objective and reliable data that allow researchers to establish functional relations between behaviour changes and treatments. The process of social validation is used alongside objective data to determine the social validity of goals, methods and outcomes as perceived by consumers. Related to the social validation of outcomes, Wolf (1978) noted that '... behavior analysts may give their opinions, and these opinions may even be supported with empirical objective behavioral data, but it is the participants and other consumers who want to make the final decision about whether a program helped solve their problems' (p. 210). Social validation, when applied from a postpositivist point of view, does recognize that the reality captured by objective data may be different from the reality perceived by the participant or other consumer. As a result, it becomes imperative to collect data on these perceptions in addition to objective behavioural data. When applied within a postpositivist paradigm, the social validation approach offers flexibility as to who may constitute an appropriate evaluator ('participants and other consumers'). Essentially, anyone (including but not limited to the AAC user) who directly or indirectly controls the viability of an AAC intervention may be an appropriate person to socially validate goals, methods and outcomes (for a detailed discussion on selecting appropriate consumers to validate interventions see Schlosser, in press). In terms of techniques, social validation within this paradigm commonly employs questionnaires, rating scales, and structured interviews. Typically, social validation has been applied only to the validation of goals, methods and outcomes. Although these are undoubtedly important steps in the intervention research process, they represent only selected steps of the more comprehensive research process. For instance, there is a considerable amount of work going into problem sensing and the literature review, which greatly influences the research question to be posed or the intervention goal to be derived. Usually, social validation seeks neither the perspectives of consumers for steps that precede the statement of goals nor the steps (e.g. problem sensing) that come after the validation of outcomes (e.g. dissemination). Social validation, when applied within the postpositivist paradigm, may thus be an approach with clear purposes but also with clear limitations as far as involving consumers *throughout* the research process.

Social validation, however, could also fit well within an emancipatory paradigm when the people asked to do the ratings are those with the least power *and* those who will be affected by the treatment (Mertens, 1998). It follows that in this paradigm persons with little or no functional speech would represent the most appropriate raters of social validity of AAC interventions. Although it would be legitimate to consult family members (they may meet the 'least power' criterion, too) and other communication partners (e.g. speech-language pathologists may not meet the 'least power' criterion) as well, the perspective of the person with little or no functional speech would clearly carry the most weight. When applied within an emancipatory paradigm, however, all steps of the research process need to be socially validated. This, however, would require a considerable extension beyond the validation of goals, methods and outcomes, typically done in social validation of AAC interventions to date (Schlosser, in press).

Participatory action research and emancipatory research

Participatory action research (PAR) and emancipatory research are discussed as two other approaches to involve consumers in the AAC research process (Balandin and Raghavendra, this volume; Bersani, this volume; Krogh, 1997). Balandin and Raghavendra (this volume) cite references that help them distinguish PAR from emancipatory research (Oliver, 1992). They argue that while PAR seeks to involve participants in the research process, only emancipatory research ensures that researchers relinquish control over the process to those with the least power and who are the most affected by the research. Others, however, equate PAR and emancipatory research and place it within the same theoretical perspective of the 'emancipatory paradigm ' – Mertens (1998) argues that PAR aims to relinquish control of the research to the marginalized groups (see also Reason, 1994). Regardless of the school of thought, the distinction between 'mere participation' and 'relinquishing control' is useful and informs our debate. The emancipatory paradigm clearly requires that the perspectives of the participating person with little or no functional speech are given the most weight, and that these perspectives need to be made known throughout the research process. Along these lines, Bersani (this volume) argues that while it is often a wide array of people who may be potential consumers who are represented in the research process, '... our ultimate obligation is to people with little or no functional speech, they are the consumers of our research products ...' . Balandin and Raghavendra (this volume) propose that AAC users should be the direct consumers as the research issues they discuss in their paper have direct bearing on them. They also acknowledge, however, that in some instances non-disabled members of the research team may be considered direct consumers. Both Balandin and Raghavendra (this volume) and Bersani (this volume) draw from their research experiences in reporting on methodological issues they encountered within the emancipatory paradigm. These papers should stimulate an increased interest among researchers and consumers to explore this paradigm further.

Focus groups

Huer and Parette (this volume) discuss methodological issues concerning the use of focus groups as a technique. Based on the participants being Hispanic families who have children using AAC, the methodological issues they raise inform the planning, implementation and analysis of focus groups with families from a diverse cultural background. Focus groups may be approached from a variety of theoretical paradigms. Focus groups may be used in conjunction with the postpositivist paradigm, for example, to develop the content of a questionnaire (Soto, 1997b). Focus groups within the interpretive/constructivist paradigm may be held with AAC users as well as stakeholders other than AAC users (see Huer and Parette, this volume). Focus groups within an emancipatory paradigm, on the other hand, require the participants to be AAC users. I am not aware of any focus group studies with AAC users as the participants. Such research would provide much needed information. For example, although we know what prominent researchers propose as an AAC research agenda (Beukelman and Ansel, 1995), we do not know what research agenda AAC users would propose. Another distinction between the two paradigms in using focus groups relates to the research process. Huer and Parette (this volume), for example, used focus groups in the data collection phase of the research process to determine the perspective of Hispanic families with children using AAC. The families were not systematically consulted during problem-sensing and formulation and other steps of the research process. This is an appropriate use of focus groups in an interpretive/constructivist paradigm. Had this same research issue been approached within an emancipatory paradigm, however, using focus groups only at one step of the research process would be considered inappropriate. Clearly, we need to see more applications of focus groups in the AAC field based on each of the theoretical paradigms, but in particular within the emancipatory paradigm.

Conclusions

Consumer perspectives in AAC research are a relatively recent phenomenon. It is therefore not surprising that consumers and researchers alike are faced with many challenging methodological issues. In the absence of any 'how-to' guidelines, the chapters in this section are invaluable toward advancing this discussion. Drawing from their own research experiences, the authors successfully discuss their perceptions of encountered methodological issues, present limitations and contemplate potential solutions, often by bringing in applications from related fields. Using the terminology distinction raised by Bersani (this volume), I am optimistic that these pioneering contributions will enable others to engage in more AAC research 'with' rather than 'on' consumers. It is hoped that the discussion of theoretical underpinnings of various approaches and techniques in this introduction facilitate and stimulate the reading of the chapters ahead.

Chapter 23
Challenging Oppression: Augmented Communicators' Involvement in AAC Research

Susan Balandin and Pammi Raghavendra

> Disabled people have come to see research as a violation of their experiences, as irrelevant to their needs and as failing to improve their material circumstances and quality of life. (Oliver, 1992, p. 105)

Traditionally research in augmentative and alternative communication (AAC) has tended to be quantitative or interpretative and has been disseminated through journals and conference presentations. Both Krogh (1997) and Bersani (Chapter 24, this volume) have identified a number of stages in the research process (e.g. formulating research ideas, assembling the research team) which could, and indeed should, involve augmented communicators. Yet, to date, there have been only a few studies reported in which augmented communicators were included as part of the research team (e.g. Alm, 1994; Balandin and Iacono, 1997; Balandin and Morgan, 1997; McGregor and Alm, 1992).

McGregor (McGregor and Alm, 1992) reported on his involvement in developing and evaluating prototypes of AAC equipment. He noted the benefits of being part of a research team. These included travel, attending conferences and increasing social networks as well as helping develop new technology. Alm (1994), in a discussion of some of the ethical issues involved in AAC research, raised practical issues that must be considered when augmented communicators are part of the research team (e.g. payment, expectations of the team members who use AAC, and issues of time and commitment). These have posed unique problems that the research team has to solve. He also noted that it may be hard for an augmented communicator to be critical of the research process. Balandin and Morgan (1997) and Balandin and Iacono (1997) reported studies in which augmented communicators assisted with the development of grant applications by advising on the research questions. The augmented communicators involved in these two studies and in the ongoing 'critical pathway' project (Raghavendra and The Steering Committee, 1998) have also advised on the development of survey instruments to be used with individuals with a disability. Despite these reports, currently, within the AAC field there is a scarcity of published studies initiated and led by augmented communicators and there is limited information on the issues that augmented communicators consider important for the AAC research agenda.

Drake (1997) suggested that it is inappropriate for people without a disability to conduct research about people with a disability, yet the AAC field abounds with such studies. Few, if any, researchers in AAC would see themselves as exploiting vulnerable groups (Swain, Heyman and Gillman, 1998), taking the role of oppressor (Oliver, 1992), or reinforcing the idea that any problems experienced by people with a disability result from their own inadequacy (Abberley, 1992). Nevertheless, such charges are being made against researchers who fail to adequately consult with and include people with a disability in research projects (Oliver, 1992; Zarb, 1992). Schlosser (1997a) noted that although there is agreement that consumers should be included in research projects, the definition of a consumer is not always clear. He noted that the profile of the consumer group may vary depending on the focus of the research project. Schlosser suggested that in AAC research the direct consumers may be augmented communicators or their natural speaking partners, whereas indirect consumers are not involved in the research study per se but may still be affected by it. In this chapter individuals with a disability, including augmented communicators, may be considered direct consumers as the research issues discussed have a direct impact on them. In addition, other non-disabled members of the research team may in some instances also be considered direct consumers, particularly if they are engaged in emancipatory or participatory research projects.

French and Swain (1997) have discussed the characteristics, similarities and differences between participatory research and emancipatory research in the field of disability. They describe participatory research as aiming '... to reflect, explore and disseminate the views, feelings and experiences of research participants from their own perspectives,' whereas, 'A major characteristic of emancipatory research is the insistence that people with a disability should control (rather than merely participate in) the entire research process from the formulation of the research question to the dissemination of the findings' (French and Swain, 1997, p. 27). Both French and Swain (1997) and Oliver (1992) noted that although it is possible to involve individuals with a disability in participatory research, emancipatory research is part of a political struggle that individuals with a disability can only take up for themselves.

The issues of who owns the agenda and who stands to gain most from research processes have been addressed in both the qualitative research literature and the literature that considers the social construct of disability (e.g. French and Swain, 1997; Oliver, 1992; Oliver, 1996a; Ramcharan and

Grant, 1994; Zarb, 1992). There appears to be agreement within this literature that individuals with a disability have a right to be included in all
aspects of research and that, until research is directed by individuals with a
disability, not only research validity but also the ideal of social equality
remain a myth (Oliver, 1992).

There can be little doubt that those involved in AAC, whether as
researchers or augmented communicators, should consider the new
paradigms of participatory and emancipatory research. Where are we in
the field of AAC? Are AAC consumers involved in the design, data collection and evaluation of the research? Are the researchers accountable to the
consumers? Are we anywhere close to where AAC consumers set a
research agenda, plan and direct the research? Some augmented communicators consider that they have their own culture (M. Allen, personal
communication, 10 July 1998; M. B. Williams, personal communication,
23 July 1998), and this must be recognized and valued by AAC researchers
if they do not wish to participate in a process of discrimination (Oliver,
1992; Stalker, 1998; Thomas and Parry, 1996). Consequently, AAC
researchers must be at pains to ensure that they avoid 'abelist' assumptions but rather participate in a process of cultural exchange and cross-
cultural interaction. Williams (1995, p. 1) defined abelism as '...
discrimination based on ability, especially discrimination against people
with disabilities'. A description of the problems encountered during a
project involving researchers from two cultures, hearing and deaf (Jones
and Pullen, 1992), has relevance for the field of AAC. It can be argued that
when natural speakers and augmented communicators work together it is
indeed cross-cultural research. In the field of AAC there are a number of
the important issues to consider if AAC research is to move towards a more
equitable position vis-a-vis augmented communicators. Our own attempts
to deal with these issues, some of which have been more successful than
others, will be discussed and illustrated with some examples. As an
example of a participatory form of research, we present an ongoing
project undertaken at Crippled Children's Association (CCA) of South
Australia Inc., which demonstrates how to involve augmented communicators from the planning stages of a project in AAC (Raghavendra and The
Steering Committee, 1998). We also share some of our experiences that
may provide guidelines to other researchers contemplating a participatory
form of research.

Setting the research agenda

Traditionally research agendas are set by the researchers. Oliver (1992)
suggested that this accords the researchers the role of elite experts, who
are in complete charge of the process and who thus perpetuate the
distinction between researchers and the researched. The disability
movement as a whole finds such a distinction oppressive. Nevertheless it

is recognized that setting the agenda for research is often problematic as it is usually governed by the requirements of the funding agency (Aspis, 1997; Oliver, 1992; Thomas and Parry, 1996).

Adults with cerebral palsy set the agenda for a recent study of ageing and cerebral palsy (Balandin and Morgan, 1997). This project developed from the concerns of a small group of individuals with cerebral palsy who were worried that their physical, mental and social well being, which included their communication skills, was deteriorating as they aged. They wanted to set a broad agenda for addressing ageing issues within the organization where they worked. They lobbied the organization for several years for a small amount of funding to conduct a preliminary survey of the experiences of adults with cerebral palsy who are ageing. Balandin was employed to work on this project with a steering committee of individuals with cerebral palsy, all of whom had a severe communication impairment.

The steering group, chaired by Morgan, had no difficulty in setting the broad agenda but experienced problems with refining the issues to be considered. They needed help with some basic research processes (e.g. ethical issues, confidentiality, aims and outcomes, data collection, and the overall logistics of conducting a study). These issues are raised by Krogh (1997) in her description of a case study research project conducted with an augmented communicator. All the individuals on the steering group considered ageing from their own perspective and had limited knowledge of any other research that had been done in the area. Balandin undertook a review of the literature and presented it to the group. This helped individuals to verify some of their own beliefs and caused them to question others. It also confirmed that it is helpful for individuals with a disability and no research background who wish to develop research projects to have access to someone with a research background who is able to support them (Oliver, 1996b).

It took some time to agree on survey questions that asked relevant questions that could be answered through a mail survey and collated to give a meaningful picture of the issues faced by adults with cerebral palsy who are ageing. Balandin, as the non-disabled member of the steering committee, experienced some difficulty in not taking over the process and directing the questions to suit her own agenda. She alerted the group to the need to be assertive about what they considered important. Oliver (1996b) emphasized that both individuals with a disability and researchers need to work together. Both Oliver (1996b) and Krogh (1997) stressed that those with a disability and researchers without a disability must be aware of the politics of power that are likely to exist, at least initially between the two groups. In Balandin and Morgan's (1997) project open discussion of this issue and regular meetings to discuss the project assisted in ensuring that no single person dominated the process. Finally, after many meetings and discussions, a number of questions addressing issues of health and health service provision for individuals with cerebral palsy were selected. The steering committee agreed that data gained through this process would assist them to identify important issues for the adults with cerebral palsy who participated in the survey (e.g. general practitioners' lack of knowledge about cerebral palsy, limited use of written material to gain knowledge of the ageing process). Setting a research agenda that augmented communicators consider important and worthy of research is problematic, not only because of funding limitations but also because there is little information on augmented communicators' research agenda.

In the 'Development of a critical pathway for the prescription and support of voice output communication aids (VOCAs) for adults with multiple disabilities in the community' project (Raghavendra and The Steering Committee, 1998), augmented communicators were neither involved in setting the initial research agenda nor in writing the research proposal and procuring funding. However, they are on a committee that is 'steering' the project and providing valuable input to it at various stages. The augmented communicators, caregivers and professionals on the committee have provided extensive input into developing tools, including a set of questions to ask augmented communicators in an interview. They have also helped to develop procedural issues (e.g. why a face-to-face interview is better than a mail survey for augmented communicators).

Recruitment of participants

Thomas and Parry (1996) noted that individuals with a disability may be encouraged to participate in a research project because they believe that it is an opportunity to 'have a voice' and implement change. Yet often, research projects involving people with a disability evaluate systems already in existence rather than challenging the system as a whole. Oliver (1992) suggested that participants with a disability may be left in exactly the same position after the research project whereas the researcher moves forward in his/her career. He advocated that researchers learn to put their skills at the disposal of their research participants with a disability so that both groups may work together to combat disabilism within an able bodied society, thereby acknowledging that both groups are mutually beneficial and support each other. Of course, participating in a research project can be a positive and rewarding experience. McGregor (McGregor and Alm, 1992) outlined the benefits and enjoyment that he had gained from participating in research projects. AAC researchers must be sensitive to the expectations of their participants and be wary of exploiting them, albeit unconsciously. They must also ensure that the project focuses on the abilities of the research participants.

There is a tendency in traditional research projects involving partici-pants with a communication impairment to focus on the limitation of the research participants rather than identifying the limits in the research methodology (Booth and Booth, 1996). Oliver (1992, 1996b) acknowledged that researchers may be constrained by factors beyond their control (e.g. funding requirements, submission guidelines) to conduct research that fits a traditional rather than a participatory research paradigm. In such instances, those conducting research in the AAC field must question what is the best and fairest way to encourage augmented communicators to participate in such projects. Zarb (1992) suggested that researchers should critically evaluate existing research as a starting point in moving towards a participatory research paradigm. He proposed that there are a number of questions that are useful to consider in order to help researchers understand what research paradigm is being used and what the benefits for people with a disability may be. The questions include (a) who controls the research; (b) how will it be conducted; (c) how are people with disabilities involved; (d) what opportunities are there for people with disabilities to criticize the research; and (e) what happens to the products of the research. Additionally, the dissemination of the results should be discussed with the participants (Zarb, 1992, p. 128). Such an evaluation at the beginning of the project would help the research participants with and without a disability to ensure that the project is beneficial to all parties. It would also safeguard against those with a disability being put in a less powerful (i.e. oppressed) position vis-a-vis the non-disabled research team members. It might also guarantee that participants with a disability continue to be part of the project throughout (Alm, 1994; McGregor and Alm, 1992) and gain acknowledgement for their participation.

In Balandin and Morgan's (1997) ageing study, the target group was adults aged 30 and over who could complete the survey from their own perspective and give additional comments if they wished. Thus, this project did not seek the opinions of formal or informal care providers or advocates, but rather wished to tap directly into the experiences of adults with cerebral palsy. Information about the project was disseminated through a variety of news sheets and by word of mouth. Some adults asked to be included. In an attempt to conduct a national study, the research steering committee contacted individuals they knew and told them about the project. The main recruitment, however, was through organizations that provided services to adults with cerebral palsy. Survey forms and letters of explanation were sent to the organizations who were asked to post the surveys out to individuals who in their opinion would be able to complete the survey or give their own responses to a scribe who could complete the survey for them. It is clear such a recruitment process could be labelled oppressive. The organizations were put in the position of experts who could choose who would or would not be offered the chance to participate. If more generous funding had been available, members of the steering committee would have conducted focus groups across Australia, provided funding for individuals with cerebral palsy to attend the groups with adequate support and collected the information directly from individuals in the groups. This was not an option. Nevertheless, in hindsight, the recruitment of participants for this project can be seen to be far from ideal. It may well have excluded individuals who could have participated and in fact, reinforced an abelist model of research. It also meant that, apart from a few individuals known personally to the steering committee, only people who chose to use the services were contacted. Thus, the recruitment process was selective and must have had some impact on the internal validity of the project. Recruitment of participants, even if the project is driven by individuals with a disability, remains problematic. It is difficult to contact individuals who are not receiving formal services and who are unlikely to read newspapers or information sheets in which projects are advertised. Local knowledge of support networks (e.g. church groups, social groups) may assist in contacting individuals who would like to participate in projects but who otherwise would not be aware of the project, although this can be very time-consuming (Bigby, 1995).

Another form of recruitment was undertaken in the development of the 'Critical Pathway Project' (Raghavendra and The Steering Committee, 1998) that is currently ongoing. Every stage of this project involves augmented communicators. Critical pathways are maps or guidelines of clinical practice that document good clinical practice, and also include the needs expressed by internal customers (i.e. clinicians) and external customers (i.e. augmented communicators). Hence, the involvement of augmented communicators in the development of critical pathways is both important and necessary. Augmented communicators who use VOCAs were invited to be on the steering committee of a project that would provide input to and 'steer' the project.

Initial consumer participation

Letters were sent to seven augmented communicators, inviting them to participate on the steering committee. The letter was written in non-technical language as augmented communicators within the organization vary in their cognitive abilities, literacy skills and world experiences. Contact was made with each augmented communicator after a week to ask whether he or she would be interested in being on the steering committee. Originally only one augmented communicator was to be on the committee, but two augmented communicators showed interest, consequently both were invited.

Consumer profiles

Both augmented communicators are males with multiple disabilities and are aged 21 and 36 years. One uses a Liberator, Blissymbols and signing, and has just completed high school studies, whereas the other uses a

Dynavox and lives in shared care accommodation and attends day centre activities. The organization provides their transport and pays their support worker costs.

Steering committee

In addition to the two augmented communicators, the steering committee consists of four caregivers from day centres and accommodation agencies, two speech pathologists, a communication assistant and the manager of the service. The steering committee was asked to:

* provide input on questions designed for the focus group;
* help with the development of questionnaires and the other evaluation tools;
* share personal experiences regarding VOCA assessment, training and use;
* read and discuss an article on VOCA;
* provide feedback on information gathered from questionnaires.

Working with consumers on the steering committee

Out of the four meetings, held once every month, one augmented communicator attended three whereas the other attended only one meeting. The different agencies involved in his service provision needed to be informed of his commitment to the steering committee. Even though letters were sent to his home and to the different agencies he missed the meetings because there were communication breakdowns regarding the meeting dates and times.

The augmented communicators' participation in the discussion was limited for the following reasons:

* One augmented communicator had never had any experience in participating in meetings before, and hence did not feel confident as he knew he was lacking skills that other people attending had.
* Both consumers' devices did not work satisfactorily.
* One hour meetings were too short.
* Even though questions had been sent on the issues that would be discussed, no answers were prepared. The interactions were limited to 'Yes' and 'No' answers.

The care workers were also quiet and hesitant and it took them at least two meetings before they felt confident and comfortable enough to talk about issues related to assessment for VOCAs, training, use and follow-up. Therefore, the fact that the two augmented communicators with severe multiple disabilities did not contribute should not have been a total surprise.

Suggestions to improve participation

Apart from their devices not working properly, the reasons for the augmented communicators' limited participation could have been due to issues such as: (a) never having spoken in a group situation before; (b) no previous experience of speaking in groups that included strangers/ authority figures; and (c) not having the personal and technical support to facilitate their group interactions.

The project is ongoing as funding for a second year has been secured. Some changes to the workings of the steering committee have been implemented in an attempt to ensure a more productive second year:

- Smaller groups – the final group consisted of 11 people when everyone was present and they were a mixed group of individuals. Currently, there are seven members including one augmented communicator and his support worker and this is more effective. Hopefully, reducing the group size will result in more productive meetings.
- Better coordination with the agencies was needed in order to make sure that the augmented communicator was at the meetings and that he had had the time and appropriate help to prepare for the meeting. The coordinator of the project now reconfirms the meeting date and time with the manager of the day centre agency a few days before the meeting.
- The coordinator also meets with the augmented communicator and his support worker an hour before a meeting for a 'practice session'. This has addressed the issue of one hour meetings being too short for the augmented communicator to prepare what he wants to say. It also allows the coordinator to check that the device is working properly.
- One augmented communicator indicated that he was bored at the meetings. Care will be taken to make sure that the language used in meetings is simple and the issues under discussion are visually supported. Those who attend the meetings must be involved in redesigning the format and presentation style to ensure that everyone is included and able to contribute. The practice session with the augmented communicator also helps to address some of these issues.

These changes have made meetings with all the members of the committee more effective and efficient. In addition to these changes, the support worker could be encouraged to use prompts to remind the augmented communicator to contribute his ideas at appropriate points in the meeting. The coordinator must be sure to provide opportunities for any augmented communicators present to raise questions or concerns pertaining to the project.

Analysis of results

Oliver (1992) indicated that the methodology of research with individuals with a disability should be built upon trust and respect, and should incorporate reciprocity between all parties involved in the project. In AAC research, data from studies are usually analysed by non-disabled researchers who then interpret the results in the light of their knowledge of augmented communicators. The importance of social validation has been recognized in AAC vocabulary research (e.g. Karlan and Lloyd, 1983; Balandin and Iacono, 1998). Schlosser (1997b) provided a much needed conceptual framework for social validation in AAC. He explored social validation issues and proposed a social validity matrix for AAC interventions that will assist in the assessment of the social validity of future AAC research projects. In many instances, attempts to socially validate the complete research process with augmented communicators fall short. For example, a recent study of the topics of conversation and perceptions of communicative interactions by augmented communicators and natural speakers (Balandin and Iacono, 1997) was developed with input from augmented communicators. However, no attempt was made to include augmented communicators in the analysis or to verify if the researchers' interpretation of the conversations were indeed consistent with augmented communicators' interpretations. Balandin and Iacono (1997) interviewed the participants after the project. They asked the augmented communicators what they thought of the project and whether they considered it to have been useful. However, they did not discuss the data with the participants or seek their opinion on how to interpret them. In such studies there are ethical considerations regarding actual data that must be taken into account. Nevertheless, the practice of interpreting data without reference to augmented communicators is consistent with much of the current AAC research practice reported in the literature.

Stalker (1998), discussing her research procedures in conducting a project focusing on choices made by men with a disability, noted that, if she had conducted a respondent validation check the participants would have had some input into the way the findings were represented. Similarly, in AAC research such checks would not only allow augmented communicators to comment on the interpretation of the results, but would also help cement a stronger, more equitable relationship between the researchers and the research participants.

In the critical pathway project (Raghavendra and The Steering Committee, 1998) results from the focus groups with access workers from day centres and accommodation agencies, and parents of augmented communicators and clinicians, were presented to the steering committee who provided suggestions on the emerging themes. The committee also provided feedback on the initial draft of a pathway and will be responsible for analysing interviews with augmented communicators.

Analysis of data by the researcher is a part of most research projects. However, Zarb (1992) suggested that it is possible to challenge the way research is usually conducted, and involve individuals with a disability in the analysis process. Involving individuals with a disability throughout the research process and recognizing conflicts of interest (e.g. the need for publications and career advancement) that occur for researchers during a research project may mitigate to some extent the fact that research analysis frequently emphasizes the powerful position of the researcher who analyses and interprets the data according to his/her own constructs of disability.

Dissemination of results

How results are disseminated often calls into question who is the main beneficiary of a research project (Drake, 1997; Ramcharan and Grant, 1994; Stalker, 1998; Swain et al., 1998). As already stated, participants usually join a research project in the belief that they and their peers will benefit from the results. Both Oliver (1992) and Swain et al. (1998) noted that it is the researcher who usually stands to gain most from the process and that the results may never be disseminated to the participants, nor may the project bring about the change for which participants hoped. Research results are frequently disseminated as published articles. This creates problems for those who do not have access to the relevant journals, or who have literacy problems. Only 43% of the participants with cerebral palsy in Balandin and Morgan's (1997) study read for information. Conference presentations are another forum for dissemination of results, yet individuals with a disability rarely make up the bulk of conference audiences. Thus, disseminating information to the people who should stand to benefit most is a vexed question. If augmented communicators are part of the research team, they may be better placed than the natural speakers to disseminate information to their peers. It is hoped that the augmented communicator on the steering committee of the critical pathway project (Raghavendra and The Steering Committee, 1998) will share his experiences and findings from the project with other augmented communicators and support workers. This will be in addition to the project coordinator's presentation of the critical pathway to train various stakeholders in the project.

The Internet, publications and conferences that focus specifically on individuals with a disability offer a forum for information to be disseminated in an appropriate format. After the ageing study (Balandin and Morgan, 1997), a number of focus groups were conducted to enable the researchers to inform participants of the results and to promote discussion of the implications of the research for the participants, their carers and service providers. A group with a focus on ageing was started by individuals with cerebral palsy as a result of this. Initially, the group met monthly and was informal. However, it has now become more structured. The group is chaired by an individual with a severe communication impairment, but also includes representatives from management and service provision who have no disability. The group is now working collaboratively and successfully with other agencies. It has managed to obtain funding to investigate some accommodation issues for adults who are ageing.

Research teams need to be aware of the importance of ensuring that augmented communicators know of the results of studies in which they have been involved. This may be done through focus groups, writing research news sheets in large print and in non-technical language and making tapes or short videos that discuss the project and findings. After the ageing study (Balandin and Morgan, 1997), Morgan was interviewed for the organization's news video that is made four times a year and seen by many adult augmented communicators across Australia.

Funding

Alm (1994) noted that funding augmented communicators who are participating in research projects presents problems if they stand to lose benefits because of increased earnings. He stated that in his centre, they overcame this problem to some extent by paying fringe benefits to augmented communicators on the research team (e.g. conference fees, generous travel allowance). While this does in some way reimburse the augmented communicators it still reinforces the fact that there are different regulations for different members of the team. We have found no satisfactory way of overcoming this issue in Australia unless we are able to employ one of the few augmented communicators working and not drawing any social benefits. Consequently, we have resorted to much the same methods as Alm (1994). In the critical pathway project (Raghavendra and The Steering Committee, 1998), the participation of the augmented communicator and the access workers on the steering committee is voluntary and only the support worker is paid by the service. Where possible we now apply for funding for augmented communicators involved in the project to attend conferences and participate in the presentation of research findings in the initial grant budget unless the funding bodies specify that this will not be considered in the budget.

Another funding issue is one of time. If a person with a severe disability undertakes a particular task on a project (e.g. clerical work), it may take much longer to complete the task. The issue then is one of payment for the task or for the time taken. We have paid for the task regardless of the time taken, and have made a group decision on the monetary worth of each task. This is not ideal, as it certainly reinforces the idea that the disability is the fault of the individual rather than of those running the research project who were unable to construct tasks in a way that was easy to complete (Oliver, 1992). The issue of matching skills to a specific task means that careful job descriptions may need to be part of the research tender. This will help ensure that individuals are not disadvantaged on the grounds of their disability when in fact they have the ability to complete the job with some modification to the work environment. In reality, certainly within Australia, ensuring that an individual with a disability has the appropriate access, assistive technology and support is problematic and frequently not feasible.

Within Australia, for example, funding for research projects in the current climate of economic changes is highly competitive. Researchers in disability often have to compete for a small pot of money with researchers from both the social science and medical fields at a national level. What chance do augmented communicators with limited research experience in initiating and leading projects have in applying for funds to conduct research? On the other hand, will funding bodies regard projects initiated by augmented communicators to be more socially valid and hence view them more favourably, particularly if an experienced researcher is on the research team but not the chief investigator? These issues need to be investigated.

Ethics

Much has been written about the ethics of research with individuals with a disability, including those with a communication impairment (Alm, Arnott and Newell, 1992; Booth and Booth, 1996; Oliver, 1992; Stalker, 1998; Swain et al., 1998; Thomas and Parry, 1996). Why do individuals with a disability participate in research projects? Krezman (personal communication, 28 July 1998) suggested that a sense of duty to one's own people as well as a search for social and psychological validation motivates many. How constrained augmented communicators feel to participate in a research project is an ethical concern. In spite of assurances that it is acceptable to refuse to participate or to withdraw from the project at any time, it is likely that many individuals participate because it is too difficult to say no. For example, in Australia, where there are few augmented communicators in employment, it may be hard for researchers to accept that a potential participant for an employment research project does not want to participate. There is a great temptation to try to wheedle a change of heart.

Participating in research can be both time-consuming (Alm, 1994) and disruptive of routines for augmented communicators. Frequently routines are built around attendant care and support services and any changes can be very inconvenient. Two of the participants in Balandin and Iacono's (1997) study cheerfully altered their routines in order to take part in the project. They both stated that they were pleased to be able to help. They were in fact helping the researchers as much as other augmentative communicators. Stalker (1998) recognized that limited life choices and the feeling of always being undervalued may result in individuals with a disability being acquiescent and unable to refuse the researchers' demands. Such individuals may attempt to maintain a friendly relationship by avoiding tension and by not suggesting that the researcher's agenda is not theirs.

It is common for individuals with a disability who are socially isolated to regard staff as friends, a feeling not necessarily reciprocated by the staff (Lutfiyya, 1991). Many augmented communicators interact more frequently with staff than with their peers. They may interact with authority figures (doctors, teachers, therapists) more than with other augmented communicators. This must be recognized as a potential cause for ethical and methodological concern as it can result in exploitation of research participants and may also invalidate results. Alm (1994) suggested that participation in a research project may provide social contact, a change from routine and the opportunity to make a contribution. He noted that some research participants may be lonely and have unrealistic expectations of the friendship that already exists on a research team.

Additional ethical considerations arise when the participants are too trusting. Swain et al. (1998) reported a study of abuse in which ethical concerns arose from the participants' willingness to disclose personal information that was either not required, or presented the researchers with a dilemma of whether they should act on it or not. They suggested that in any research project ethical issues need constant re-evaluation throughout the project.

Within our own experience of research with augmented communicators on the team, and indeed with augmented communicators as participants, two of the main issues have centred on confidentiality and informed consent. Augmented communicators are a relatively small group in Australia, consequently it is harder to maintain the anonymity of research participants.

It is beyond the scope of this chapter to discuss issues of informed consent for participation in a project. Both government departments and ethics committees have procedures and guidelines on developing letters of consent and explanations of a project for participants which must be adhered to before a project may be undertaken. The participants in the projects discussed in this chapter were all able to give informed consent.

How often material is used (e.g. video material), what is said about it, and how frequently we gain the permission of the participants to show it (Alm, 1994) remains an ethical issue. Interpreting research results becomes an ethical issue in the light of the disability movement's current view that interpretative research is negative and oppressive to individuals with a disability (Oliver, 1992; Zarb, 1992). Ensuring that augmented communicators set the agenda and are actively involved in the analysis of the material goes some way to ensure that the research serves the augmented communicators' agenda as well as the researchers, but this is not always easy to facilitate. Swain et al. (1998) stressed that respect for the individual is part of the ethics of research. Involving individuals with a disability in the planning of the research methodology, including data collection, interpretation of results and dissemination of information after the project, is a means of realizing respect and maintaining an equal balance of power. In research studies where tape recordings are used (e.g. Balandin and Iacono, 1997) confidentiality may be at risk if a number of people have access to the data. In addition, self-disclosure on audiotape or videotape may mean that the researcher may have to make decisions on whether to use the material or not (Alm, 1994).

Conclusions

Participatory research that involves disabled people in a meaningful way is perhaps a prerequisite to emancipatory research in the sense that researchers can learn from disabled people and vice versa, and that it paves the way for researchers to make themselves 'available' to disabled people (Zarb, 1992, p. 128).

It is important to ask whether research into augmented communicators' views will really empower individuals (Thomas and Parry, 1996). The Critical Pathways Project (Raghavendra and The Steering Committee, 1998) and other AAC research projects would benefit from a critical evaluation utilizing the questions developed by Zarb (1992). The field of AAC is moving slowly towards using different research paradigms that will help ensure that augmented communicators have a more equal voice in the research process.

Although there are studies in which augmented communicators are part of a research team, as yet the agenda for research has not been set by augmented communicators. Projects that involve communicators with various abilities in a participatory form of research are relatively new, and consequently, are a learning experience for everyone involved. It is important to share information on these projects so that the AAC research field may benefit as a whole. Those working in the field of AAC are committed to empowering those who use AAC and to facilitating their inclusion within society without suffering discrimination. Thus, it is important to recognize that empowerment is a political struggle. Professionals in AAC must be prepared to give up their expert status and work together with augmented communicators to assist them in a battle against abelism. It is clear that some difficulties are more easily surmounted than others. Nevertheless, the field of AAC research is now actively attempting to ensure that augmented communicators are included as research partners in projects and will hopefully encourage and support augmented communicators to conduct emancipatory research in the future.

Acknowledgement

We are grateful to all the augmented communicators who participated in the research projects that we have discussed. Special thanks to John Morgan who was a patient, tolerant and generous co-researcher.

Chapter 24
Nothing About Me Without Me: A Proposal for Participatory Action Research in AAC

HANK BERSANI JR

Nothing about me without me

This is the new slogan of many disability rights activists in the USA. People with disabilities are wearing buttons, t-shirts and bumper stickers on the backs of their wheelchairs that proclaim 'Nothing about me without me'. The message is clear: people are telling us that if they are to be the subject of an activity, they need to be a part of that activity. They explain that when staff meet to discuss a participant in a programme (student in school, or an adult in a service programme), the individual needs to be at the table and participating in the discussion. Similarly, these advocates assert that even if they themselves are not being discussed as individuals, that if people with disabilities are being discussed, planned for, etc., they (disability activists) should be at the table as well. Many fields seem comfortable discussing people with disabilities in their absence in a way that would not seem reasonable with other groups. Imagine a meeting about the needs of female professors, with no women in the room, or a discussion about the concerns of black families with only whites partici- pating in the discussion. Imagine a discussion of the needs and interests of people with communication impairments with only people who are good natural speakers at the table. Balandin and Raghavendra (Chapter 23, this volume) call for AAC researchers to 'consider new paradigms of participa- tory and emancipatory research'.

Research is not a value-free zone

Why should well trained professional researchers consult with people with disabilities, who have communication impairments, who may have no research training or experience and may have not read the current liter- ature on a given line of inquiry? The answers may be found in values.

Some assert that research can and must be value-free, that the scientific method is 'the pursuit of objective knowledge' (Neale and Liebert, 1973, p. 2). In fact, there is also recognition of the limits of so-called objectivity. Kerlinger, while touting the objectivity of science, also admits the value of subjective opinion. He urges people with disabilities to

> ... discuss, argue, debate, and even fight about research. Take a stand. Be opinionated. (1973, p. viii)

In reality, no research enterprise can proceed in the absence of a value base. Value decisions are made when research priorities are set. Values affect the decision about who will and who will not be studied. Value decisions drive what is and is not funded. Values affect which manuscripts are and are not accepted for publication, and which sentences will be edited out of the final manuscript. Blumer, while explaining the nature of symbolic interaction research, states:

> The first premise is that human beings act toward things on the basis of the meaning the things have for them. (1969, p. 2)

The image of value-fee research is a myth. Participatory action research (PAR) offers an alternative research paradigm that includes divergent values, especially the values of the individuals being studied (Santelli et al., in press; Turnbull and Turnbull, 1996).

Efforts can be made to balance different value perspectives in research. In some of my early AAC research, my co-researcher and I often held differing hopes and assumptions about the outcomes of a series of studies. The goal was not to have value-free research, but to prevent values from skewing research. Suggestions from the other are often reviewed sceptically as an opportunity for the other to take some advantage by swaying the study to the other's point of view. To keep the research objective, one needs to be clear about interests, and represent competing interests. If values do drive the research enterprise, then whose values should be represented, balanced or counterbalanced?

Although there are many interests to be balanced in any research endeavour, the one addressed here is the obligation to include the interests of the group of individuals being studied, the participants, or consumers. Many people who use AAC are now calling for greater participation in the field (Williams, 1995, 1996) and they are saying to us, 'Nothing about me without me!'

Lessons from the field of mental retardation

Ironically, in the area of cognitive disability attention is directed to 'giving a voice' to people with disabilities; that is, assisting the world in seeing things from the point of view of the person with the disability

(Bersani, 1996). While it may be tempting to see PAR as an idealized concept, but less than essential, like the proverbial 'icing on the cake', Whitney-Thomas (1996) argues that PAR is an essential aspect of offering quality services to people with disabilities, including those with cognitive impairments.

Wolfensberger (1972) first described what he called 'consumer representation' in mental retardation services. He indicated that people with mental retardation need to be directly represented on both governing and advisory boards of services for people with mental retardation. Wolfensberger and Glenn (1973) went on to call for what they refer to as 'consumer participation' in the evaluation of human services:

> Consumer participation in human services ... is viewed not only as a valuable force in bringing about adaptive change ... but also increasingly as a civil right. (Wolfensberger and Glenn, 1973, p. 48)

In Maryland, people with developmental disabilities are participating in participatory action research, evaluating the quality of services to people with mental retardation and other developmental disabilities (Bonham et al., 1998).

In a recent policy paper by the President's Committee on Mental Retardation (1996) recommendations in the area of research included:

> People with disabilities should be involved and fully supported in all facets of research, including learning how research is conducted.
> Key stakeholders and people from different fields, including self-advocates should be brought together to work toward greater involvement in research with findings in which they have a vested interest. (p. 62)

Heller et al. (no date) offer a variety of concrete suggestions for ways that people with disabilities can assist in a research project, ranging from 'Be a subject in a research study' to 'Help researchers better understand the information they find from research'. Their manual is written for people with disabilities including people with cognitive impairments as a way of promoting PAR in the field of developmental disabilities. It is also noteworthy that two of the four authors themselves have developmental disabilities.

Arguably, if 'a voice' can be given to people with cognitive impairments, and if the participation of people with mental retardation can be valued, then one should be able to find at least as many ways to value the research voice of people who use AAC.

The question that needs to be addressed is *'How can we best include the expertise and values of augmented speakers in as many levels of research on augmentative and alternative communication (AAC) as possible?'*

Word selection: defining terms

Defining 'consumers'

What does the term 'consumer' mean in the field of AAC research? This discussion will use the terms 'consumer' and 'participant' to identify the people who are most often referred to as 'subjects' of the research as well as other individuals who use augmentative communication to whom the research might also apply. For example, in a study on rate enhancement in people with cerebral palsy (CP), the 'subjects' would have CP, and would in the PAR model be participants. Other consumers of the study might also be other people with CP, or other people whose communication rate may be increased by the results of the study, even if they do not themselves have CP. In this sense, there is often a wide array of people who are potential consumers who might be represented in the research process.

Patient patients

Participants, or representatives of participants, may have specific ideas concerning the words researchers use in writing about their research, and especially the terms used to describe those participants. Again, in the field of mental retardation people who have grown up with the label 'mentally retarded' say that they find it disrespectful, and akin to the term 'nigger'. They ask to find more positive ways to describe them. Recently, a colleague was conducting an AAC therapy session with a man, developing a communication book with him. When interrupted by a telephone call, she told the caller she could not speak now, as she was with a 'patient'. The man (clearly upset) communicated his displeasure at being called a patient. A discussion ensued while the pair patiently worked to develop a mutually agreeable terminology for the relationship.

Being a subject is subjective

In research, a parallel discussion is needed. How does one refer to the people in AAC-related studies and those to whom the studies might apply? Are they merely 'subjects', or does that term needlessly restrict their role. What does it matter if people are named 'participants', 'subjects', 'patients' or 'consumers'? Consumer activist Ralph Nader has pointed out that there is power in being seen as a consumer and is generally credited with developing the concept of 'consumers' rights'. Although the consumers of research include other researchers, teachers, students and policy makers, researchers' ultimate obligation is to people with communication impairments; they are the consumers of AAC research products.

Proposed prepositions

'On', 'for', 'with', all seem like innocent enough terms. However, in daily life it can easily be seen that if a spouse or supervisor was reviewing information 'for' someone, 'on' someone or 'with' someone, each situation would convey a very different meaning. The people AAC researchers talk about emphasize that the words that are chosen do make a difference (Williams, 1995, 1996). In recent years several sets of guidelines were developed for writing about people with disabilities, including one by the Research and Training Center on Independent Living for Underserved Populations (1996).

Research done 'on' a subject (or a material, or a concept) implies a very passive relationship being acted upon. Only minimal protections and rights apply to subjects who are researched 'on' whom the research is conducted.

Research done 'for' an individual or group clearly implies a role of consumer, a more active status, with additional rights and interests beyond the rights of research subjects. Diligent researchers ask consumers of their research for suggestions to improve the quality and quantity of knowledge being sought on their behalf.

Research done 'with' an individual or group denotes a more active, even equal status – a partnership. Truly participatory AAC research will adequately reflect the concerns and values of AAC consumers in each step in the research process. One may have different values, but one needs to take into account differences so that the research remains balanced.

Researchers must select terms with care. After all, the identity of the field, revolves around the central assertion of the importance of communication. One must ask *'Are we conducting research 'on' augmented speakers, 'for' them, or 'with' them?'*

Clearly there are times when it is appropriate to conduct research 'on' a given topic. That is not being disputed here. The question is, are there opportunities to expand the nature of the research by making augmented speakers more active consumers and participants in research?

Augmented beginnings

Augmentative communication has made progress as a field, and as an organization the International Society on Augmentative and Alternative Communication (ISAAC) has reflected this progress in *Augmentative and Alternative Communication (AAC)*, the journal of the organization. Lloyd and Kangas (1988) proposed a list of key words for indexing articles appearing in *AAC*. In that draft, the terms 'consumer' and 'participatory' were not mentioned. Two years later (Lloyd and Kangas, 1990) the list included the term 'consumer', but still lacks the term 'participatory', which means that even if the focus was on the issue of participation, the key words in the journal indexing would not reflect this. Schlosser and

Braun (1992) offer five indices of efficacy. One index is social evaluation and within social evaluation, is subjective evaluation, which includes 'the opinions of persons who have a special position due to their expertise or their relationship to the client' (p. 38). Although Schlosser and Braun do not explicitly mention it, Schlosser (1997a) clarifies that people in a special position because of their closeness to the client include the individual and other people with similar needs.

Smith-Lewis and Ford (1987) report a case study of a woman called Dawn. Their conclusion is most appropriate here.

> By disregarding the perspective of the user, an extremely valuable source is omitted from the decision-making process. (p. 16)

Research is like a chess match

No two research projects follow the exact same plan. However, for the purposes of this paper a minimum of 20 common research steps can be identified from the development of an idea, to the dissemination of results, as presented in Table 24.1. This process is not often as linear in

Table 24.1. Stages of research

Openings
Formulate research ideas and or pet theories
Set a research agenda
Narrow the inquiry
Review and interpret extant literature
Seek informal suggestions from colleagues
Identify available participant pools
Develop the research questions(s) or null hypotheses
Select a methodology
Develop/select research instruments/data collection approach
Assemble the research team
File with the Human Subjects Committee/Institution Review Board
Serve on the Human Subjects review/Institution Review Board
Seek funding opportunities
Write grant application
Review grant applications/funding requests

Middle game
Collect data
Analyse data
Interpret results

Endgame
Write manuscripts for publication
Review manuscript submissions for publication
Incorporate research into training

---

real life as it is in theory. The research enterprise is like a chess match, it is important to set out a course of action well in advance, and it is important to be prepared to change course as circumstances change. In chess, experts refer to three stages: openings, middle game and endgame. The list of stages of a research inquiry can be broken into the same three stages.

Openings

The first and largest cluster of research activities are those that occur before the research is actually conducted. This includes setting research priorities, and reflecting upon the information gained and questions left unanswered by previous research. Although an idealized vision of this process including researchers and graduate students sitting around a coffee pot reflecting, positing, challenging and refining may only occur in imagination, the fact is that a research plan is nurtured, and evolves over time. Some studies rely methodologically on posing hypotheses to be tested, others may use focus groups or qualitative research techniques to formulate research questions based on the points of view of people from outside of the research team. How are participants involved in the opening stage of research? What are the opportunities for further participation? From a PAR point of view, when AAC research is read, it is fair to ask to what extent were people who use AAC involved in the development of the research questions, the selection of instruments, the collection of data, data analysis, interpretation and dissemination.

There are formal research options such as pilot studies and focus groups. However, in order to be fully participatory, this stage of inquiry needs to include people with disabilities as clearly equal partners with faculty members, graduate students and research consultants. (Maybe even researchers and professionals who themselves have disabilities.) Extant research needs to be reviewed and interpreted by the people the research was done 'on'. Future research questions need to come from people who the research will be done 'for'. Ideas for the next steps in research need to come from the people with disabilities who will be researched 'with'.

Some of the steps at this stage will require changes on the parts of organizations and institutions, rather than individual researchers themselves. Truly participatory disability research would require that people with disabilities sit on Human Subjects Committees, and peer review panels for grant applications, and as manuscript reviewers for refereed journals. Individual researchers may not be able to effect this sort of institutional change themselves. However, it is important to identify this as an opportunity and a need. Further, it is an obligation to seek out consumers who could participate on such committees, to identify the supports they would need, and to promote their inclusion.

The middle game

In the middle game, the actual research is done. This includes collecting and analysing the data and making preliminary interpretations of the results. Opportunities for consumer participation here range from serving on advisory committees to management teams that actually oversee and manage research centres to being employed as data collectors. Researchers committed to PAR may be able to establish advisory committees and even hire data collectors who are consumers. However, in many research settings, institutional changes may be needed to support the efforts of researchers interested in promoting PAR. Researchers need to encourage their institutions to establish an infrastructure that is conducive to PAR.

The endgame

After the research is done, it is time to explain to the world (or at least to interested parties) the results and the implications of the findings. Researchers dedicated to PAR will find ways to involve people with disabilities in interpreting results, conducting training to disseminate results, writing manuscripts and so on. Individual researchers will again need institutional assistance in the endgame. Truly participatory research will require that editorial review boards of refereed journals include consumers on review panels, and that conference planning committees include consumers as voting members when deciding which research is given plenary session status, which is offered a poster session, and which research is rejected altogether.

Who holds the proxy?

By definition, the participants in much of AAC research are people with impaired communication. Many also have significant cognitive impairments. In the event that the participants in a specific study, or line of inquiry, are people with severe, multiple disabilities, the researcher is not excused from the obligation of implementing consumer participation. Heller et al. (no date) point out that meaningful participation of people with disabilities often requires support, that this support needs to be individualized, that it may include changes in the pace of meetings, the language used, and the need for special consideration around meeting times, transportation, etc.

In some instances, it may be difficult or impossible to involve as collaborators those who are exactly like the 'subjects' in the study. In studying non-speaking three-year-old children, for example, it may be difficult and impractical to call on other non-speaking three-year-old children as co-researchers to contribute to the process. Clearly a proxy is needed. The only question then is 'Who holds the proxy for this group?' Historically, AAC research has turned to family members, staff or advocate allies to serve as proxies for people with communication disabilities. The fact is that they are almost always naturally speaking adults, with very few experiences in common with the true consumers. A more meaningful proxy would be to turn to other people with similar (but not exactly the same) kinds of disabilities, or less severe manifestations of the disability. A better proxy from the PAR point of view would be adults who are now competent communicators, who were themselves non-speaking three-year-olds at one time. Likewise, if the research is to focus on people with significant intellectual impairment, the proxy might be individuals who might have been assumed to have severe intellectual impairments before their access to communication technology.

Hey, Buddy, can you paradigm?

Participatory action research represents a fundamental paradigm shift in research. The implications of this research are presented in Table 24.2. The individual with a disability moves from being a powerless subject being experimented 'on', to a powerful participant conducting research 'with' the researcher. A shift from being a student to being a teacher. Subjects are expected to *follow* directions, participants are expected to help formulate the directions. Subjects are controlled, while co-researchers share in control. The role shifts from being passive and being acted on to an active role of taking action. The view of the individual with a disability shifts from one who is a 'victim who suffers from' a given disability, to being an expert on that disability. In short, they shift from being a patient to being a researcher. Finally, the individual moves from being the 'problem' being studied, to a part of the solution being sought.

Table 24.2. Reflections of the paradigm shift from traditional AAC research to PAR-based AAC research

From	To
Beneficiary	Benefactor
Powerless	Powerful
Survivor	Leader
Student	Teacher
Patient	Staff member
Controlled	Controller
Following directions	Giving directions
Client	Staff
Subject	Participant
Victim	Researcher

No tokens!

Participation of people with disabilities in research, especially those with communication or cognitive impairments, always opens the possibility of tokenism. When people with disabilities do participate in research, is it tokenism or is it meaningful participation? If the individual is filling a designated slot to be filled with little or no concern for their ability to contribute, it might be tokenism. If the needed support is not present, it is almost ensured that the participation will be superficial at best. Similarly, if the participants are called upon to give advice, but have no actual control, no vote or veto power, the real value of their contribution is greatly diminished.

If people with disabilities fill valued roles comparable to the professionals on the team, and are given support in accordance with their needs, they then are clearly participants. A word of caution about accommodating to the needs of participants with disabilities. There is a growing consciousness of the degree to which the needs of professionals and other collaborators are accommodated. If a valued researcher cannot meet early mornings, then adjustments are made. If a colleague requests materials in advance via e-mail, it is accommodated. This is the same level of recognition that people with disabilities are asking for.

Levels of support

Different people will need different levels of support in order to maximize the meaning of their participation. Sometimes, to support consumers, researchers will need to speak more slowly in meetings and may need to teach new team members the research jargon and acronyms insiders depend on. Other consumers, in order to participate more fully, will need access to agenda items in advance so that they can store responses to anticipated discussion topics. Effective consumer participation often requires financial as well as intellectual commitments. To gain the meaningful participation by people who use AAC, there often will be added expenses of long distance telephone calls, specialized transportation and personal assistants for people who need them. Researchers need to incorporate these expenses into the cost of doing business, and funding bodies need to see these expenses as essential direct costs.

A matter of compensation

The fact of the matter is that most participants in the research process are compensated for their efforts. Most have a financial interest of some kind in the work. Many are rewarded with academic promotion for their research, some publish books and sell them to others, and some are paid as consultants. Even the lowly graduate assistant is paid a token stipend and hopes for mention in an acknowledgement, or the prized co-author position. What is compensation for a person with a disability who participates in research? In the USA, many cannot receive financial compensation because it could result in the loss of their disability benefits, including health insurance. Some are interested in publishing, but few have jobs where 'publish or perish' is a reality. Participation in research by consumers is valuable to other researchers and to the research itself. It is not just a good idea, it is of intrinsic value. Ways need to be found to offer reciprocal value to these experts who assist from their personal expertise.

Action implications for ISAAC

The paradigm shift to PAR requires changes from individual researchers. It also requires change on the part of organizations. As an organization, several action steps appear to be appropriate to ISAAC, as listed in Table 24.3. The organization can have several levels of action. Members can be encouraged to make the shift to the PAR paradigm. The organizers of a biennial, international congress can influence members and others who would speak at and attend conferences by making conferences more participatory in nature. The publishers of the major journal in the field can shape the future of research in the field by revising authors' guidelines, and review practices to support research that is truly participatory.

Table 24.3. Ways ISAAC could support participatory action research

Develop a policy statement to encourage the participation of consumers in every stage of AAC research.

Include 'participatory' as a key word for indexing publications in *AAC*.

Feature consumer-led research discussions at conferences.

Assign consumers to editorial review positions in *AAC*.

Encourage authors to include information about the level and variety of consumer participation in manuscripts submitted for publication.

Establish a minimal threshold of consumer participation for research to be considered ethical.

Identify a list of augmented speakers who are prepared to participate in research nationally and internationally.

Develop and publish a list of suggestions to support augmented speakers to serve as co-researchers.

Urge funding bodies to include people with disabilities, including people who use AAC, as reviewers on funding proposals.

Encourage Institutional Review Boards/Human Subjects Committees to include people with disabilities on their committees.

Offer regular training sessions to prepare augmented speakers for new roles in research.

Develop specific guidelines for researchers on how to support to people who use AAC to maximize their ability to contribute.

Personal change comes first

There are any number of changes that ISAAC should support that would create a research environment that is more supportive of participatory action research. However, for individual researchers, there is an ethical imperative to begin today, and not wait for the organizational structure to be in place. In fact, it is likely that the best way to change the organization in the long run is to change individual research practices starting today. Not all AAC researchers are bound by the ASHA (American Speech-Language-Hearing Association) code of ethics, but each one can still take guidance from one of the core principles in that code:

> Individuals shall honor their responsibility to hold paramount the welfare of persons they serve professionally. (ASHA, 1998, p. 43)

There is no doubt that research is more expedient with just an inner circle of research colleagues, but then, as the old adage says 'Nothing worthwhile comes easy.' No one ever suggested that PAR was easy, just important.

Acknowledgement

The author would like to acknowledge the gracious assistance of his colleagues, Melanie Fried-Oken PhD, for sharing her professional insights, and Ms Janice Staehely for contributing valuable insights from her life experience as an augmented speaker.

Chapter 25
Examining the Perspectives of Families: Issues Related to Conducting Cross-cultural Research

M**ARY** B**LAKE** H**UER AND** H**OWARD** P. P**ARETTE** J**R**

Augmentative and alternative communication (AAC) service delivery programmes are expanding to previously underserved populations. Increasingly, consumers with communication needs are being identified across different cultural communities. The changing demographics of AAC users are reflected in recent literature (Huer, 1994; Soto, Huer and Taylor, 1997). The manner in which clients and their families view the intervention process affects outcomes of the service delivery (Parette and Brotherson, 1996). How consumers perceive healthcare professionals, feel about their disabilities, understand and can identify the various barriers to communication determines the success or failure of any prescribed AAC intervention.

When researchers are interested in interviewing individuals regarding their perceptions, feelings, reactions and knowledge bases about a given topic, they may employ qualitative research strategies (Patton, 1990; Taylor and Bogdan, 1984). Qualitative research methods employ a range of approaches (e.g. focus groups, participant observations and in-depth interviews). Useful information has been gathered about consumer perspectives through such methods. For example, Smith-Lewis and Ford (1987) reported one consumer's beliefs, feelings, attitudes and life experiences during an in-depth interview. In 1990, Huer and Lloyd summarized the perspectives from 165 different consumers through an analysis of published accounts. These records of 'conversations' and consumer perspectives provided invaluable information about attitudes towards professionals, communication partners and aided techniques.

Qualitative research approaches warrant careful planning and preparation before, during and after an investigation. These approaches, however, do yield interesting results, particularly when used in studies of families of AAC consumers. The purpose of this chapter is to discuss four methodological issues that emerged during the planning and implementation of one study using cross-cultural interviewing via focus groups: (a) selecting an appropriate research methodology, (b) preparing for cross-cultural focus group research, (c) the limitations and strengths of focus groups, and (d) the reliability checks necessary in order to validate the perspectives of families as well as researchers.

Rationale for selection of the study

By the year 2020, the largest non-European American population of AAC consumers (460 000) in the USA is projected within the Hispanic community (Soto, Huer and Taylor, 1997). Given estimates of population growth during the next 30 years, it is quite likely that service practitioners will be providing strategies to persons who are Spanish speaking. A review of the literature reveals the scarcity of information pertaining to therapy strategies, graphic symbols and communication aids which reflect the Hispanic culture. Therefore, the investigators wished to design a study which examined the perspectives of families within a Hispanic community. Specifically, the purpose of the study was to examine the perception of disability and communication issues within a Mexican-American community, using qualitative research approaches. During the course of the study several methodological issues emerged which had to be resolved. The research approach, as finally conducted, was selected for presentation and discussion within this chapter as an example of one research method which may be used for studying perspectives of consumers.

Selecting an Appropriate Research Methodology

A qualitative research methodology was selected for the study (Brotherson and Goldstein, 1992; Glaser and Strauss, 1967; Goetz and LeCompte, 1984; Krueger, 1988; Patton, 1990; Taylor and Bogdan, 1984). The research approach incorporated a series of focus groups with families within a Mexican-American community in southern California. Focus groups are useful for researchers to gain a holistic understanding of the nature and perception of intervention services provided to children with disabilities and their families (Bogden and Biklen, 1992; Brotherson, 1994; Glesne and Peshkin, 1992). Proponents of focus group approaches, however, have not discussed their methodological applications to culturally diverse families.

A deeper understanding of the various human-made systems of 'meaning' which exist across cultural communities is necessary if practitioners are to achieve the primary objective of the AAC intervention process – to seek strategies which facilitate communication between partners. Since culture permeates who and what an individual perceives, and what people like to communicate about, practitioners must take time to acquire greater knowledge about the cultures of the individuals they serve (Battle, 1998; Lynch and Hanson, 1992; Roseberry-McKibbin, 1995).

There are several ways to learn about other cultures. One strategy is to have informal conversations with a person or persons in a community different from one's own. Another way is to observe people from differing cultural backgrounds in environments where typical communicative interactions occur, e.g. in the home, lunch room or market place (Soto et al., 1997). If possible, it is always beneficial to ask individual persons within a given community to evaluate or comment regarding the professional services they have already received or anticipate receiving in the future. It is appropriate to ask clients about their feelings, reactions to, and perceptions about AAC practices (Parette et al., 1996). Multiple perspectives provide professionals with several differing viewpoints from which to gain a greater understanding of a community different from their own.

Summaries describing Hispanic culture, lifestyles, family values, and communication styles and patterns are readily available to persons interested in human communication (Battle, 1998; Bennett, 1988; Curt, 1984; Dodd, Nelson and Peralez, 1988; Grossman, 1984; Langdon, 1992; Lynch and Stein, 1987; Marin and Marin, 1991). However, summaries describing the potential impact of culture on AAC practices are not (Cronen and Mercaitis, 1998; Hetzroni and Harris, 1996; Huer, 1997a,b,c; Soto et al., 1997). Therefore, it was necessary to learn as much as possible about the possible impact of culture on the practice of AAC. In particular, it was important to review the literatures regarding the Hispanic community, as the focus of the study was on Mexican-American families.

Preparing for conducting cross-cultural research

The US Department of Education has funded a Special Project (Parette and VanBiervliet, 1995) to conduct focus groups and structured interviews with Hispanic families to understand their issues regarding AAC decision-making. The funded project represented a preliminary effort to determine the perspectives of families with regard to their experiences within an AAC service delivery programme.

Selecting and training a moderator

The moderator of the focus groups (first author), a speech-language pathologist, received special training from a national expert skilled in focus group/structured interview methodologies. This training was a part of preparation for a larger study (Parette et al., 1996) which examined the impact of culture on family decision-making in AAC. The training was extensive, and telephone follow-up was conducted between the moderator and trainer. The moderator had previous experience in qualitative research methodology (Huer and Lloyd, 1990), and in examining first person perspectives of AAC users. Also, the moderator lived in southern California and was the Project Director of a federally funded personnel preparation training grant which focused on AAC across cultures. The moderator was familiar with the Mexican-American community through personal and professional experiences. However, the moderator did not speak Spanish. Therefore, it was necessary to plan for an interpreter.

Ideally, in most qualitative approaches, the families and the moderator should speak the same language and share the same culture. However, in the present investigation the 'ideal' was not possible. Therefore, specific preparations were made to approximate the ideal, and to minimize the effects resulting from communication styles and patterns introduced through the use of two languages from two linguistic communities, and two cultures.

Developing a questioning probe

Based on literature reviews that suggested potential areas of concern related to AAC decision-making, an interview protocol was developed for use with each focus group and structured family interview. During each focus group, the moderator was instructed to utilize a set of probe questions to direct the interview. Table 25.1 includes the initial probe questions that were selected before the interviews. During the moderator

Table 25.1. Probe questions for family focus groups and structured interviews

What are (were) your goals or expectations for the AAC device that your child will receive (received)?

Have your goals or expectations about the potential of the AAC device changed since your child has been using the device?

Describe in what ways they have changed (if a device is present)?

In what ways, if any, has or might the AAC device affect/ed your family?

Other probe questions for use, as appropriate:

Do you see it affecting (or has it affected) roles that you must assume?

Do you think it would affect organization of the home environment?

Do you think it would affect relationships with family members?

Do you think it would affect demands placed on your time?

Do you think it would affect levels of stress that you currently experience?

Do you think it would affect your relationship with others in the community?

Do you think it would affect your ability to take your child into the community, to eat at restaurants, or other social or recreational activities?

What have been your greatest concerns in working with professionals in getting your child's AAC device?

What should the role of professionals be when trying to work with you to get your child an AAC device?

What about AAC devices were important to you but not considered by professionals?

If you could tell professionals how to work better with families when trying to identify AAC devices for children, what would you say?

How, if at all, are the values and beliefs of professionals different from yours? How did these differences affect what happened when decisions were being made about devices?

If there anything else about this subject that I haven't asked you about?

training, instruction was provided regarding the need to be sensitive to issues that might emerge during discussions that deviated from the probe questions. The moderator, though guided by the probe questions, was encouraged to introduce open-ended elaboration, as appropriate.

The literature reviews identified issues which might pertain to the process of the AAC intervention. Several expert panel members reviewed the probe questions before the interviews in preparation for the data collection phase of the study. The focus group moderator would not be obligated to use all of the questions, but the questions would be available to guide the families through presumed critical issues relevant to the provision of services to children having disabilities. The final format selected was a focus group format where the moderator led a general discussion and probed into topics which the families introduced.

Working with an interpreter

Because the moderator was English-speaking and the families would be speaking Spanish, it was necessary to select an interpreter. Soto, Huer and Taylor (1997) suggest two criteria for the selection of an interpreter: (a) the interpreter should be '*bilingual* (i.e. proficient in both the language of the family and the service provider); and (b) *bicultural* (i.e. able to understand and appreciate the culture of both parties, and able to convey the subtle nuances of each)' (p. 411). Additionally, the investigators searched for an interpreter who was familiar with the intervention process and professional jargon used in the clinical process, and perceived as trustworthy by the families participating in the focus groups (Erickson and Iglesias, 1986; Hanson, 1992). The interpreter selected for the present study was a speech-language pathologist with extensive experience. Although her culture was European American and her first language was English, she was in a 12-year bicultural marriage with a Mexican-American man with a large family whose first language was Spanish. She earned her PhD from Temple University, within the Hispanic Emphasis Program in Philadelphia. She had 24 years as a bilingual speaker, with a score of 4.0 on a 5.0 scale from the Foreign Service Institute (FSI) Exam in Spanish. In addition, she had served as the bilingual diagnostician for two school districts in California, completing over 100 assessments in Spanish. Given the interpreter's extensive training with the California State Department of Education and her Volunteer Service to America (VISTA) experiences with Mexican nationals as well as with Puerto Rican children in a Head Start programme, the investigators suggested that the two criteria established by Soto et al. (1997) were met. Not only did the interpreter possess the skills necessary for working with Spanish-speaking families, she also had worked on an AAC personal preparation training grant (Huer, 1993) and was somewhat familiar with the professional jargon in the field of AAC. Therefore, the researchers felt that the preparations for the interviews were as close to the ideal as possible given the circumstances.

Gaining access

Permission to conduct the study within a public elementary school district located within a predominately Mexican-American community in southern California was requested. While securing approval from the school district, the moderator and interpreter spoke with researchers, as well as community liaisons to develop trust and rapport within the community.

Selecting focus group participants

After intensive correspondence with the administration within the school district, permission was granted, and the participants were invited to the school for a day. Four criteria were established for selection of the participants. The participants were: (a) members of the Mexican-American community; (b) parents of children who had been evaluated for an AAC device, but had not yet received a device; (c) parents having children who had already received an AAC device; and (d) parents available to attend the focus group on the school site on the day scheduled. A total of seven family members participated during two focus group interviews: four family members of children with AAC devices (Alpha Talkers); and three family members of children who expected to receive AAC devices, but had not yet received them.

Special arrangements

Special ethnic foods were served. All families received a small stipend and gifts of food for their participation. The focus groups were conducted during a 1-day, 8-hour, social occasion with refreshments and breaks.

Data collection

As the data collection phase of the study began, the moderator noted that changes needed to be incorporated into the process. Even though careful preparations had been included in the planning for the interviews, a few adjustments were necessary during data collection. Soto et al. (1997) discussed the necessity to understand verbal as well as non-verbal forms of communication that may be utilized by particular cultural groups. As the moderator began the interviews, it immediately became apparent that the structured interview format, and the list of probe questions which had been prepared for the families, tended to create a sense of discomfort. The nature of focus groups, i.e. discussions with a moderator, was unfamiliar to the participants. The preferred conversational styles of the participants were observed by the moderator. It was interesting to note that the moderator and interpreter, in planning for the interviews, had focused on a style which is described as low-context. On the one hand, the answers to the probe questions were expected to be verbal and linguistic in communication style, with less reliance on gestures and environmental clues. But, on the other hand, the families' preferred conversational styles were high-context. That is, in communities where the conversational style is closely linked to context, there is heavy reliance on non-verbal cues and gestures. In addition, there is an expectation of more formality between the families and the moderator than would be observed between persons within communities where the conversational style is not linked so closely to contextual cues. Sensing the difference between the conversational styles of the moderator and participants, the moderator adapted her style to one that appeared to be more comfortable for the families (Soto et al., 1997). In addition, she modified the wording of the probe questions (see Table 25.2) and reduced the amount of paperwork initially planned. The moderator began the interviews by asking the families to simply 'Tell her about their children.'

Table 25.2. Modified probe questions asked during the focus groups

---

I would like for you to tell me a little bit about your child.
How does your child talk to you?
If your child does not speak to you, how does he communicate with his aunt and other relatives and with strangers and other people?
Can you tell me some stories about when your son used his communication device and with whom?
Would your son demonstrate the use of his device for me?
How has this device been used within your family?
How does your child feel about the device?
Are there any problems with the device that you worry about or that we can make better to help you or your child to use it?
When the school made the recommendations to you, did you feel included in the selection of the device and pictures?
Does the fact that the therapy is in English make it difficult at home with your friends and family?
Has this device changed the communication in your home?
Is there anything you could tell us so that we could be more helpful in the future?

Thus, during the data collection stage of this project the moderator balanced the need to maintain adequate research stability and integrity of protocol and procedures with respect for differences in family culture and comfort levels. It was a fine line between gaining the family voice and adhering to the research agenda. The families were initially not comfortable during the focus groups. Several of the probe questions were not used, as they did not fit in the flow of the conversations. Sometimes it appeared as if participants were fearful of 'government', especially when asked personal information such as that necessary to complete the demographic questionnaires. During these occasions, videotaping and completion of questionnaires ceased, as it appeared that too much paperwork hindered the participant's willingness to speak. As appropriate, some of the paperwork pertaining to demographic information was set aside till the end of the focus groups.

The moderator conducted the focus groups at the school site. The interpreter was present during both focus groups. The moderator and interpreter were aware of the need to be culturally sensitive during each of the 2-hour interviews which were arranged at a time and day on the elementary school campus, a convenient location for the family members. Several of the families took time off work, viewing the interviews as important and allowing for as much time as necessary. Two graduate students assisted the moderator in audiotaping and videotaping the interviews. One of the graduate students was a Mexican-American man who also assisted in the translations and interpretations as necessary throughout the interviews. The interpreter assisted the participants with the completion of questionnaires and consent forms.

Content analysis

After the data collection, the interviews were transcribed in English. The transcripts for each of the focus groups (a total of seven persons) were analysed simultaneously because the purpose of the research was to collect perspectives of Mexican-American families, not to compare the perspectives of families without AAC devices to those with devices. The videotapes were viewed and transcriptions read and reread during the content analysis/theme development phases. Following a methodology similar to that reported by Smith-Lewis and Ford (1987), a 'constant comparative method of data analysis' (p. 14) was employed during the analysis of the transcripts. The content was analysed as the issues and themes emerged from the family voices (Johnson and Montague, 1992; Patton, 1990).

The typed transcripts (English translations) were analysed following procedures traditionally utilized. Passages in the typed, English transcripts were marked with notations about the topic of the text. After reading and rereading the families' words, synthesis statements were written. Following established qualitative analysis procedures (Patton, 1990; Taylor and Bogdan, 1984; Tesch, 1990), the investigators employed the constant comparative approach of continued reading and rereading of the transcripts in order to identify major themes or issues for families. Quotations which reflected similar topics were grouped during the topical thematic analysis. The frequency of each topic was noted and compared with the frequency of occurrence of other topics to determine whether all of the participants expressed the same view or had different opinions. By repeatedly returning to the data, the investigators selected and represented the perceptions of the participants rather than their own presuppositions (Huer and Lloyd, 1990; Smith-Lewis and Ford, 1987). Issues were organized and integrated into the major themes that emerged. After reaching a point of saturation, the final themes were presented to members within the Mexican-American community for stakeholder reviews. The final step was to select quotes summarizing the themes on which everyone agreed.

Reliability and validity checks on perspectives

Several different techniques were incorporated into the research approach in order to ensure that the data reported were valid and reliable. Brotherson and Goldstein (1992) have noted that issues of credibility of data need to be addressed to enhance rigour of design. Credibility pertains to the integrity and congruence between constructed realities of the families and those realities identified by the research team (Guba, 1981). Comparing multiple perspectives from researchers, families, and expert outsiders completed data triangulation (Brotherson and Goldstein, 1992). Interrater reliability for theme categorization was determined utilizing specific quotations within the data.

The recurring process of presenting information and checking interpretations by different individuals was included during the analysis in order to check the credibility of the research. Persons from a Hispanic community who did not participate in the focus groups gave feedback and reflection on the findings of the study (e.g. Does this summary reflect what you think was said? Do you have any additional comments?). Member checks resulted in clarifying concepts and perspectives. Finally, comparisons of the results and the literature were used to further strengthen the credibility of the findings.

Summary and future directions

Focus group approaches, as evidenced by the example included within this chapter, provide the opportunity for researchers to gain new insight into consumer perspectives because the researcher is afforded the opportunity to listen to the stories of families first-hand. During focus groups, direct exchanges of feelings, perceptions and opinions are shared by family members. The researcher has the opportunity to clarify, ask additional questions, and to paraphrase the messages for acceptance or denial by the participants themselves because the researcher is close to the data source during the data collection process. Similarly, the families are more involved within this research approach. In fact, the messages provided by the families, and what the families choose to talk about, directly influence the outcomes of the research.

At the same time, focus group approaches are not without limitations. Several methodological issues encountered when preparing for the interviews with families were noted within this chapter, e.g. securing an interpreter, eliminating probe questions during the interviews, and attending to the conversational styles while attempting to adhere to probe questions. Even with careful preparations, modifications had to be made during each phase of the research. These findings are in agreement with several authors who have expertise on cultural and linguistic diversity who state that during preparation for meeting families it is important to modify procedures when working with non-English proficient individuals (Erickson and Iglesias, 1986; Kayser, 1998; Soto et al., 1997).

In addition to changes in data collection and analysis, there were other issues which emerged in this approach. For example, the strategy of 'story-telling' was much more comfortable for the participants than was a more structured interview format. This was an excellent example of how the existing professional literature is inadequate in its delineation of appropriate interviewing strategies for Hispanic populations. Discussions of 'low' versus 'high' context cultures (e.g. Lynch and Hanson, 1992) typically fail to provide the level of specificity needed for focus group research, emphasizing the usefulness of the findings of this study for future researchers.

Given that focus group methodology fails to provide generalizable findings to larger populations, its utility may lie solely with providing researchers with perspectives unique to families who participate in the process. Such information would be advantageous for intervention planning. Also, when conducting interviews, whether cross-culturally or within one culture, it is not always possible to completely eliminate bias between the researcher and the consumer. That is, there is a 'social desirability' factor in which the families will want to please or meet the expectations of the professional (Gloria Soto, personal communication, 27 August 1998). These limitations, in the authors' opinions, are overcome by the wealth of information which may be collected using focus group approaches. The use of reliability and validity checks, as previously discussed, are introduced to counterbalance the issues pertaining to sample size and social desirability.

Future, well-controlled studies should be conducted which incorporate the methods discussed within this chapter. Family members need to be included during the initial design of the study, as well as during the analysis and interpretation as a check and balance on the outcomes of the process. Far too few studies pertaining to the perspectives of consumers are available, in contrast to the numbers of consumers who are receiving AAC services. As future demographic projections indicate that practitioners will be serving an increasingly cultural and linguistically diverse population, many more cross-cultural studies will be necessary to learn about the perceptions of families from within other communities.

In summary, focus group approaches are useful for examining the perspectives of families of consumers who utilize augmentative and alternative communication. With careful preparation, interviews between family members and professionals will yield meaningful information for practitioners setting up AAC interventions. The need for planning before conducting consumer research, however, cannot be overstated.

Establishing a research plan for examining consumer perspectives across cultures involves attending to several critical methodological issues such as:

1. understanding the rationale for the study;
2. selecting a research approach;
3. preparing before meeting the family members;
4. determining the process through which the data will be collected;
5. securing any necessary training, or competencies before beginning the study;
6. working with interpreters, where applicable;
7. including experts, and representatives from the community in pre-planning;
8. securing permission for use of human subjects;
9. incorporating reliability and validity checks on perspectives; and
10. building in flexibility to maintain research integrity with respect for differences in family culture and comfort levels.

Researchers who incorporate these guiding principles into their work will find that they will gain greater insight into the perspectives of families each time they collect data. The perspectives of consumers are too important to be overlooked, or limited by inappropriate and limited research methodologies.

References

Aaron, P. G., Keetay, V., Boyd, M., Palmatier, S. and Wacks, J. (1998). Spelling without phonology: A study of deaf and hearing children. Reading and Writing: An Interdisciplinary Journal, 10, 1–22.

Abberley, P. (1992). Counting us out: A discussion of the OPCS disability surveys. Disability, Handicap and Society, 7, 139–155.

Adams, M. J. (1990). Beginning to Read. Cambridge, MA: MIT Press.

Affleck, G., Tennen, H., Rowe, J., Roscher, B. and Walker, L. (1989). Effects of formal support on mother's adaptation to hospital to home transition of high-risk infants: The benefits and costs of helping. Child Development, 60, 488–501.

Ahlsén, E. (1998, July). Aphasia and text writing. Paper presented at the Second European Conference of Writing, Speech and Context, University of Nottingham, Nottingham, UK.

Allaire, J., Gressard, R., Blackman, J. and Hostler, S. (1991). Children with severe speech impairments: Caregiver survey of AAC use. Augmentative and Alternative Communication, 7, 248–255.

Allen, W. T. (1998). Read My Lips: It's My Choice. St Paul, MN: Minnesota Governor's Council on Developmental Disabilities.

Alm, N. (1994). Ethical issues in AAC research. In J. Brodin and E. Björk Åkesson (Eds), Methodological Issues in Research in Augmentative and Alternative Communication. Proceedings of the Third ISAAC Research Symposium (pp. 98–104). Jönköping, Sweden, Jönköping University Press.

Alm, N., Arnott, J. L. and Newell, A. F. (1992). Prediction and conversational momentum in an augmentative communication system. Communications of the ACM, 35(5), 46–57.

Alm, N. and Newell, A. F. (1996). Being an interesting conversation partner. In S. von Tetzchner and M. H. Jensen (Eds), Augmentative and Alternative Communication: European Perspectives (pp. 171–181). London: Whurr.

American Speech-Language-Hearing Association. (1998). Code of ethics. Asha, 40 (Suppl. 18).

Angelo, D. (1998). Amish study illuminates use of AAC on rare disorder. In J. K. Jensen, M. J. Montesano and M. Moore (Eds), ASHA Leader, 3(23), 9.

Angelo, D., Jones, S. and Kokoska, S. (1995). Family perspective on augmentative and alternative communication: Families of young children. Augmentative and Alternative Communication, 11, 193–201.

Angelo, D., Kokoska, S. and Jones, S. (1996). Family perspective on augmentative and alternative communication: Families of adolescents and young adults. Augmentative and Alternative Communication, 12, 13–20.

Arnott, J. L. (1990). The communication prosthesis: A problem of human–computer integration. In Proceedings of European Conference on the Advancement of Rehabilitation Technology (ECART1) (section 3.1.1–3.1.5). Hoensbroek, The Netherlands: ECART.

Arnott, J., Hannan, J. M. and Woodburn, R. J. (1993). Linguistic prediction for disabled users of computer-mediated communication. In The Swedish Handicap Institute (Ed.), Proceedings of the European Conference on the Advancement of Rehabilitation Technology (ECART2) (section 11.1). Stockholm: Kommentus.

Aslin, R. N., Jusczyk, P. W. and Pisoni, D. B. (1998). Speech and auditory processing during infancy: Constraints and precursors to language. In W. Damon, D. Kuhn and R. S. Siegler (Eds), Handbook of Child Psychology: Vol. 2. Cognition, Perception, and Language (5th edn, pp. 147–198). London: Wiley.

Aspis, S. (1997). Self-advocacy for people with learning difficulties: Does it have a future? Disability and Society, 12, 647–654.

Atkinson, M. (1992). Children's Syntax: An Introduction to Principles and Parameters Theory. Oxford, UK: Blackwell.

Bailey, B. R. and Downing, J. (1994). Using visual accents to enhance attending to communication symbols for students with severe multiple disabilities. RE:view, 26, 101–118.

Bailey, D., Buysse, V. and Palsha, S. (1990). Self ratings of professional knowledge and skills in early intervention. Journal of Special Education, 23, 423–435.

Bailey, D. B. and Simeonsson, R. J. (1984). Critical issues underlying research and intervention with families of young handicapped children. Journal of the Division for Early Childhood, 9, 38–48.

Bailey, D. B. and Simeonsson, R. J. (1988). Assessing needs of families with handicapped infants. Journal of Special Education, 22, 117–127.

Baker, A. (1998, August). Me Tarzan, you Jane: Can you communicate without language? The linguistic perspective. Presented at the Eighth Biennial Conference of the International Society for Augmentative and Alternative Communication, Dublin, Ireland.

Baker, B. (1982). Minspeak. Byte, 9, 186–202.

Baker, B. (1987). Semantic compaction for sub-sentence vocabulary units compared to other encoding and prediction systems. In Proceedings of the Tenth Annual Conference on Rehabilitation Technology (pp. 118–120). Washington, DC: RESNA.

Baker, C. (1995). A Parents' and Teachers' Guide to Bilingualism. Clevedon, UK: Multilingual Matters.

Balandin, S. and Iacono, T. (1997). Impact of a socially valid vocabulary on interactions between employees with severe communication impairment and their non-disabled peers (Research report 1). Canberra, Australia: Australian Government Publishing.

Balandin, S. and Iacono, T. (1998). A few well chosen words. Augmentative and Alternative Communication, 14, 147–161.

Balandin, S. and Morgan, J. (1997). Adults with cerebral palsy: What's happening? Journal of Intellectual and Developmental Disability, 22, 109–124.

Ball, J. E. and Ling, D. T. (1995). Spoken language processing in the persona conversational assistant. In P. Dalsgaard and L. B. Larsen (Eds), Proceedings of ESCA Workshop on Spoken Dialogue Systems (pp. 109–112). Aalborg, Denmark: ESCA and Center for Person Communication.

Ball, L. J., Marvin, C. A., Beukelman, D. R., Lasker, J. and Rupp, D. (1998). Generic small talk use by preschool children. In Proceedings of ISAAC '98 Conference (pp. 170–171). Dublin, Ireland: ISAAC/Ashfield Publications.

Bandura, A. (1992). Social cognitive theory. In R. Vasta (Ed.), Six Theories of Child Development (pp. 1–60). London: Jessica Kingsley.

Barnett, S. and Bax, M. (1996). Communication and young adults with cerebral palsy (Report for SCOPE). London.

Barnett, S. and Woll, B. (1998). Towards a sociolinguistic perspective on augmentative and alternative communication. Augmentative and Alternative Communication, 14, 200–211.

Barron, R. (1986). Word recognition in early reading: A review of the direct and indirect access hypothesis. Cognition, 24, 93–119.

Basil, C. (1992). Social interaction and learned helplessness in severely disabled children. Augmentative and Alternative Communication, 8, 188–199.

Basil, C. (1994). Family involvement in the intervention process. In J. Brodin and E. Björck-Åkesson (Eds), Methodological Issues in Research in Augmentative and Alternative Communication. Proceedings of the Third ISAAC Research Symposium (pp. 89–95). Jönköping, Sweden: Jönköping University Press.

Bates, E., Bretherton, I. and Snyder, L. (1988). From First Words to Grammar. Cambridge, UK: Cambridge University Press.

Bateson, G. (1972). Steps to an Ecology of Mind. New York: Ballantine.

Batshaw, M. L. and Perret, Y. M. (1992). Children With Handicaps: A Medical Primer (3rd edn). Baltimore: Paul H. Brookes.

Battle, D. E. (Ed.). (1998). Communication Disorders in Multicultural Populations (2nd edn). Boston: Butterworth-Heinemann.

Bedrosian, J. L. (1997). Language acquisition in young AAC system users: Issues and directions for future research. Augmentative and Alternative Communication, 13, 179–185.

Beeferman, D., Berger, A. and Lafferty, J. (1997). A model of lexical attraction and repulsion. In Proceedings of the 35th Annual Meeting of the Association for Computational Linguistics and the 8th Conference of the European Chapter of the ACL (pp. 373–380). Madrid, Spain: Association for Computational Linguistics.

Begun, A. L. (1996). Family systems and family-centered care. In P. Rosin, A. D. Whitehead, L. I. Tuchman, G. S. Jesien, A. L. Begun and L. Irwin (Eds), Partnerships in Family-centered Care: A Guide to Collaborative Early Intervention (pp. 33–64). Baltimore: Paul H. Brookes.

Bennett, A. T. (1988). Gateways to powerlessness: Incorporating Hispanic deaf children and families into formal schooling. Disability, Handicap and Society, 3, 119–151.

Berger, K. S. and Thompson, R. A. (Eds). (1996). The Developing Person Through Childhood. New York: Worth.

Berko, R. M., Wolvin, A. D. and Wolvin, D. R. (1977). Communication: A Social and Career Focus. Boston: Houghton Mifflin.

Berninger, V. W. (1987). Global, component, and serial processing of printed words in beginning reading. Journal of Experimental Child Psychology, 43, 387–418.

Berninger, V. and Gans, B. (1986). Language profiles in nonspeaking individuals of normal intelligence with cerebral palsy. Augmentative and Alternative Communication, 2, 45–50.

Bernstein, B. (1971, 1975). Class, Codes, and Control (Vols 1, 2). London: Routledge and Kegan Paul.

Bersani, H. (1996). Leadership in developmental disabilities: Where we've been, where we are, and where we're going. In G. Dybwad and H. Bersani (Eds), New Voices: Self-advocacy by People with Disabilities. Cambridge, MA: Brookline Books.

Bersani, H. A., Fried-Oken, M., Anctil, T. and Staehely, J. (1998, August). Warning: High school transition can be hazardous to your AAC! Seminar presented at the Eighth Biennial Conference of the International Society for Augmentative and Alternative Communication, Dublin, Ireland.

Beukelman, D. R. and Ansel, B. M. (1995). Research priorities in augmentative and alternative communication. Augmentative and Alternative Communication, 11, 131–134.

Beukelman, D. R. and Mirenda, P. (1992). Augmentative and Alternative Communication: Management of Severe Communication Disorders in Children and Adults. Baltimore: Paul H. Brookes.

Bickley, C. and Hunnicutt, S. (1993). A voice-accessed predictive knowledge-based engineering system. In M. Binion (Ed.), Proceedings of the RESNA International '93 Conference (pp. 148–150). Washington, DC: RESNA.

Bickley, C., Hunnicutt, S. and Lamel, L. (1993). Alternative strategies for creating AutoCAD drawings. In S. Hunnicutt, B. Granström and K.-E. Spens (Eds), Proceedings of an ESCA Workshop: Speech and Language Technology for Disabled Persons (pp. 103–106). Stockholm: ESCA and KTH, Department of Speech Communication and Music Acoustics.

Bickley, C., Jones, C. S., Wang, J., Tan, H. Z., Ebert, R. and Horowitz, D. M. (1993). Case study of voice control of AutoCAD. In the Swedish Handicap Institute (Ed.), Proceedings of the European Conference on the Advancement of Rehabilitation Technology (ECART2) (section 7.3). Stockholm: Kommentus.

Bigby, C. (1995). Is there a hidden group of older people with intellectual disability and from whom are they hidden? Lessons from a recent case finding study. Australia and New Zealand Journal of Developmental Disabilities, 20, 15–24.

Bijou, S. W. (1992). Behavior analysis. In R. Vasta (Ed.), Six Theories of Child Development (pp. 61–84). London: Jessica Kingsley.

Billeaud, F. (1993). Communication Disorders in Infants and Toddlers: Assessment and Intervention. Boston: Andover.

Birenbaum, A. (1971). The mentally retarded child in the home and the family life cycle. Journal of Health and Social Behavior, 12, 55–65.

Bishop, D. (1982). Test of Reception of Grammar. Manchester, UK: University of Manchester, Department of Psychology.

Bishop, D. (1997). Uncommon Understanding: Development and Disorders of Language Comprehension in Children. East Sussex, UK: Psychology Press.

Bishop, D. V. M. and Robson, J. (1989a). Accurate non-word spelling despite congenital inability to speak: Phoneme-grapheme conversion does not require subvocal articulation. British Journal of Psychology, 80, 1–13.

Bishop, D. V. M. and Robson, J. (1989b). Unimpaired short-term memory and rhyme judgements in congenitally speechless individuals: Implications for the notion of articulatory coding. Quarterly Journal of Experimental Psychology, 41A, 124–140.

Bishop, K., Rankin, J. and Mirenda, P. (1994). Impact of graphic symbol use on reading acquisition. Augmentative and Alternative Communication, 10, 113–125.

Björck-Åkesson, E., Granlund, M. and Olsson, C. (1996). Collaborative problem solving in communication intervention. In S. von Tetzchner and M. H. Jensen (Eds), Augmentative and Alternative Communication: European Perspectives (pp. 324–341). London: Whurr.

Björck-Åkesson, E. and Lindsay, P. (Eds). (1997). Communication... Naturally: Theoretical and Methodological Issues in Augmentative and Alternative Communication. Proceedings of the Fourth ISAAC Research Symposium. Västerås, Sweden: Mälardalen University Press.

Blackstone, S. (1990). Early prevention of severe communication disorders. Augmentative Communication News, 3(1), 1–3.

Blackstone, S. (1994). What is and who is a family? Augmentative Communication News, 7(6), 1–8.

Blackstone, S. (1995). Outcomes in AAC. Augmentative Communication News. 7(1), 1–8.

Blackstone, S. (1997). The intake's connected to the input. Augmentative Communication News, 10(1), 1–3.

Blackstone, S. and Pressman, H. (1995). Outcomes in AAC conference report: Alliance '95. Monterey, CA: Augmentative Communication.

Blackstone, S. and Williams, M. (1994). Family involvement in the AAC intervention process: Conceptual and methodological issues. In J. Brodin and E. Björck-Åkesson (Eds), Methodological Issues in Research in Augmentative and Alternative Communication. Proceedings of the Third ISAAC Research Symposium (pp. 82–88). Jönköping, Sweden: Jönköping University Press.

Bleile, K. (1998). Where words come from: The origins of expressive language. In R. Paul (Ed.), Exploring the Speech-language Connection (pp. 119–138). Baltimore: Paul H. Brookes.

Blischak, D. M. and Lloyd, L. L. (1996). Multimodal augmentative and alternative communication: Case study. Augmentative and Alternative Communication, 12, 37–46.

Blischak, D. M., Lloyd, L. L. and Fuller, D. R. (1997). Terminology issues. In L. L. Lloyd, D. R. Fuller and H. H. Arvidson (Eds), Augmentative and Alternative Communication: A Handbook of Principles and Practices (pp. 38–42). Boston: Allyn and Bacon.

Blischak, D., Loncke, F. and Waller, A. (1997). Intervention for persons with developmental disabilities. In L. L. Lloyd, D. R. Fuller and H. H. Arvidson (Eds), Augmentative and Alternative Communication: A Handbook of Principles and Practices (pp. 299–339). Boston: Allyn and Bacon.

Blischak, D. M. and Wasson, C. (1997). Sensory impairments. In L. L. Lloyd, D. R. Fuller and H. H. Arvidson (Eds), Augmentative and Alternative Communication: A Handbook of Principles and Practices (pp. 254–279). Boston: Allyn and Bacon.

Blockberger, S. (1994). From efficacy to effectiveness in AAC intervention. Unpublished manuscript, University of British Columbia, Vancouver, British Columbia, Canada.

Blockberger, S. (1995). AAC intervention and early conceptual and lexical development. Journal of Speech-Language Pathology and Audiology, 19, 221–232.

Blockberger, S. (1998, August). Grammatical morphology acquisition by children unable to speak. Presented at the Eighth Biennial Conference of the International Society for Augmentative and Alternative Communication, Dublin, Ireland.

Bloom, L. (1973). One Word at a Time. The Hague, The Netherlands: Mouton.

Bloom, L. and Lahey, M. (1978). Language Development and Language Disorders. New York: Wiley.

Bloomberg, K., Karlan, G. R. and Lloyd, L. L. (1990). The comparative translucency of initial lexical items represented by five graphic symbol systems. Journal of Speech and Hearing Research, 33, 717–725.

Blumer, H. (1969). Symbolic Interactionism: Perspective and Method. Englewood Cliffs, NJ: Prentice Hall.

Bogden, R. and Biklen, S. K. (1992). Qualitative Research for Education: An Introduction to Theory and Methods (2nd edn). Boston: Allyn and Bacon.

Bonham, G. S., Piza, L. M., Marchand, C. B., Harris, C., White, D. and Schalock, R. L. (1998). Ask Me! The Quality of Life of Marylanders with Developmental Disabilities Receiving DDA Funded Supports. Annapolis, MD: The Arc of Maryland.

Booth, T. and Booth, W. (1996). Sounds of silence: Narrative research with inarticulate subjects. Disability and Society, 11, 55–69.

Bowlby, J. (1988). Developmental psychiatry comes of age. American Journal of Psychiatry, 145, 1–10.

Boyes-Braem, P. (1973). A Study of the Acquisition of the Dez in American Sign Language. Manuscript, University of California at Berkeley.

Braine, M. (1988). Modelling the acquisition of linguistic structure. In Y. Levy, I. Schlesinger and M. Braine (Eds), Categories and Processes in Language Acquisition (pp. 217–260). Hillsdale, NJ: Erlbaum.

Brett, E. M. (1983). The blind retarded child. In K. Wybar and D. Taylor (Eds), Pediatric Ophthalmology: Current Aspects (pp. 113–122). New York: Marcel Dekker.

Bronfenbrenner, U. (1979). The Ecology of Human Development. Cambridge, MA: Harvard University Press.

Bronfenbrenner, U. (1992). Ecological systems theory. In R. Vasta (Ed.), Six Theories of Child Development (pp. 187–249). London: Jessica Kingsley.

Brotherson, M. J. (1994). Interactive focus group interviewing: A qualitative research method in early intervention. Topics in Early Childhood Special Education, 14, 101–118.

Brotherson, M. J. and Goldstein, B. L. (1992). Quality design of focus groups in early childhood special education research. Journal of Early Intervention, 16, 334–342.

Brown, P. F., DellaPietra, S. A., DellaPietra, V. J., Lai, J. C. and Mercer, R. L. (1992). An estimate of an upper bound for the entropy of English. Computational Linguistics, 18(1), 31–40.

Brown, R. (1973). A First Language: The Early Stages. Cambridge, MA: Harvard University Press.

Bruder, M. (1997). The effectiveness of specific educational/developmental curricula for children with established disabilities. In M. Guralnick (Ed.), Effectiveness of Early Intervention (pp. 523–548). London: Paul H. Brookes.

Bryant, P. E., MacLean, M., Bradley, L. L. and Crossland, J. (1990). Rhyme and alliteration, phoneme detection, and learning to read. Developmental Psychology, 26, 429–438.

Bryen, D. N., Slesaransky, G. and Baker, D. B. (1995). Augmentative communication and empowerment supports: A look at outcomes. Augmentative and Alternative Communication, 11, 79–88.

Bulwer, S. (1644). Chirologia or the Natural Language of the Hand. London.

Burnett, J. K., Klabunde, C. R. and Britell, C. W. (1991). Voice and head pointer operated electronics computer assisted design workstations for individuals with severe upper extremity impairments. In J. J. Presperin (Ed.), Proceedings of the 14th Annual Conference (RESNA '91) (pp. 48–49). Washington, DC: RESNA.

Byrne, B. (1992). Studies in the acquisition procedure for reading: Rationale, hypotheses, and data. In P. B. Gough, L. C. Ehri and R. Treiman (Eds), Reading Acquisition (pp. 1–34). Hillsdale, NJ: Erlbaum.

Byrne, B. and Carroll, M. (1989). Learning artificial orthographies: Further evidence of a nonanalytic acquisition procedure. Memory and Cognition, 17, 311–317.

Byrne, B. and Fielding-Barnsley, R. (1989). Phonemic awareness and letter knowledge in the child's acquisition of the alphabetic principle. Journal of Educational Psychology, 81, 313–321.

Calculator, S. (1988). Promoting the acquisition and generalization of conversation skills by individuals with severe disabilities. Augmentative and Alternative Communication, 4, 94–103.

Calculator, S. (1997). Fostering early language acquisition and AAC use: Exploring reciprocal influences between children and their environments. Augmentative and Alternative Communication, 13, 149–157.

Calculator, S. (in press). AAC outcomes for children and youth with severe disabilities: When seeing is believing. Augmentative and Alternative Communication.

Calderon, R. and Greenberg, M. (1997). The effectiveness of early intervention for deaf children and children with hearing loss. In M. Guralnick (Ed.), Effectiveness Of Early Intervention (pp. 455–482). London: Paul H. Brookes.

Carlberger, A. (1998). Lexicons and grammar for speech recognition in an engineering design program (ICAD). In P. Branderud and H. Traunmüller (Eds). Proceedings of Fonetik 98, the Eleventh Swedish Phonetics Conference (pp. 172–175). Stockholm: Stockholm University, Department of Linguistics.

Carlberger, A., Carlberger, J., Magnuson, T., Palazuelos-Cagigas, S., Hunnicutt, S. and Aguilera-Navarro, S. (1997a). Profet, a new generation of word prediction: An evaluation study. In A. Copestake, S. Langer and S. Palazuelos-Cagigas (Eds), Natural Language Processing for Communication Aids. Proceedings of the Workshop at the 35th Annual Meeting of the Association for Computational Linguistics and the 8th Conference of the European Chapter of the ACL (pp. 23–28). Madrid, Spain: Association for Computational Linguistics.

Carlberger, A., Lewin, E., Nord, L., Rosengren, E., Ström, N., Carlson, R. and Hunnicutt, S. (1997b). ENABL – Access to design by speech recognition. In R. Bannert, M. Heldner, K. Sullivan and P. Wretling (Eds), Phonum: Vol. 4. Proceedings of Fonetik 97, the Tenth Swedish Phonetics Conference (pp. 89–92). Umeå, Sweden: Umeå University, Department of Phonetics.

Carlberger, J. (1997). Design and implementation of a probabilistic word prediction program. Unpublished master's thesis, KTH, Stockholm, Sweden.

Carlson, R. and Hunnicutt, S. (1995). The natural language component – STINA. In STL-QPSR 1 (Technical Report, pp. 29–48). Stockholm: KTH, Department of Speech Communication and Music Acoustics.

Carlson, R. and Hunnicutt, S. (1996). Generic and domain-specific aspects of the Waxholm NLP and Dialog modules. In H. T. Bunnell and W. Idsardi (Eds), Proceedings of ICSLP-96, Fourth International Conference on Spoken Language Processing (pp. 677–680). Wilmington, DE: Applied Science and Engineering Laboratories, Alfred I. duPont Institute.

Carpenter, B. (1998). Defining the family: Towards a critical framework for families of children with disabilities. European Journal of Special Needs Education, 13, 180–188.

Carpenter, B. and Herbert, E. (1994, Summer). The peripheral parent: Research issues and reflections on the role of fathers in early intervention. PMLD Link, 19, 16–25.

Carpenter, B. and Herbert, E. (1997). Fathers: Are we meeting their needs? In B. Carpenter (Ed.), Families in Context: Emerging Trends in Family Support and Early Intervention (pp. 50–61). London: David Fulton.

Carter, D., Kaja, J., Neumeyer, L., Rayner, M., Weng, F. and Wirén, M. (1996). Handling compound nouns in a Swedish speech-understanding system. In H. T. Bunnell and W. Idsardi (Eds), Proceedings of ICSLP-96, Fourth International Conference on Spoken Language Processing (pp. 26–29). Wilmington, DE: Applied Science and Engineering Laboratories, Alfred I. duPont Institute.

Castro-Caldas, A., Petersson, K. M., Reis, A., Stone-Elander, S. and Ingvar, M. (1998). The illiterate brain. Brain, 121, 1053–1063.

Cheepen, C. (1988). The Predictability of Informal Conversation. London: Pinter.

Chomsky, N. (1965). Aspects of the Theory of Syntax. Cambridge, MA: MIT Press.

Chomsky, N. (1986). Knowledge of Language. New York: Praeger.

Clark, C. R. (1984). A close look at the standard Rebus system and Blissymbolics. Journal of the Association for Persons with Severe Handicaps, 9, 37–48.

Clark, E. (1995). Language acquisition: The lexicon and syntax. In J. Miller and P. Eimas (Eds), Speech, Language, and Communication: Handbook of Perception and Cognition (2nd edn, Vol. 11, pp. 303–337). San Diego, CA: Academic Press.

Clark, E. and Hecht, B. (1983). Comprehension, production, and language acquisition. Annual Review of Psychology, 34, 325–349.

Clark, R., Hutcheson, S. and van Buren, P. (1974). Comprehension and production in language acquisition. Journal of Linguistics, 10, 39–54.

Claypool, T., Ricketts, I., Gregor, P., Booth, L. and Palazuelos, S. (1998). Learning rates of a Tri-Gram based Gaelic word predictor. In Proceedings of the Eighth Biennial Conference of the International Society for Augmentative and Alternative Communication (pp. 178–179). Dublin, Ireland: ISAAC/Ashfield Publications.

Clibbens, J. (1997). Relevance theory and augmentative and alternative communication. In M. Groefsema (Ed.), Proceedings of the University of Hertfordshire Relevance Theory Workshop (pp. 73–77). Chelmsford, UK: Peter Thomas and Associates.

Cochran, M. and Woolever, F. (1983). Beyond the deficit model: The empowerment of parents with information and information supports. In I. E. Sigel and L. M. Laosa (Eds), Changing Families (pp. 225–245). New York: Plenum Press.

Cole, R. A., Mariani, J., Uszkoreit, H., Zaenen, A. and Zue, V. (1995). Survey of the State of the Art in Human Language Technology [On-line]. Available: http://www.clres.com/surveys.html

Collins, S. (1996). Referring expressions in conversations between aided and natural speakers. In S. von Tetzchner and M. H. Jensen (Eds), Augmentative and Alternative Communication: European Perspectives (pp. 89–100). London: Whurr.

Columbo, J. and Bundy, R. S. (1981). A method for the measurement of infant auditory selectivity. Infant Behavior and Development, 4, 219–223.

Cooper, R. and Fuller, D. R. (1996) Differences in preschool children's learning of black-on-white versus white-on-black graphic symbols. Unpublished manuscript, University of Arkansas at Little Rock, University of Arkansas for Medical Sciences at Little Rock.

Copestake, A. (1996). Applying natural language processing techniques to speech prostheses. In Proceedings of the AAAI Fall Symposium on Developing Assistive Technology for People with Disabilities (pp. 5–12). Menlo Park, CA: American Association for Artificial Intelligence.

Copestake, A. (1997). Augmented and alternative NLP techniques for augmentative and alternative communication. In A. Copestake, S. Langer and S. Palazuelos-Cagigas (Eds), Natural Language Processing for Communication Aids. Proceedings of the Workshop at the 35th Annual Meeting of the Association for Computational Linguistics and the 8th Conference of the European Chapter of the ACL (pp. 37–42). Madrid, Spain: Association for Computational Linguistics.

Copestake, A. and Flickinger, D. (1998a). Evaluation of NLP technology for AAC using logged data. Presented at the ISAAC Research Symposium, Dublin, Ireland.

Copestake, A. and Flickinger, D. (1998b). Enriched language models for flexible generation in AAC systems. In Proceedings of the Technology and Persons with Disabilities Conference (CSUN-98). Northridge, CA: California State University Center on Disabilities. Available: http://www.dinf.org/csun_98/csun98.htm

Copestake, A., Langer, S. and Palazuelos-Cagigas, S. (Eds). (1997). Natural Language Processing for Communication Aids. Proceedings of the Workshop at the 35th

Annual Meeting of the Association for Computational Linguistics and the 8th Conference of the European Chapter of the ACL. Madrid, Spain: Association for Computational Linguistics.

Costello, J. M. (1998, November). AAC intervention with the temporarily non-speaking patient in the pediatric ICU: The children's hospital-Boston Model. Presented at the Annual Convention of the American Speech-Language-Hearing Association, San Antonio, TX.

Crain, S. (1987). On performability: Structure and process in language understanding. Clinical Linguistics and Phonetics, 1, 127–145.

Crain, S. and Fodor, J. (1993). Competence and performance in child language. In E. Dromi (Ed.), Language and Cognition: A Developmental Perspective (pp. 141–171). Norwood, NJ: Ablex.

Cress, C. (1998, August). Communication milestones for young non speaking children: Assessment and intervention strategies. Presented at the Eighth Biennial Conference of the International Society for Augmentative and Alternative Communication, Dublin, Ireland.

Cronen, M. and Mercaitis, P. (1998). Augmentative and alternative communication for persons with severe speech impairments and severe speech and physical impairments. In C. Seymour and E. Nober (Eds), Introduction to Communication Disorders: A Multicultural Approach (pp. 205–224). Boston: Butterworth-Heinemann.

Crowe, T. (1993). Time use of mothers with young children: The impact of a child's disability. Developmental Medicine and Child Neurology, 35, 621–630.

Culp, D., Ambrosi, D., Berniger, T. and Mitchell, J. (1986). Augmentative communication aid use – A follow-up study. Augmentative and Alternative Communication, 2, 19–24.

Cunningham, A. E. (1990). Explicit versus implicit instruction in phonemic awareness. Journal of Experimental Child Psychology, 50, 429–444.

Cunningham, A. E. and Stanovich, K. E. (1990). Assessing print exposure and orthographic processing skill in children: A quick measure of reading experience. Journal of Educational Psychology, 82, 733–740.

Curt, C. J. N. (1984). Nonverbal Communication in Puerto Rico. Cambridge, MA: Lesley College, Evaluation, Dissemination, and Assessment Center.

Cushler, C., Badman, A., Demasco, P. and McCoy, K. (1996). A communication aid enhanced with semantic parsing. In Proceedings of the Seventh Biennial Conference of the International Society for Augmentative and Alternative Communication (pp. 493–494). Vancouver, British Columbia, Canada: ISAAC.

Dahlgren Sandberg, A. (1996). Literacy abilities in nonvocal children with cerebral palsy. Doctoral thesis, Göteborg University, Göteborg, Sweden.

Dahlgren Sandberg, A. and Hjelmquist, E. (1996a). A comparative, descriptive study of reading and writing skills among non-speaking children: A preliminary study. European Journal of Disorders of Communication, 31, 289–308.

Dahlgren Sandberg, A. and Hjelmquist, E. (1996b). Phonologic awareness and literacy abilities in nonspeaking preschool children with cerebral palsy. Augmentative and Alternative Communication, 12, 138–153.

Dahlgren Sandberg, A. and Hjelmquist, E. (1997). Language and literacy in nonvocal children with cerebral palsy. Reading and Writing: An Interdisciplinary Journal, 9, 107–133.

Dahlstrom, E. (1989). Theories and ideology of family function, gender relations and human reproduction. In K. Boh, M. Back, C. Clason, M. Pankratora, J. Qvortup, B. G. Sgritta and K. Aerness (Eds), Changing Patterns of European Family Life. London: Routledge.

Daneman, M. (1991). Individual differences in reading skills. In R. Barr, M. L. Kamil, P. Mosenthal and P. D. Pearson (Eds), Handbook of Reading Research (pp. 512–538). New York: Longman.

Darragh, J. J. and Witten, I. H. (1992). The Reactive Keyboard. Cambridge, UK: Cambridge University Press.

Deci, E. L. (1975). Intrinsic Motivation. New York: Plenum Press.

de Houwer, A. (1995). Bilingual language acquisition. In P. Fletcher and B. MacWhinney (Eds), Handbook of Child Language (pp. 219–250). London: Blackwell.

DeLoache, J. S., Pierroutsakos, S. L., Uttal, D. H., Rosengren, K. and Gottlieb, A. (1998). Grasping the nature of pictures. Psychological Science, 9, 205–210.

DeLoache, J. S., Uttal, D. H. and Pierroutsakos, S. L. (1998). The development of early symbolization: Educational implications. Learning and Instruction, 8, 325–339.

Demasco, P. W. and McCoy, K. F. (1992). Generating text from compressed input: An intelligent interface for people with severe motor impairments. Communications of the ACM, 35(5), 68–78.

DeRuyter, F. (1994). Assistive technology usage outcomes: A preliminary report. Paper presented at RESNA, Nashville, TN.

DeRuyter, F. (1997). The importance of outcome measures for assistive technology service delivery systems. Technology and Disability, 6, 89–104.

DeRuyter, F. (1999). A longitudinal study of factors contributing to assistive technology outcomes. Manuscript in preparation.

DeRuyter, F., Doyle, M. and Kennedy, M. (1990). Who is doing what for the nonspeaking person with traumatic brain injury? Presented at the Fourth Biennial Conference of the International Society for Augmentative and Alternative Communication, Stockholm, Sweden.

DeRuyter, F. and Kennedy, M. (1990). Augmentative communication following traumatic brain injury. In D. R. Beukelman and K. M. Yorkston (Eds), Communication Disorders Following Traumatic Brain Injury. Austin, TX: Pro-Ed.

DeRuyter, F., Kennedy, M. and Doyle, M. (1990). Augmentative communication and stroke rehabilitation: Who is doing what and do the data tell the whole story? Presented at the National Stroke Rehabilitation Conference, Boston, MA.

de Villiers, J., Bibeau, L., Ramos, E. and Galty, J. (1993). Gestural communication in oral deaf mother–child pairs: Language with a helping hand? Applied Psycholinguistics, 14, 319–347.

Devlin, S. (1997). Creating an augmentative reading aid for aphasic people. In Proceedings of the British Aphasiology Society Biennial International Conference. Manchester, UK: University of Manchester.

Dodd, J. M., Nelson, J. R. and Peralez, E. (1988). Understanding the Hispanic student. The Rural Educator, 10(2), 8–13.

Drake, R. F. (1997). What am I doing here? Disability and Society, 12, 643–645.

Dunst, C. J. (1990). Family support principles: Checklists for the program builder. (Family Systems Intervention Monograph Series, 2 [5]).

Dunst, C. J. (1997). Conceptual and empirical foundations of family-centered practice. In R. J. Illback, C. T. Cobb and H. M. Joseph, Jr. (Eds), Integrated Services for Children and Families (pp. 75–91). Washington, DC: American Psychological Association.

Dunst, C., Cushing, P. and Vance, S. (1985). Response-contingent learning in profoundly handicapped infants: A social systems perspective. Analysis and Intervention in Developmental Disabilities, 5, 33–47.

Dunst, C. J., Johanson, C., Trivette, C. M. and Hamby, D. (1991). Family oriented early intervention policies and practices: Family-centered or not? Exceptional Children, 58, 115–126.

Dunst, C., Trivette, C. and Deal, A. (1988). Enabling and Empowering Families: Principles and Guidelines for Practice. Cambridge, MA: Brookline Books.

Dye, R., Alm, N., Arnott, J. L., Harper, G. and Morrison, A. (1998). A script-based AAC system for transactional encounters. Journal of Natural Language Engineering, 4(1), 57–72.

EAGLES Group. (1995). Evaluation of natural language processing systems: Final report [On-line]. Available: http://www.issco.unige.ch/projects/ewg96/ewg96.html

Ehri, L. C. (1987). Learning to read and spell words. Journal of Reading Behavior, 19, 5–31.

Ehri, L. C. (1992). Reconceptualizing the development of sight word reading and its relationship to recoding. In P. B. Gough, L. C. Ehri and R. Treiman (Eds), Reading Acquisition (pp. 107–143). Hillsdale, NJ: Erlbaum.

Ehri, L. C. and Wilce, L. S. (1980). The influence of orthography on readers' conceptualization of the phoneme structure of words. Applied Psycholinguistics, 1, 371–385.

Ejerhed E., Källgren, G., Wennstedt, O. and Åström, M. (1992). The linguistic annotation system of the Stockholm-Umeå Corpus Project (Report No. DGL-UUM-R-33). Umeå, Sweden: University of Umeå, Department of General Linguistics.

Elbers, L. (1995). Production as a source of input for analysis: Evidence from the developmental course of a word-blend. Journal of Child Language, 22, 47–71.

Elbers, L. and Wijnen, F. (1992). Effort, production skill and language learning. In C. A. Ferguson, L. Menn and C. Stoel-Gammon (Eds), Phonological Development: Models, Research, Implications (pp. 337–368). Timonium, MD: York Press.

Elbro, C. (1994). Dyslexia in adults: Evidence for deficits in non-word reading and in the phonological representation of lexical items. Annals of Dyslexia, 44, 205–226.

Elbro, C. (1996). Early linguistic abilities and reading development: A review and a hypothesis. Reading and Writing: An Interdisciplinary Journal, 8, 453–485.

Elman, J., Bates, E., Johnson, M., Karmiloff-Smith, A., Parisi, D. and Plunkett, K. (1996). Rethinking Innateness: A Connectionist Perspective on Development. Cambridge, MA: MIT Press.

Engwis, P. and Sweeney, L. A. (1997). Perspectives on life and communicating: A dynamic family interview. In E. Björck-Åkesson and P. Lindsay (Eds), Communication... Naturally: Theoretical and Methodological Issues in Augmentative and Alternative Communication. Proceedings of the Fourth ISAAC Research Symposium (pp. 231–240). Västerås, Sweden: Mälardalen University Press.

Erickson, J. G. and Iglesias, A. (1986). Assessment of communication disorders in non-English proficient children. In O. L. Taylor (Ed.), Nature of Communication Disorders in Culturally and Linguistically Diverse Populations (pp. 181–217). San Diego, CA: College-Hill Press.

Ervin-Tripp, S. (1979). Children's turn-taking. In E. Ochs and B. Schieffelin (Eds), Developmental Pragmatics (pp. 91–414). London: Academic Press.

Fairbanks, G. (1954). Systematic research in experimental phonetics: 1. A theory of the speech mechanism as a servo-mechanism. Journal of Speech and Hearing Disorders, 19, 133–139.

Ferguson, C. A. (1978). Learning to pronounce: The earliest stages of phonological development in the child. In F. D. Minifie and L. L. Lloyd (Eds), Communicative and Cognitive Abilities – Early Behavioral Assessment (pp. 273–297). Baltimore: University Park Press.

Ferrier, L., Fell, H., Mooraj, Z., Delta, H. and Moscoe, D. (1996). Baby-Babble Blanket: Infant interface with automatic data collection. Augmentative and Alternative Communication, 12, 110–119.

File, P. and Elder, L. (1997). Using NLP in the design of a conversation aid for non-speaking children. In A. Copestake, S. Langer and S. Palazuelos-Cagigas (Eds), Natural Language Processing for Communication Aids. Proceedings of the Workshop at the 35th Annual Meeting of the Association for Computational Linguistics and the 8th Conference of the European Chapter of the ACL (pp. 43–46). Madrid, Spain: Association for Computational Linguistics.

File, P., Todman, J., Alm, N., Elder, L. and Smith, H. (1995). PICTALK: A conversation aid for nonspeaking, nonreading people. Journal of Rehabilitation Sciences, 8, 47.

Fisher, C., Hall, G., Rakowitz, S. and Gleitman, L. (1994). When it is better to receive than give: Syntactic and conceptual constraints on vocabulary growth. Lingua, 92, 333–375.

Fodor, J. (1983). The Modularity of the Mind. Cambridge, MA: Bradford.

Fogel, A. and Thelen, E. (1987). Development of early expressive and communicative action: Reinterpreting the evidence from a dynamic systems perspective. Developmental Psychology, 23, 747–761.

Foorman, B. R., Jenkins, L. and Francis, D. J. (1993). Links among segmenting, spelling, and reading words in first and second grades. Reading and Writing: An Interdisciplinary Journal, 5, 1–15.

Fraiberg, S. (1977). Insights from the Blind. New York: Basic Books.

French, S. and Swain, J. (1997). Changing disability research: Participating and emancipatory research with disabled people. Physiotherapy, 83(1), 26–32.

Frith, U. (1985). Beneath the surface of developmental dyslexia. In K. E. Patterson, J. C. Marshall and M. Coltheart (Eds), Surface Dyslexia (pp. 301–330). London: Erlbaum.

Fuller, D. R. (1988). Effects of translucency and complexity on the associative learning of Blissymbols by cognitively normal children and adults. (Doctoral dissertation, Purdue University, 1987). Dissertation Abstracts International, 49, 710B.

Fuller, D. R. (1997). Initial study into effects of translucency and complexity on the learning of Blissymbols by children and adults with normal cognitive abilities. Augmentative and Alternative Communication, 13, 30–39.

Fuller, D. R. and Lloyd, L. L. (1987). A study of physical and semantic characteristics of a graphic symbol system as predictors of perceived complexity. Augmentative and Alternative Communication, 3, 26–35.

Fuller, D. R. and Lloyd, L. L. (1991). Towards a common usage of iconicity terminology. Augmentative and Alternative Communication. Augmentative and Alternative Communication, 7, 215–220.

Fuller, D. R. and Lloyd, L. L. (1997). Symbol selection. In L. L. Lloyd, D. R. Fuller and H. H. Arvidson (Eds), Augmentative and Alternative Communication: A Handbook of Principles and Practices (pp. 214–225). Boston: Allyn and Bacon.

Fuller, D. R., Lloyd, L. L. and Schlosser, R. W. (1992). Further development of an augmentative and alternative communication symbol taxonomy. Augmentative and Alternative Communication, 8, 67–74.

Fuller, D. R., Lloyd, L. L. and Schlosser, R. W. (1997). What do we know about graphic AAC symbols, and what do we still need to know about them? In E. Björck-Åkesson and P. Lindsay (Eds), Communication... Naturally: Theoretical and Methodological Issues in Augmentative and Alternative Communication. Proceedings of the Fourth ISAAC Research Symposium (pp. 113–125). Västerås, Sweden: Mälardalen University Press.

Fuller, D. R., Lloyd, L. L. and Stratton, M. M. (1997). Aided AAC symbols. In L. L. Lloyd, D. R. Fuller and H. H. Arvidson (Eds), Augmentative and Alternative Communication: A Handbook of Principles and Practice (pp. 48–79). Boston: Allyn and Bacon.

Furrow, D., Nelson, K. and Benedict, H. (1979). Mothers' speech to children and syntactic development: Some simple relationships. Journal of Child Language, 6, 423–442.

Gamradt, J. (1998). Survey of Support Available for an Augmentative Communication Device. Madison, WI: Communication Development Program-Trace Center.

Gangkofer, M. (1990). Bilder lesen muss man lernen: Grundschüler deuten BLISS-Symbole [To read images must be learned: Preschoolers interpret Blissymbols]. In H. Brügelmann and H. Balhorn (Eds), Das Gehirn, sein Alfabet und andere Geschichten (pp. 169–177). Konstanz, Germany: Fraude.

Garay-Vitoria, N. and Abascal, J. G. (1997). Word prediction for inflected languages: Application to Basque language. In A. Copestake, S. Langer and S. Palazuelos-Cagigas (Eds), Natural Language Processing for Communication Aids. Proceedings of the Workshop at the 35th Annual Meeting of the Association for Computational Linguistics and the 8th Conference of the European Chapter of the ACL (pp. 29–36). Madrid, Spain: Association for Computational Linguistics.

Garcia, E. E. (1994). Addressing the challenges of diversity. In S. L. Kagan and B. Weissbourd (Eds), Putting Families First (pp. 243–275). San Francisco, CA: Jossey-Bass.

Gibbon, D., Moore, R. and Winsky, R. (Eds). (1998). Spoken language systems assessment. In Handbook of Standards and Resources for Spoken Language Systems: Vol. III. Berlin, Germany: Mouton.

Gibson, E. J. (1969). Principles of Perceptual Learning and Development. New York: Meredith Corporation.

Glaser, B. G. and Strauss, A. L. (1967). The Discovery of Grounded Theory Strategies for Qualitative Research. New York: Aldine.

Gleick, J. (1987). Chaos: Making a New Science. New York: Penguin Books.

Gleitman, L. and Gleitman, H. (1992). A picture is worth a thousand words, but that's the problem: The role of syntax in vocabulary acquisition. Current Directions in Psychological Science, 1, 31–35.

Gleitman, L., Newport, E. and Gleitman, H. (1984). The current status of the motherese hypothesis. Journal of Child Language, 11, 43–79.

Glesne, C. and Peshkin, A. (1992). Becoming Qualitative Researchers: An Introduction. White Plains, NY: Longman.

Godbert, E., Mouret, P., Pasero, R. and Rolbert, M. (1997). A software for language education and rehabilitation of autistic-like children. In A. Copestake, S. Langer and S. Palazuelos-Cagigas (Eds), Natural Language Processing for Communication Aids. Proceedings of the Workshop at the 35th Annual Meeting of the Association for Computational Linguistics and the 8th Conference of the European Chapter of the ACL (pp. 59–64). Madrid, Spain: Association for Computational Linguistics.

Goetz, J. P. and LeCompte, M. D. (1984). Ethnography and Qualitative Design in Education Research. New York: Academic Press.

Goldbart, J. (1994). Opening the communication curriculum to students with PMLDs. In J. Ware (Ed.), Educating Children with Profound and Multiple Learning Difficulties (pp. 15–62). London: David Fulton.

Goldbart, J. (1998, August). Pressing levers or picking locks: Should we train people to use language or allow them to acquire it? The case for a developmental approach. Presented at the Eighth Biennial Conference of the International Society for Augmentative and Alternative Communication, Dublin, Ireland.

Goldin-Meadow, S. (1995). When does gesture become language? A study of gesture used as a primary communication system by deaf children of hearing parents. In K. R. Gibson and T. Ingold (Eds), Tools, Language and Cognition in Human Evolution (pp. 63–85). New York: Cambridge University Press.

Goldin-Meadow, S., Butcher, C., Mylander, C. and Dodge, M. (1994). Nouns and verbs in a self-styles gesture system: What's in a name? Cognitive Psychology, 27, 259–319.

Goldin-Meadow, S. and McNeill, D. (in press). The role of gestures and mimetic representation in making language the province of speech. In M. Corballis and S. Lea (Eds), Evolution of the Hominid Mind. Oxford, UK: Oxford University Press.

Goldin-Meadow, S. and Mylander, C. (1990). Beyond the input given: The child's role in acquisition of language. Language, 66, 323–355.

Golinkoff, R., Mervis, C. and Hirsh-Pasek, K. (1994). Early object labels: The case for a developmental lexical principles framework. Journal of Child Language, 21, 125–155.

Goossens, C. A. (1984). The relative iconicity and learnability of verb referents differentially represented as manual signs, Blissymbolics, and Rebus symbols: An investigation with moderately retarded individuals. (Doctoral dissertation, Purdue University, 1983). Dissertation Abstracts International, 45, 809A.

Goossens, C. (1998, August). Engineering circle time. Presented at the Eighth Biennial Conference of the International Society for Augmentative and Alternative Communication, Dublin, Ireland.

Goswami, U. and Bryant, P. (1990). Phonological Skills and Learning to Read. London: Erlbaum.

Gottardo, A. (1995). Syntactic and phonological processing in children with language impairments, children with reading disabilities and normally achieving children. Unpublished doctoral dissertation, University of Toronto, Toronto, Ontario, Canada.

Granlund, M. and Björck-Åkesson, E. (1996a). Inservice training of preschool consultants in family-oriented intervention – Training process and outcome. British Journal of Developmental Disabilities, XLII, 1–24.

Granlund, M. and Björck-Åkesson, E. (1996b, August). Learning collaborative problem solving in family centered intervention. Seminar presented at the Seventh Biennial Conference of the International Society for Augmentative and Alternative Communication, Vancouver, British Columbia, Canada.

Granlund, M., Björck-Åkesson, E. and Carlhed, C. (1999). The impact of early intervention on the family system. Manuscript in preparation.

Granlund, M., Blackstone, S. and Norris, L. (1997). Measuring the outcome of AAC intervention: Defining outcomes. In E. Björck-Åkesson and P. Lindsay (Eds), Communication... Naturally: Theoretical and Methodological Issues in Augmentative and Alternative Communication. Proceedings of the Fourth ISAAC Research Symposium (pp. 203–216). Västerås, Sweden: Mälardalen University Press.

Granlund, M. and Steénson, A.-L. (1998). Team över tid [A longitudinal study of teams]. In M. Granlund (Ed.), Barn med Flera Funktionsnedsättningar i Särskolan (pp. 265–382). Stockholm: Stiftelsen ALA.

Grossman, H. (1984). Educating Hispanic Students: Cultural Implications in Instruction, Classroom Management, Counseling and Assessment. Springfield, IL: Thomas.

Grove, N. (1995). An analysis of the linguistic skills of signers with learning disabilities. Unpublished doctoral dissertation, University of London, Institute of Education, London.

Grove, N. (1997). Gesture, language and multimodality: Implications for research and practice. In E. Björk Åkesson and P. Lindsay (Eds), Communication... Naturally: Theoretical and Methodological Issues in Augmentative and Alternative Communication. Proceedings of the Fourth ISAAC Research Symposium (pp. 92–101). Västerås, Sweden: Mälardalen University Press.

Grove, N., Clibbens, J., Barnett, S. and Loncke, F. (1997). Constructing theoretical models of augmentative and alternative communication. In E. Björck-Åkesson and P. Lindsay (Eds), Communication... Naturally: Theoretical and Methodological Issues in Augmentative and Alternative Communication. Proceedings of the Fourth ISAAC Research Symposium (pp. 48–66). Västerås, Sweden: Mälardalen University Press.

Grove, N., Dockrell, J. and Woll, B. (1996). The two-word stage in manual signs: Language development in signers with intellectual impairments. In S. von Tetzchner and M. H. Jensen (Eds), Augmentative and Alternative Communication: European Perspectives (pp. 101–118). London: Whurr.

Grove, N. and Smith, M. (1997, November). Input–output asymmetries: Language development in AAC. The ISAAC Bulletin, (50), 1–3.

Guba, E. G. (1981). Criteria for assessing the trustworthiness of naturalistic inquiries. Educational Communication and Technology Journal, 29, 75–92.

Guba, E. G. and Lincoln, Y. S. (1994). Competing paradigms in qualitative research. In N. K. Denzin and Y. S. Lincoln (Eds), The Handbook of Qualitative Research (pp. 105–117). Thousand Oaks, CA: Sage.

Guenthner, F., Krüger-Thielmann, K., Pasero, R. and Sabatier, P. (1993). Communication aids for handicapped persons. In The Swedish Handicap Institute (Ed.), Proceedings of the European Conference on the Advancement of Rehabilitation Technology (ECART2) (section 1.4). Stockholm: Kommentus.

Guenthner, F., Krüger-Thielmann, K., Pasero, R. and Sabatier, P. (1994). Guided composition of text used in communication aids for handicapped persons. In ISAAC '94 Conference Book and Proceedings (pp. 474–478). Maastricht, The Netherlands: ISAAC.

Guenthner, F., Langer, S., Krüger-Thielmann, K., Pasero, R. and Sabatier, P. (1993). KOMBE: Communication Aids for the Handicapped (Report 92–55). Munich, Germany: CIS.

Guess, D., Rues, J., Roberts, S. and Siegel-Causey, E. (1993). Extended Analysis of Behavior State, Environmental Venets, and Related Variables Among Students with Profound Disabilities – Final report. Lawrence, KS: University of Kansas.

Guess, D. and Sailor, W. (1993). Chaos theory and the study of human behavior: Implications for special education and developmental disabilities. Journal of Special Education, 27, 16–34.

Guralnick, M. (1997). Effectiveness of Early Intervention. London: Paul H. Brookes.

Gustason, G., Pfetzing, D. and Zawolkow, E. (1980). Signing Exact English (3rd edn). Los Alamitos, CA: Modern Signs Press.

Habermas, J. (1984). The Theory of Communicative Action (Vol. 1). Boston: Beacon Press.

Hanson, M. J. (1992). Ethnic, cultural, and language diversity in intervention settings. In E. W. Lynch and M. J. Hanson (Eds), Developing Cross-cultural Competence: A Guide for Working with Young Children and Their Families (pp. 3–18). Baltimore: Paul H. Brookes.

Hanzlik, J. (1990). Nonverbal interaction patterns of mothers and their infants with cerebral palsy. Education and Training in Mental Retardation, 25, 333–343.

Harris, D. and Vanderheiden, G. (1980). Enhancing the development of communication interaction. In R. Schiefelbusch (Ed.), Nonspeech Language and Communication: Analysis and Intervention (pp. 227–257). Baltimore: University Park Press.

Harris, M. (1992). Language Experience and Early Language Development: From Input to Uptake. Cambridge, MA: MIT Press.

Hart, E. and Risley, T. (1995). Meaningful Differences in the Everyday Experience of Young American Children. Baltimore: Paul H. Brookes.

Hayes, C. (1996). The effects of translucency and complexity on the acquisition and retention of Blissymbols by elderly individuals. Independent Research Project, University of Arkansas at Little Rock, University of Arkansas for Medical Sciences at Little Rock.

Hazen, N. L. and Black, B. (1989). Preschool peer communications skills: The role of social status and interaction context. Child Development, 60, 867–876.

Heim, M. J. M. and Baker-Mills, A. E. (1996). Early development of symbolic communication and linguistic complexity through augmentative and alternative communication. In S. von Tetzchner and M. H. Jensen (Eds), Augmentative and Alternative Communication: European Perspectives (pp. 232–248). London: Whurr.

Heim, M. J. M. and Jonker, V. M. (1996). Communicative development of nonspeaking children and their communication partners. Manuscript in preparation.

Heller, T., Miller, A., Nelis, T. and Pederson, E. (no date). Getting Involved in Research and Training Projects: A Guide for Persons with Disabilities. Chicago: University of Illinois at Chicago.

Henry, A. D. and Coster, W. J. (1997). Competency beliefs and occupational role behavior among adolescents: Explication of the personal causation construct. American Journal of Occupational Therapy, 51, 267–276.

Hern, S., Lammers, J. and Fuller, D. R. (1996). The effects of translucency, complexity, and other variables on the acquisition of Blissymbols by institutionalized individuals with mental retardation. Unpublished manuscript, University of Arkansas at Little Rock, University of Arkansas for Medical Sciences at Little Rock.

Hetzroni, O. E. and Harris, O. L. (1996). Cultural aspects in the development of AAC users. Augmentative and Alternative Communication, 12, 52–58.

Higginbotham, D. J. (1992). Evaluation of keystroke savings across five assistive communication technologies. Augmentative and Alternative Communication, 8, 258–272.

Hinde, R. A. (1992). Ethological and relationships approaches. In R. Vasta (Ed.), Six Theories of Child Development (pp. 251–285). London: Jessica Kingsley.

Hjelmquist, E. (1991). Methodological approaches to AAC and other 'technologies' of communication from a developmental perspective. In E. Björck-Åkesson and J. Brodin (Eds), Methodological Issues in Research in Augmentative and Alternative Communication (pp. 124–128). Stockholm: The Swedish Handicap Institute.

Hjelmquist, E. (1997). Issues of representation in alternative language development. In E. Björck-Åkesson and P. Lindsay (Eds), Communication... Naturally: Theoretical and Methodological Issues in Augmentative and Alternative Communication. Proceedings of the Fourth ISAAC Research Symposium (pp. 19–25). Västerås, Sweden: Mälardalen University Press.

Hjelmquist, E. and Dahlgren Sandberg, A. (1996). Sounds and silence: Interaction in aided language use. In S. von Tetzchner and M. H. Jensen (Eds), Augmentative and Alternative Communication: European Perspectives (pp. 137–154). London: Whurr.

Hjelmquist, E., Dahlgren Sandberg, A. and Hedelin, L. (1994). Linguistics, AAC and metalinguistics in communicatively handicapped adolescents. Augmentative and Alternative Communication, 10, 169–183.

Hockett, C. F. (1958). A Course in Modern Linguistics. New York: MacMillan.

Hooper, J. and Lloyd, L. L. (1988). An investigation of element explanation on the ability of preschool children to learn Blissymbols. Unpublished manuscript, Purdue University, West Lafayette, IN.

Huer, M. B. (1993). A master's program in speech-language pathology with special emphasis in augmentative and alternative communication and multiculturalism (1994–1999). Grant funded through the US Department of Education, Preparation of Personnel/Careers in Special Education, CFDA 84.029B (No. H029B40232).

Huer, M. B. (1994, November). Diversity now: Multicultural issues in AAC. Miniseminar presented at the Annual Convention of the American Speech-Language-Hearing Association, New Orleans, LA.

Huer, M. B. (1997a). Augmentative and alternative communication. In T. A. Crowe (Ed.), Applications of Counseling in Speech-Language Pathology and Audiology (pp. 335–362). Baltimore: Williams & Wilkins.

Huer, M. B. (1997b). Culturally inclusive assessments for children using augmentative and alternative communication (AAC). Journal of Children's Communication Development, 19(1), 23–24.

Huer, M. B. (1997c). Looking through color lenses: Cultural strategies for AAC. Advance for Directors in Rehabilitation, 6(6), 37–40.

Huer, M. B. (1998, August). Examining perceptions of graphic symbol sets across cultures: Implications for the practice of augmentative and alternative communication. Paper presented at the International Society for Augmentative and Alternative Communication Research Symposium, Dublin, Ireland.

Huer, M. B. and Lloyd, L. L. (1990). AAC users' perspectives on augmentative and alternative communication. Augmentative and Alternative Communication, 6, 242–249.

Hugunin, J. and Zue, V. (1997). On the design of effective speech-based interfaces for desktop applications. In G. Kokkinakis, N. Fakotakis and E. Dermatas (Eds), Proceedings of the Fifth European Conference on Speech Communication and Technology (EuroSpeech '97) (pp. 1335–1338). Patras, Greece: ESCA and University of Patras.

Hunnicutt. S. (1986). Bliss symbol-to-speech conversion: 'Blisstalk'. Journal of the American Voice I/O Society, 3, 19–38.

Hunt-Berg, M. (1998, August). Children's use of pointing cues in aided language intervention. Paper presented at the Eighth Biennial Conference of the International Society for Augmentative and Alternative Communication, Dublin, Ireland.

Hunt-Berg, M. and Schick, B. (1995, December). Learning graphic symbols: Do children have a categorical bias? Presented at the Annual Convention of the American Speech-Language-Hearing Association, Orlando, FL.

Hymes, D. H. (1972). On communicative competence. In J. B. Pride and J. Holmes (Eds), Sociolinguistics (pp. 269–293). Harmondsworth, UK: Penguin.

Iacono, T. A. and Duncum, J. (1995). Comparison of sign alone and in combination with an electronic communication device in early language intervention: Case study. Augmentative and Alternative Communication, 11, 249–259.

Iacono, T., Mirenda, P. and Beukelman, D. (1993). Comparison of unimodal and multimodal AAC techniques for children with intellectual disabilities. Augmentative and Alternative Communication, 9, 83–94.

Iverson, J. M. and Thal, D. J. (1998). Communicative transitions: There is more to the hand than meets the eye. In A. M. Wetherby, S. F. Warren and J. Reichle (Eds), Transitions in Prelinguistic Communication (pp. 59–86). Baltimore: Paul H. Brookes.

Jackendoff, R. S. (1987). Consciousness and the Computational Mind. Cambridge, MA: MIT Press.

Jackendoff, R. S. (1990). Semantics and Cognition. Cambridge, MA: MIT Press.

Jefferson, G. (1984). On stepwise transition from talk about trouble to inappropriately next-positioned matters. In J. Atkins and J. Heritage (Eds), Structures of Social Action-Studies in Conversation Analysis (pp. 191–222). London: Cambridge University Press.

Johnson, L. J. and LaMontagne, M. (1994). Program evaluation. The key to quality programming. In L. J. Johnson, R. J. Gallagher, M. J. LaMontagne, J. B. Jordan, J. J. Gallagher, P. L. Hutinger and M. B. Karnes (Eds), Meeting Early Intervention

Challenges. Issues from Birth to Three (2nd edn, pp. 185–216). Baltimore: Paul H. Brookes.

Johnson L. J. and Montague, M. J. (1992). Using content analysis to examine the verbal or written communication of stakeholders within early intervention. Journal of Early Intervention, 17, 73–79.

Johnson, M., Dziurawiec, S., Ellis, H. and Morton, J. (1991). Newhorns' preferential tracking of face-like stimuli and its subsequent decline. Cognition, 40, 1–19.

Johnson-Laird, P. N. (1983). Mental Models: Towards a Cognitive Science of Language, Inference, and Consciousness. Cambridge, MA: Harvard University Press.

Jones, K. R. and Cregan, A. (1986). Sign and Symbol Communication for Mentally Handicapped People. London: Croom Helm.

Jones, L. and Pullen, G. (1992). Cultural differences: Deaf and hearing researchers working together. Disability, Handicap and Society, 7, 198–192.

Jonker, V. M. and Heim, M. J. M. (1994). Implementation of an intervention programme for non-speaking children and their partners: In-service training. In ISAAC'94 Conference Book and Proceedings. Hoensbroek, The Netherlands: ISAAC.

Juel, C., Griffith, P. L. and Gough, P. B. (1986). Acquisition of literacy: A longitudinal study of children in first and second grade. Journal of Educational Psychology, 78, 243–255.

Jusczyk, P. (1997). The Discovery of Spoken Language. Cambridge, MA: MIT Press.

Kaiser, A., Hemmeter, M. L. and Hester, P. (1997). The facilitative effects of input on children's language development: Contributions from studies of enhanced milieu teaching. In L. Adamson and M. A. Romski (Eds), Communication and Language Acquisition: Discoveries from Atypical Development (pp. 267–294). Baltimore: Paul H. Brookes.

Kangas, K. A. and Lloyd, L. L. (1998). Augmentative and alternative communication. In G. H. Shames, E. H. Wiig and W. A. Secord (Eds), Human Communication Disorders: An Introduction (5th edn, pp. 510–551). Boston: Allyn and Bacon.

Karlan, G. R. and Lloyd, L. L. (1983). Considerations in the planning of communication intervention: Selecting a lexicon. Journal of the Association for the Severely Handicapped, 8, 13–25.

Karmiloff-Smith, A. (1992). Beyond Modularity: A Developmental Perspective on Cognitive Science. London: MIT Press.

Karmiloff-Smith, A. (1997, November). Is abnormal development necessarily a window on normal language acquisition? Keynote address presented at the Boston University Conference on Language Development, Boston, MA.

Kayser, H. (1998). Hispanic cultures and language. In D. Battle (Ed.), Communication Disorders in Multicultural Populations (2nd edn, pp. 157–195). Boston: Butterworth-Heinemann.

Kerlinger, F. N. (1973) Foundations of Behavioral Research. New York: Holt, Rinehart & Winston.

Kielhofner, G. (Ed.). (1995). A Model of Human Occupation: Theory and Application (2nd edn). Baltimore: Williams & Wilkins.

Kiersuk, T., Smith, A. and Cardillo, J. (1994). Goal Attainment Scaling: Applications, Theory, and Measurement. London: Erlbaum.

Klima, E. and Bellugi, U. (1979). The Signs of Language. London: Harvard University Press.

Knapp, M. (1995). How shall we study comprehensive, collaborative services for children and families? Educational Researcher, 24, 5–16.

Knowles, W. and Masidlover, M. (1982). Derbyshire Language Scheme. Derbyshire, UK: Derbyshire County Council.

Kolers, P. and Roediger, H. (1984). Procedures of mind. Journal of Verbal Learning and Verbal Behavior, 23, 425–449.

Kosslyn, S. M. (1983). Ghosts in the Mind's Machine. New York: W. W. Norton.

Koul, R. (1995). Comparison of graphic symbol learning in individuals with aphasia and right hemisphere brain damage. (Doctoral dissertation, Purdue University, 1994). Dissertation Abstracts International, 56(02), 770B.

Koul, R. and Lloyd, L. L. (1998). Comparison of graphic symbol learning in individuals with aphasia and right hemisphere brain damage. Brain and Language, 62, 398–421.

Kraat, A. (1985). Communication Interaction Between Aided and Natural Speakers: A State of the Art Report. Toronto, Ontario, Canada: Canadian Rehabilitation Council for the Disabled.

Kraat, A. and Brune, P. (1998, August). Transitioning through Batman, The White House and Bones: A case study. Paper presented at the Eighth Biennial Conference of the International Society for Augmentative and Alternative Communication, Dublin, Ireland.

Krogh, K. (1997). Incorporating consumer perspectives into research methodology. In E. Björck-Åkesson and P. Lindsay (Eds), Communication... Naturally: Theoretical and Methodological Issues in Augmentative and Alternative Communication. Proceedings of the Fourth ISAAC Research Symposium (pp. 192–202). Västerås, Sweden: Mälardalen University Press.

Krueger, R. A. (1988). Focus Groups: A Practical Guide for Applied Research. Newbury Park, CA: Sage.

Kumin. L. (1994). Communication Skills in Children with Down Syndrome: A Guide for Parents. Rockville, MD: Woodbine House.

Langdon, H. W. (1992). The Hispanic population: Facts and figures. In H. W. Langdon and L. L. Cheng (Eds), Hispanic Children and Adults with Communication Disorders (pp. 20–56). Rockville, MD: Aspen.

Langer, S. and Hickey, M. (1997). Automatic message indexing and full text retrieval for a communication aid. In A. Copestake, S. Langer and S. Palazuelos-Cagigas (Eds), Natural Language Processing for Communication Aids. Proceedings of the Workshop at the 35th Annual Meeting of the Association for Computational Linguistics and the 8th Conference of the European Chapter of the ACL (pp. 9–16). Madrid, Spain: Association for Computational Linguistics.

Langer, S. and Hickey, M. (1998). Using semantic lexicons for full text message retrieval in a communication aid. Journal of Natural Language Engineering, 4(1), 41–56.

Lehmann, S. and Oepen, S. (1996). TSNLP – Test suites for natural language processing in COLING-96. In Proceedings of the 16th International Conference on Computational Linguistics. Copenhagen, Denmark. Available: http://cl-www.dfki.uni-sb.de/tsnlp/publications.html#coling96

Le Pévédic, B. and Maurel, D. (1996). La prédiction d'une catégorie grammaticale dans un système d'aide à la saisie pour handicapés [The prediction of grammatical categories in an input prediction system for handicapped]. In Actes de la 21ème Conférence sur le Traitement Automatique du Langage Naturel (TALN). Marseille, France.

Levelt, W. J. (1993). Speaking: From Intention to Articulation. Cambridge, MA: MIT Press.

Lewin, E. (1997). The broker architecture [On-line]. Available: http://www.speech.kth.se/proj/broker

Lieven, E., Pine, J. and Baldwin, G. (1997). Lexically-based learning and early grammatical development. Journal of Child Language, 24, 187–219.

Light, J. (1989). Toward a definition of communicative competence for individuals using augmentative and alternative communication systems. Augmentative and Alternative Communication, 5, 137–144.

Light, J. (1997). 'Lets go star fishing': Reflections on the contexts of language learning for children who use aided AAC. Augmentative and Alternative Communication, 13, 158–171.

Light, J. (1999). Do augmentative and alternative communication interventions really make a difference? The challenges of efficacy research. Augmentative and Alternative Communication, 15(1), 13–24.

Light, J., Collier, B. and Parnes, P. (1985a). Communicative interaction between young non-speaking physically disabled children and their primary caregivers: Part 1 – Discourse patterns. Augmentative and Alternative Communication, 1, 74–83.

Light, J., Collier, B. and Parnes, P. (1985b). Communicative interaction between young nonspeaking physically disabled children and their primary caregivers: Part II – Communicative function. Augmentative and Alternative Communication, 1, 98–107.

Light, J. and Kelford-Smith, A. (1993). The home literacy experiences of preschoolers who use augmentative communication systems and of their nondisabled peers. Augmentative and Alternative Communication, 9, 10–25.

Lindblom, B. (1990). On the communication process: Speaker–listener interaction and the development of speech. Augmentative and Alternative Communication, 6, 220–230.

Linell, P. (1982). The Written Language Bias in Linguistics. Linköping, Sweden: University of Linköping.

Livingstone, S. (1983). Levels of development in the language of deaf children: ASL grammatical processes, SE structures and semantic features. Sign Language Studies, 37, 345–386.

Lloyd, L. L. (1990). AAC visions and needs for the next decade. In B. Mineo (Ed.), Augmentative and Alternative Communication in the Next Decade: Visions Conference Proceedings (pp. 65–68). Wilmington, DE: University of Delaware, Alfred I. duPont Institute.

Lloyd, L. L. (1994, November). Multicultural issues in augmentative and alternative communication. Paper presented at the Annual Convention of the American Speech-Language-Hearing Association, New Orleans, LA.

Lloyd, L. L. and Blischak, D. M. (1992). AAC terminology: Policy and issues update. Augmentative and Alternative Communication, 8, 104–109.

Lloyd, L. L. and Fuller, D. R. (1986). Toward an augmentative and alternative communication symbol taxonomy: A proposed superordinate classification. Augmentative and Alternative Communication, 2, 165–171.

Lloyd, L. L. and Fuller, D. R. (1990). The role of iconicity in augmentative and alternative communication symbol learning. In W. I. Fraser (Ed.), Key Issues in Mental Retardation Research (pp. 295–306). London: Routledge.

Lloyd, L. L., Fuller, D. R. and Arvidson, H. H. (Eds). (1997a). Augmentative and Alternative Communication: A Handbook of Principles and Practices. Boston: Allyn and Bacon.

Lloyd, L. L., Fuller, D. R. and Arvidson, H. H. (1997b). Introduction and overview. In L. L. Lloyd, D. R. Fuller and H. H. Arvidson (Eds), Augmentative and Alternative Communication: A Handbook of Principles and Practices (pp. 1–17). Boston: Allyn and Bacon.

Lloyd, L. L., Fuller, D. R., Loncke, F. and Bos, H. (1997). Introduction to AAC symbols.

In L. L. Lloyd, D. R. Fuller and H. H. Arvidson (Eds), Augmentative and Alternative Communication: A Handbook of Principles and Practices (pp. 43–47). Boston: Allyn and Bacon.

Lloyd, L. L. and Kangas, K. A. (1988). AAC terminology policy and issues. Augmentative and Alternative Communication, 4, 54–57.

Lloyd, L. L. and Kangas, K. A. (1990). AAC terminology policy and issues update. Augmentative and Alternative Communication, 6, 167–170.

Lloyd, L. L. and Karlan, G. R. (1983). Nonspeech communication symbol selection considerations. In Proceedings of the XIX Congress of the International Association of Logopaedics and Phoniatrics (Vol. III, pp. 1155–1160). Edinburgh, Scotland: University of Edinburgh.

Lloyd, L. L. and Karlan, G. R. (1984). Non-speech communication symbols and systems: Where have we been and where are we going? Journal of Mental Deficiency Research, 28, 3–20.

Lloyd, L. L., Karlan, G. H. and Nail-Chiwetalu, B. (1994). Translucency values for 910 Blissymbols. Unpublished manuscript, Purdue University, West Lafayette, IN.

Lloyd, L. L. and Kiernan, C. (1984). Graphic symbols: An overview. In Proceedings of the Second International Conference on Rehabilitation Engineering (ICRE-II): Special Sessions (pp. 34–37). (Combined with the Seventh Annual RESNA Conference), Ottawa, Ontario, Canada.

Lloyd, L., Quist, R. and Windsor, J. (1990). A proposed augmentative and alternative communication model. Augmentative and Alternative Communication, 6, 172–183.

Locke, J. (1995). Development of the capacity for spoken language. In P. Fletcher and B. MacWhinney (Eds), Handbook of Child Language (pp. 278–302). London: Blackwell.

Locke, J. (1996). Why do infants begin to talk? Language as an unintended consequence. Journal of Child Language, 23, 251–268.

Locke, J. (1997). A theory of neurolinguistic development. Brain and Language, 58, 265–326.

Locke, J. (1998). Are developmental language disorders primarily grammatical? Speculations from an evolutionary model. In R. Paul (Ed.), Exploring the Speech-Language Connection (pp. 53–72). Baltimore: Paul H. Brookes.

Loncke, F., Blischak, D., McNeill, D., Vander Beken, K. and Verbanck, I. (1997, November). Gesture analysis as a resource for multimodal communication intervention. Paper presented at the Annual Convention of the American-Speech-Language-Hearing Association, Boston, MA.

Loncke, F. and Bos, H. (1997). Unaided AAC symbols. In L. L. Lloyd, D. R. Fuller and H. H. Arvidson (Eds), Augmentative and Alternative Communication: A Handbook of Principles and Practices (pp. 80–106). Boston: Allyn and Bacon.

Loncke, F., Vander Beken, K. and Lloyd, L. L. (1997). Toward a theoretical model of symbol processing and use. In E. Björck-Åkesson and P. Lindsay (Eds), Communication... Naturally: Theoretical and Methodological Issues in Augmentative and Alternative Communication. Proceedings of the Fourth ISAAC Research Symposium (pp. 102–112). Västerås, Sweden: Mälardalen University Press.

Love, R. and Webb, W. (1996). Neurology for the Speech-Language Pathologist (3rd edn). Newton, MA: Butterworth-Heinemann.

Luftig, R. L. and Bersani, H. A., Jr. (1985a). An initial investigation of translucency, transparency, and component complexity of Blissymbolics. Journal of Childhood Communication Disorders, 8, 191–209.

Luftig, R. L. and Bersani, H. A., Jr. (1985b). An investigation of two variables influencing Blissymbol learnability with non handicapped adults. Augmentative and Alternative Communication, 1, 32–37.

Lundberg, I., Frost, J. and Petersen, O. (1988). Effects of an extensive program for stimulating phonological awareness in preschool children. Reading Research Quarterly, 23, 263–284.

Lutfiyya, Z. M. (1991). A feeling of being connected: Friendships between people with and without learning difficulties. Disability, Handicap and Society, 6, 233–245.

Lynch, E. W. and Hanson, M. J. (Eds) (1992). Developing Cross-cultural Competence: A Guide for Working with Young Children and Their Families. Baltimore: Paul H. Brookes.

Lynch, E. W. and Stein, R. (1987). Parent participation by ethnicity: A comparison of Hispanic, Black and Anglo families. Exceptional Children, 54, 105–111.

Magnuson, T. (1998). Linguistic evaluation of Profet II: A pilot project. In Proceedings of the Eighth Biennial Conference of the International Society for Augmentative and Alternative Communication (pp. 479–480). Dublin, Ireland: ISAAC/Ashfield Publications.

Mann, V. A. (1986). Phonological awareness: The role of reading experience. Cognition, 24, 65–92.

Marin, G. and Marin, B. (1991). Hispanics: Who are they? In G. Marin and B. Marin (Eds), Research with Hispanic Populations (pp. 1–17). Beverly Hills, CA: Sage.

Markman, E. (1992). Constraints on word learning: Speculations about their nature, origins, and domain specificity. In M. Gunnar and M. Maratsos (Eds), Modularity and Constraints in Language and Cognition (pp. 1–24). Hillsdale, NJ: Erlbaum.

Martinsen, H., Nordeng, H. and von Tetzchner, S. (1985). Tegnspråk.(Sign Language). Oslo: Universitetsforlaget.

Martinsen, H. and von Tetzchner, S. (1996). Situating augmentative and alternative communication intervention. In S. von Tetzchner and M. H. Jensen (Eds), Augmentative and Alternative Communication: European Perspectives (pp. 37–48). London: Whurr.

Mathy, P. (1998). Outcomes of AAC intervention in ALS. Augmentative Communication News, 11(1, 2), 6–7.

Mayberry, R. (1993). First-language acquisition after childhood differs from second-language acquisition: The case of American Sign Language. Journal of Speech and Hearing Research, 36, 1258–1270.

Mayberry, R. (1994). The importance of childhood to language acquisition: Evidence from American Sign Language. In J. Goodman and H. Nusbaum (Eds), The Development of Speech Perception: The Transition from Speech Sounds to Spoken Words (pp. 57–90). Cambridge, MA: MIT Press.

McCollum, J. and Hemmeter, M.-L. (1997). Parent–child interaction intervention when children have disabilities. In M. Guralnick (Ed.), Effectiveness of Early Intervention. London: Paul H. Brookes.

McConachie, H., Jolleff, N. and Clarke, M. (1998). The Castle Project. London: University College London Medical School, Institute of Child Health. Manuscript in preparation.

McConkey, R. (1994). Early intervention: Planning futures, shaping years. Mental Handicap Research, 7, 4–15.

McCoy, K. F. (1997). Simple NLP techniques for expanding telegraphic sentences. In A. Copestake, S. Langer and S. Palazuelos-Cagigas (Eds), Natural Language Processing for Communication Aids. Proceedings of the Workshop at the 35th Annual Meeting of the Association for Computational Linguistics and the 8th Conference of the European Chapter of the ACL (pp. 17–22). Madrid, Spain: Association for Computational Linguistics.

McCoy, K., Demasco, P., Gong, Y., Pennington, C. and Rowe, C. (1989). Toward a communication device which generates sentences. In Proceedings of the 12th Annual RESNA Conference (pp. 145–146). Washington, DC: RESNA.

McCoy, K. F., Demasco, P. W., Jones, M. A., Pennington, C. A., Vanderheyden, P. B. and Zickus, W. M. (1994). A communication tool for people with disabilities: Lexical semantics for filling in the pieces. In Proceedings of the First Annual ACM Conference on Assistive Technologies (ASSETS94) (pp. 107–114). New York: Association for Computing Machinery.

McCoy, K. F. and Masterman, L. N. (1997). A tutor for teaching English as a second language for deaf users of American Sign Language. In A. Copestake, S. Langer and S. Palazuelos-Cagigas (Eds), Natural Language Processing for Communication Aids. Proceedings of the Workshop at the 35th Annual Meeting of the Association for Computational Linguistics and the 8th Conference of the European Chapter of the ACL (pp. 47–54). Madrid, Spain: Association for Computational Linguistics.

McDonald, E. T. (1980). Teaching and Using Blissymbolics. Toronto, Ontario, Canada: Blissymbolics Communication Institute.

McDonald, J. (1997). Language acquisition: The acquisition of linguistic structure in normal and special populations. Annual Review of Psychology, 48, 215–241.

McGregor, A. and Alm, N. (1992). Thoughts of a nonspeaking member of an AAC research team. Augmentative and Alternative Communication, 8, 153.

McIntire, M. (1977). The acquisition of American Sign Language hand configurations. Sign Language Studies, 16, 247–266.

McLaughlin, M. L. (1984). Conversation: How Talk Is Organized. Beverly Hills, CA: Sage.

McNaughton, D. (1994). Measuring parent satisfaction with early childhood intervention programs: Current practices, problems, and future perspectives. Topics in Early Childhood Special Education, 14, 26–48.

McNaughton, S. (1985). Communicating with Blissymbolics. Toronto, Ontario, Canada: Blissymbolics Communication Institute.

McNaughton, S. (1990). A vision for the nineties: The decade for AAC users. In B. Mineo (Ed.), Augmentative and Alternative Communication in the Next Decade: Visions Conference Proceedings (pp. 5–12). Wilmington, DE: University of Delaware, Alfred I. duPont Institute.

McNaughton, S. (1993). Graphic representational systems and literacy learning. Topics in Language Disorders, 13(2), 58–75.

McNaughton, S. (1998a). Learning from a pilot study: Graphic symbols and reading acquisition. In Proceedings of the Eighth Biennial Conference of the International Society for Augmentative and Alternative Communication (pp. 132–133). Dublin, Ireland: ISAAC/Ashfield Publications.

McNaughton, S. (1998b). Reading acquisition of adults with severe congenital speech and physical impairments: Theoretical infrastructure, empirical investigation, educational application. Unpublished doctoral dissertation, University of Toronto, Toronto, Ontario, Canada.

McNaughton, S. and Lindsay, P. (1995). Approaching literacy with AAC graphics. Augmentative and Alternative Communication, 11, 212–228.

McNaughton, S., Mann, G., Harrington, K. and Harrington, R. (1988, October). Learning from those who know. Presented at the Third Biennial Conference of the International Society for Augmentative and Alternative Communication, Anaheim, CA.

McNeill, D. (1985). So you think gestures are nonverbal? Psychological Review, 92, 350–371.

McNeill, D. (1992). Hand and Mind. What Gestures Reveal About Thought. Chicago: University of Chicago Press.

McTear, M. (1985). Children's Conversations. Oxford, UK: Blackwell.

Merriman, W., Marazita, J. and Jarvis, L. (1995). Children's disposition to map new words onto new referents. In M. Tomasello (Ed.), Beyond Names for Things: Young Children's Acquisition of Verbs (pp. 147–185). Hillsdale, NJ: Erlbaum.

Merriman, W. and Tomasello, M. (1995). Introduction: Verbs are words too. In M. Tomasello (Ed.), Beyond Names for Things: Young Children's Acquisition of Verbs (pp. 1–20). Hillsdale, NJ: Erlbaum.

Mertens, D. M. (1998). Research Methods in Education and Psychology: Integrating Diversity with Quantitative and Qualitative Approaches. Thousand Oaks, CA: Sage.

Mervis, C. and Bertrand, J. (1993). Acquisition of early object labels: The roles of operating principles and input. In A. Kaiser and D. Gray (Eds), Enhancing Children's Communication: Research Foundations for Interventions (pp. 287–316). Baltimore: Paul H. Brookes.

Mervis, C. and Bertrand, J. (1997). Developmental relations between cognition and language: Evidence from Williams syndrome. In L. Adamson and M. A. Romski, (Eds), Communication and Language Acquisition: Discoveries from Atypical Development (pp. 75–106). Baltimore: Paul H. Brookes.

Miles, M. and Huberman, M. (1994). Qualitative Data Analysis. London: Sage.

Millen, N. (1996). Friends + Relations = FAMILY. Communicating Together, 13(2), 9–11.

Miller, L. (1990). The roles of language and learning in the development of literacy. Topics in Language Disorders, 10(1), 1–24.

Millikin, C. C. (1997). Symbol systems and vocabulary selection strategies. In S. L. Glennen and D. C. DeCoste, Handbook of Augmentative and Alternative Communication (pp. 97–148). San Diego, CA: Singular Publishing Group.

Mills, A., van den Bogaerde, B. and Coerts, J. (1994). Language input, interaction and the acquisition of Sign Language of the Netherlands. In B. van den Bogaerde, H. Knoors and M. Verrips (Eds), Language Acquisition with Non-native Input: The Acquisition of SLN (pp. 51–70). (Amsterdam Series in Child Language Development). Amsterdam: Instituut voor Algemene Tallwetenschap.

Mineo Mollica, B. and Peischl, D. (1997, August). Selecting picture-based language representations for AAC. Presented at the National Convention of the United States Society for Augmentative and Alternative Communication, Baltimore, MD.

Mirenda, P. (1997). Supporting people with challenging behavior through AAC. The ISAAC Bulletin, (48), 1–3.

Mirenda, P. and Mathy-Laikko, P. (1989). Augmentative and alternative communication applications for persons with severe congential communication disorders: An introduction. Augmentative and Alternative Communication, 5, 3–13.

Mirfin-Veitch, B. and Bray, A. (1997). Grandparents: Part of the family. In B. Carpenter (Ed.), Families in Context (pp. 76–88). London: David Fulton.

Mirfin-Veitch, B., Bray, A. and Watson, M. (1996). 'They really do care': Grandparents as informal support sources for parents of children with disabilities. New Zealand Journal of Disability Studies, 2, 136–148.

Mirfin-Veitch, B., Bray, A. and Watson, M. (1997). 'We're just that sort of family': Intergenerational relationships in families of children with disabilities. Family Relations, 46.

Mizuko, M. I. (1986). Iconicity and initial learning of three symbol systems in normal three year old children. Doctoral dissertation, University of Wisconsin, Madison.

Mizuko, M. I. and Reichle, J. (1989). Transparency and recall of symbols among intellectually handicapped adults. Journal of Speech and Hearing Disorders, 54, 627–633.

Mohay, H. (1990). The interaction of gesture and speech in the language development of two profoundly deaf children. In V. Volterra and C. Erting (Eds), From Gesture to Language in Hearing and Deaf Children (pp. 187–204). Berlin: Springer-Verlag.

Mollica, B. M. (1997). Representing the way to language learning and expression. ASHA Special Interest Division 12 – Augmentative and Alternative Communication, 6(4), 3–4.

Moon, C., Cooper, R. and Fifer, W. (1993). Two-day old infants prefer their native language. Infant Behavior and Development, 16, 495–500.

Morais, J., Alegria, J. and Content, A. (1987). The relationships between segmental analysis and alphabetic literacy: An interactive view. European Bulletin of Cognitive Psychology, 7, 415–438.

Morrison, A. and Martin, A. (1998). Evaluating the effectiveness of word prediction. In Proceedings of the Eighth Biennial Conference of the International Society for Augmentative and Alternative Communication (pp. 230–231). Dublin, Ireland: ISAAC/Ashfield Publications

Mundy, P. and Gomes, A. (1997). A skills approach to early language development: Lessons from research on developmental disabilities. In L. Adamson and M. A. Romski (Eds), Communication and Language Acquisition: Discoveries from Atypical Development (pp. 107–134). Baltimore: Paul H. Brookes.

Musselwhite, C. R. (1982). A comparison of three symbolic communication systems. Unpublished doctoral dissertation, West Virginia University, Morgantown.

Musselwhite, C. R. and Ruscello, D. (1984). Transparency of three communication symbol systems. Journal of Speech and Hearing Research, 27, 436–443.

Nail-Chiwetalu, B. J. (1992). The influence of symbol and learner factors on the learnability of Blissymbols by students with mental retardation. (Doctoral dissertation, Purdue University, 1991). Dissertation Abstracts International, 53, 1125A.

Nakamura, K., Newell, A. F., Alm, N. and Waller, A. C. (1998). How do members of different language communities compose sentences with a picture-based communication system? A cross-cultural study of picture-based sentences constructed by English and Japanese speakers. Augmentative and Alternative Communication, 14, 71–80.

Neale, J. M. and Liebert, R. M. (1973). Science and Behavior: An Introduction to Methods Research. Englewood Cliffs, NJ: Prentice-Hall.

Nelson, K. (Ed.). (1986). Event Knowledge: Structure and Function in Development. Hillsdale, NJ: Erlbaum.

Nelson, K. (1996). Language in Cognitive Development. Cambridge, MA: Cambridge University Press.

Nelson, N. W. (1992). Performance is the prize: Language competence and performance among AAC users. Augmentative and Alternative Communication, 8, 3–18.

Nelson, R. O. (1977). Assessment and therapeutic functions of self-monitoring. In I. Hersen, R. Eisler and P. Miller (Eds), Progress in Behavior Therapy (pp. 263–308). New York: Wiley.

Neville, H. (1997, November). Specificity and plasticity in human brain development. Presented at the Annual Convention of the American Speech-Language-Hearing Association, Boston, MA.

Ninio, A. and Snow, C. (1988). Language acquisition through language use: The functional sources of children's early utterances. In I. M. Schlesinger and M. Braine (Eds), Categories and Processes in Language Acquisition (pp. 1–30). Hillsdale, NJ: Erlbaum.

Norges Døveforbund. (1988). Norsk Tegnordbok. Bergen, Norway: Døves Förlag.

O'Keefe, B. (1997). Measurement methods for quality of life outcomes for AAC treatment. In E. Björck-Åkesson and P. Lindsay (Eds), Communication ... Naturally: Theoretical and Methodological Issues in Augmentative and Alternative

Communication. Proceedings of the Fourth ISAAC Research Symposium, (pp. 184–191). Västerås, Sweden: Mälardalen University Press.

Oliver, M. (1992). Changing the social relations of research production. Disability, Handicap and Society, 7, 101–114.

Oliver, M. (1996a). Re-defining disability: A challenge to research. In J. Swain, V. Finkelstein, S. French and M. Oliver (Eds), Disabling Barriers – Enabling Environments (pp. 61–67). London: Sage.

Oliver, M. (1996b). Understanding Disability. London: Macmillan.

Olson, D. R. (1997, January). The symmetries between what is taught and what children learn. Paper presented at the Ontario Institute for Studies in Education, University of Toronto, Toronto, Ontario, Canada.

Orlinsky, D. and Howard, K. (1986). Process and outcome in psychotherapy. In D. Orlinsky and K. Howard (Eds), Handbook of Psychotherapy and Behavior Change (pp. 311–381). London: Wiley.

Oxley, J. D. (1996, August). Developmental characteristics of IntroTalker use by nondisabled preschool-aged children. Presented at the Seventh Biennial Conference of the International Society for Augmentative and Alternative Communication, Vancouver, British Columbia, Canada.

Oxley, J. D. and Norris, J. A. (1997). Metamemory and memory implicated in the use of certain voice output communication aids. Manuscript submitted for publication.

Padden, C. (1983). The Deaf community and the culture of Deaf people. In C. Baker and R. Battison (Eds), Sign Language and the Deaf Community: Essays in Honor of William C. Stokoe (pp. 89–103). Silver Springs, MD: National Association of the Deaf.

Paget, K. D. (1992). Parent involvement in early childhood services. In M. Gettinger, S. N. Elliot and T. R. Kratochwill (Eds), Preschool and Early Childhood Treatment Directions. Hillsdale, NJ: Erlbaum.

Paivio, A. (1971). Imagery and Verbal Processes. New York: Holt, Rinehart & Winston.

Paivio, A. (1986). Mental Representations: A Dual Coding Approach. Oxford, UK: Oxford University Press.

Palazuelos, S., Aguilera, S., Claypool, T., Ricketts. I. and Gregor, P. (1998). Comparison of two word prediction systems using five European languages. In Proceedings of ISAAC '98 Conference (pp. 192–193). Dublin, Ireland: ISAAC/Ashfield Publications.

Palazuelos, S., Aguilera, S., Ricketts, I., Gregor, P. and Claypool, T. (1998). Artificial neural networks applied to improving linguistic word prediction. In Proceedings of ISAAC '98 Conference (pp. 193–194). Dublin, Ireland: ISAAC/Ashfield Publications.

Palazuelos-Cagigas, S. E. and Aguilera-Navarro, S. (1996). Report on word prediction for Spanish. Deliverable WP7T3D.2IR of VAESS: Voices, attitudes and emotions in speech synthesis. TIDE N. 1174.

Palazuelos-Cagigas, S., Godino-Llorente, J. and Aguilera-Navarro, S. (1997). Comparison between adaptive and non-adaptive word prediction methods in a word processor for motorically handicapped non-vocal users. In Proceedings of the Conference of the Association for the Advancement of Assistive Technology in Europe (AAATE) (pp. 158–162). Thessalonica, Greece: Association for the Advancement of Assistive Technology in Europe.

Parette, H. P. (1994, October). Family functioning and AAC device prescriptive practices. Presented at DEC Early Childhood Conference on Children with Special Needs, St Louis, MO.

Parette, H. P. and Brotherson, M. J. (1996). Family participation in assistive technology assessment for young children with mental retardation and developmental disabilities. Education and Training in Mental Retardation and Developmental Disabilities, 31, 29–43.

Parette, H. P., Stuart, S., Huer, M. B., Hoge, D. R., Hostetler, S., Dunn, N., Brotherson, M. J., VanBiervliet, A. and Wommack, J. (1996, November). Qualitative methodology and AAC decision making with families across cultures. Paper presented at the Annual Convention of the American Speech-Language-Hearing Association, Seattle, WA.

Parette, H. P. and VanBiervliet, A. (1995). Culture, families, and augmentative and alternative communication (AAC) impact: A multimedia instructional program for related services personnel and family members. Grant funded by the US Department of Education, Office of Special Education and Rehabilitative Services (No. H029K50072).

Parette, H.P., VanBiervliet, A. and Huer, M.B. (1998, August). Technology for decision-making with families across cultures. Presented at the Eighth Biennial Conference of the International Society for Augmentative and Alternative Communication, Dublin, Ireland.

Patterson, K. E., Marschall, J. C. and Coltheart, M. (1985). Surface Dyslexia: Neurological and Cognitive Studies of Phonological Reading. Hillsdale, NJ: Erlbaum.

Patton, M. (1978). Utilization-focused Evaluation. Beverly Hills, CA: Sage.

Patton, M. Q. (1990). Qualitative Evaluation and Research Methods (2nd edn). Newbury Park, CA: Sage.

Paul, R. (1997). Facilitating transitions in language development for children using AAC. Augmentative and Alternative Communication, 13, 141–148.

Paul, R. (1998). Communicative development in augmented modalities: Language without speech? In R. Paul (Ed.), Exploring the Speech-Language Connection (pp. 139–162). Baltimore, MD: Paul H. Brookes.

Persson, J. and Brodin, H. (1996). Prototype tool for assistive technology cost and utility evaluation (EU-Tide Study). Linköping, Sweden: Linköping University.

Petitto, L. (1987). On the autonomy of language and gesture: Evidence from the acquisition of personal pronouns in American Sign Language. Cognition, 27, 1–52.

Petitto, L. A. (1988). Language in the prelinguistic child: An essay. In J. Kessel (Ed.), The Development of Language and Language Researchers (pp. 187–221). Hillsdale, NJ: Erlbaum.

Petitto, L. (1993). Modularity and constraints in early lexical acquisition: Evidence from children's early language and gesture. In P. Bloom (Ed.), Language Acquisition: Core Readings (pp. 95–126). London: Harvester Wheatsheaf. (Original work published 1992)

Petitto, L. and Marentette, P. (1991). Babbling in the manual mode: Evidence for the ontogeny of language. Science, 251, 1483–1496.

Piaget, J. (1959) The Language and Thought of the Child (3rd edn). London: Routledge.

Pine, J. and Lieven, E. (1993). Reanalysing rote-learned phrases: Individual differences in the transition to multi-word speech. Journal of Child Language, 20, 551–571.

Pinker, S. (1982). A theory of mental representation of lexical-interpretative grammars. In J.W. Bresman (Ed.), The Mental Representation of Grammatical Relations (pp. 53–63). Cambridge, MA: MIT Press.

Pinker, S. (1984). Language Learnability and Language Development. Cambridge, MA: Harvard University Press.

Pinker, S. (1994). The Language Instinct: The New Science of Language and Mind. London: Allan Lane.

Pinker, S. (1995). Facts about human language relevant to its evolution. In J.-P. Changeux and J. Chavaillon (Eds), Origins of the Human Brain (pp. 262–283). New York: Oxford University Press.

Platt, C. B. and MacWhinney, B. (1983). Error assimilation as a mechanism in language learning. Journal of Child Language, 10, 401–414.

President's Committee on Mental Retardation (1996). Voices and visions: Building leadership for the 21st century. Washington, DC: US Department of Health and Human Services.

Quist, R. W., van Balkom, H., Lloyd, L. L., Welle-Donker Gimbrére, M. and Vander Beken, K. (1998, August). Translucency values of Blissymbols across cultures. In Proceedings of the Eighth Biennial Conference of the International Society for Augmentative and Alternative Communication [Abstract] (pp. 138–139). Dublin, Ireland: ISAAC/Ashfield Publications.

Radford, A. (1990). Syntactic Theory and the Acquisition of English Syntax. Oxford, UK: Blackwell.

Raghavendra, P., Collsey, B., Hardy, M. and McDonald, F. (1998). Development of a critical pathway for VOCA use by adults with disabilities in the community. Paper presented at the Fourth National Conference of AGOSCI, Perth, Australia.

Ramcharan, P. and Grant, G. (1994). Setting one agenda for empowering persons with a disadvantage in the research process. In M. Rioux and M. Bach (Eds), Disability Is Not Measles: New Research Paradigms in Disability (pp. 227–244). North York, Ontario, Canada: L'Institut Roeher Institute.

Rankin, J., Harwood, K. and Mirenda, P. (1994). Influence of graphic symbol use on reading comprehension. Augmentative and Alternative Communication, 10, 269–281.

Rappaport, J. (1987). Terms of empowerment/exemplars of prevention: Toward a theory for community psychology. American Journal of Community Psychology, 15, 121–148.

Rayner, K. (1976). Developmental changes in word recognition strategies. Journal of Educational Psychology, 68, 323–329.

Rayner, K. and Pollatsek, A. (1989). The Psychology of Reading. Englewood Cliffs, NJ: Prentice-Hall.

Reason, P. (1994). Three approaches to participative inquiry. In N. K. Denzin and Y. S. Lincoln (Eds), The Handbook of Qualitative Research (pp. 324–339). Thousand Oaks, CA: Sage.

Reich, P. and Shein, F. (1990). VOICI: A voice output intelligent communication system [Abstract]. Augmentative and Alternative Communication, 6, 104. Paper presented at the Fourth Biennial Conference of the International Society for Augmentative and Alternative Communication, Stockholm, Sweden.

Reilly, J. S., McIntire, M. and Bellugi, U. (1990). The acquisition of conditionals and ASL: Grammatical facial expressions. Applied Psycholinguistics, 11, 369–392.

Remington, B. and Clarke, S. (1993a). Simultaneous communication and speech comprehension. Part 1: Comparison of two methods of teaching expressive signing and speech comprehension skills. Augmentative and Alternative Communication, 9, 36–48.

Remington, B. and Clarke, S. (1993b). Simultaneous communication and speech comprehension. Part II: Comparison of two methods of overcoming selective attention during expressive sign training. Augmentative and Alternative Communication, 9, 49–60.

Research and Training Center on Independent Living for Underserved Populations (1996). Guidelines for Reporting and Writing about People with Disabilities. Lawrence, KS: Author.

Rimé, B. and Schiatura, L. (1991). Gesture and speech. In R. S. Feldman and B. Rimé (Eds), Fundamentals of Non-verbal Behavior (pp. 239–282). Cambridge, UK: Cambridge University Press.

Romski, M. A. and Sevcik, R. A. (1991). Patterns of language learning by instruction: Evidence from nonspeaking persons with mental retardation. In N. S. Krasnegor, D. M. Rumbaugh, R. L. Schiefelbush and M. Studdert-Kennedy (Eds), Biological and Behavioral Determinants of Language Development (pp. 429–445). Hillsdale, NJ: Erlbaum.

Romski, M. A. and Sevcik, R. A. (1992). Developing augmented language in children with severe mental retardation. In S. F. Warren and J. Reichle (Eds), Causes and Effects in Communication and Language Intervention (pp. 113–130). Baltimore: Paul H. Brookes.

Romski, M. A. and Sevcik, R. A. (1996). Breaking the Speech Barrier: Language Development Through Augmented Means. Baltimore: Paul H. Brookes.

Romski, M., Sevcik, R. and Adamson, L. (1997a, November). Comprehension profiles of preschoolers with disabilities who are not speaking. Presented at the Annual Convention of the American Speech-Language-Hearing Association, Boston, MA.

Romski, M. A., Sevcik, R. A. and Adamson, L. B. (1997b). Framework for studying how children with developmental disabilities develop language through augmented means. Augmentative and Alternative Communication, 13, 172–178.

Roseberry-McKibbin, C. (1995). Multicultural Students with Special Language Needs Oceanside, CA: Academic Communication Associates.

Roth, F. P. and Casset-James, E. (1989). The language assessment process: Clinical implications for individuals with severe speech impairments. Augmentative and Alternative Communication, 5, 165–172.

Rowland, C. (1998, August). Me Tarzan, you Jane: Can you communicate without language? Presented at the Eighth Biennial Conference of the International Society for Augmentative and Alternative Communication, Dublin, Ireland.

Ryan, J. (1977). The silence of stupidity. In J. Morton and J. C. Marshall (Eds), Psycholinguistic Series: Vol. 1. Developmental and Pathological (pp. 99–124). London: Elek Science.

Ryan, R. M., Deci, E. L. and Grolnick, W. S. (1995). Autonomy, relatedness and the self: Their relation to development and psychopathology. In D. Cicchetti and D. J. Cohen (Eds), Developmental Psychopathology: Vol. 1. Theory and Methods. New York: Wiley.

Sameroff, A. J. and Fiese, B. H. (1990). Transactional regulation and early intervention. In S. J. Meisels and J. P. Shonkoff (Eds), Handbook of Early Childhood Intervention (pp. 119–149). New York: Cambridge University Press.

Sanders, D. A. (1976). A model for communication. In L. L. Lloyd (Ed.), Communication Assessment and Intervention Strategies (pp. 1–32). Baltimore: University Park Press.

Santelli, B., Singer, G. H., DiVenere, N., Ginsberg, C. and Powers, L. E. (in press). Participatory action research: Reflections on critical incidents in a PAR project. JASH.

Schalock, M., Fredericks, B., Dalke, B. and Alberto, P. (1994). The house that traces built: A conceptual model of service delivery systems and implications for change. Journal of Special Education, 28, 203–223.

Schank, R. (1982). Dynamic Memory: A Theory of Reminding and Learning in Computers and People. Cambridge, UK: Cambridge University Press.

Schank, R. and Abelson, R. (1977). Scripts, Plans, Goals and Understanding. Hillsdale, NJ: Erlbaum.

Scherer, M. (1993). Living in the State of Stuck. Cambridge, MA: Brookline Books.

Schlosser, R. W. (1995). Effectiveness of initial element teaching in a storytelling context on Blissymbol acquisition and generalization. Journal of Speech and Hearing Research, 36, 979–995.

Schlosser, R. W. (1996, August). Social validation of interventions in augmentative and alternative communication: A proposed conceptual framework. Presented at the International Society for Augmentative and Alternative Communication Research Symposium, Vancouver, British Columbia, Canada.

Schlosser, R. (1997a). Methods and strategies for assessing the perspectives of consumers in AAC research. In E. Björck-Åkesson and P. Lindsay (Eds), Communication... Naturally: Theoretical and Methodological Issues in Augmentative and Alternative Communication. Proceedings of the Fourth ISAAC Research Symposium (pp. 166–183). Västerås, Sweden: Mälardalen University Press.

Schlosser, R. W. (1997b). Social validation of intervention research in augmentative and alternative communication: A proposed conceptual framework. In E. Björck-Åkesson and P. Lindsay (Eds), Communication ... Naturally: Theoretical and Methodological Issues in Augmentative and Alternative Communication. Proceedings of the Fourth ISAAC Research Symposium (pp. 166–183). Västerås, Sweden: Mälardalen University Press.

Schlosser, R. W. (in press). Social validation of interventions in augmentative and alternative communication. Augmentative and Alternative Communication..

Schlosser, R. W. and Braun, U. (1992). Toward a comprehensive efficacy evaluation of AAC intervention. In D. J. Gardner-Bonneau (Ed.), Methodological Issues in Research in Augmentative and Alternative Communication. Toronto, Ontario, Canada: International Association for Augmentative and Alternative Communication.

Schlosser, R. W., Lloyd, L. L. and McNaughton, S. (1997). Graphic symbol selection in research and practice: Making the case for a goal-driven process. In E. Björck-Åkesson and P. Lindsay (Eds), Communication... Naturally: Theoretical and Methodological Issues in Augmentative and Alternative Communication. Proceedings of the Fourth ISAAC Research Symposium (pp. 126–141). Västerås, Sweden: Mälardalen University Press.

Schorr, G. (1983). Visual impairment. In J. Blackman (Ed.), Medical Aspects of Developmental Disabilities in Children Birth to Three (pp. 227–231). Iowa City, IA: University of Iowa, University Hospital School, Department of Pediatrics.

Schweigert, P. and Rowland, C. (1992). Early communication and micro technology: Instructional sequence and case studies of children with severe multiple disabilities. Augmentative and Alternative Communication, 8, 273–286.

Scollon, R. (1976). Conversations With a One Year Old. Honolulu, HI: University of Hawaii Press.

Scollon, R. (1979). A real early stage: An unzippered condensation of a dissertation on child language. In E. Ochs and B. Schieffelin (Eds), Developmental Pragmatics (pp. 215–227). London: Academic Press.

Scott, A. (1998). Positive outcomes. Advance, 8(32), 7–9.

Seligman, M. (1991).Grandparents of disabled grandchildren: Hopes, fears and adaptation. Families in Society, 24, 147–152.

Seligman, M. (1992). Learned Optimism. New York: Simon and Schuster.

Selman, R.L. (1980) The Growth of Interpersonal Understanding. New York: Academic Press.

Severinson-Eklund, K. and Kollberg, P. (1995). Computer tools for tracing the writing process: From keystroke records to S-notation. In G. Rijaarsdam, M. Couzijn and H. van den Bergh (Eds), Current Research in Writing: Theories, Models and Methodology (pp. 526–541). Amsterdam: Amsterdam University Press.

Shannon, C. E. and Weaver, W. W. (1949). The Mathematical Theory of Communication. Urbana, IL: University of Illinois.

Share, D. L. (1995). Phonological recoding and self-teaching: Sine qua non of reading acquisition. Cognition, 55, 151–218.

Share, D. L., Jorm, A. F., MacLean, R. and Matthews, R. (1984). Sources of individual differences in reading achievement. Journal of Educational Psychology, 76, 466–477.

Shepard, R. N. and Cooper, L. A. (1986). Mental Images and Their Transformations. Cambridge, MA: MIT Press.

Siegel, L. S. (1993). The development of reading. Advances in Child Development and Behavior, 24, 63–97.

Silverman, F. (1995). Communication for the Speechless (3rd edn). Boston: Allyn and Bacon.

Simeonsson, R. (1995). Intervention in communicative disability: Evaluation issues and evidence. In J. Rönnberg and E. Hjelqvist (Eds), Communicative Disability: Compensation and Development (pp. 79–96). Linköping, Sweden: Linköping University.

Singleton, J., Goldin-Meadow, S. and McNeill, D. (1995). The cataclysmic break between gesticulation and sign: Evidence against an evolutionary continuum of manual communication. In K. Emmorey and J. Reilly (Eds), Sign, Gesture and Space (pp. 287–312). Hillsdale, NJ: Erlbaum.

Sinteff, B. (1998). Applying vocabulary search strategies in augmentative communication: DynaVox and DynaMyte products. In Proceedings of the Technology and Persons with Disabilities Conference (CSUN-98). Northridge, CA: California State University Center on Disabilities. Available: http://www.dinf.org/csun_98/csun98.htm

Siple, P. and Fischer, S. D. (Eds). (1991). Theoretical Issues in Sign Language Research: Vol. 2. Psychology. Chicago: University of Chicago Press.

Sjölander, K., Beskow, J., Gustafson, J., Lewin, E., Carlson, R. and Granström, B. (1998). Web-based educational tools for speech technology. In R. H. Mannell and J. Robert-Riber (Eds), Proceedings of ICSLP '98 (pp. 3217–3220). Canberra, Australia: Australian Speech Science and Technology Association.

Slater, A. and Butterworth, G. (1997). Perception of social stimuli. Face perception and imitation. In G. Bremner, A. Slater and G. Butterworth (Eds), Infant Development (pp. 223-245). Hove, East Sussex, UK: Psychology Press.

Slobin, D. (1985). The Cross-linguistic Study of Language Acquisition: The Data. Hillsdale, NJ: Erlbaum.

Smith, B. R. and Leinonen, E. (1992). Clinical Pragmatics. London: Chapman and Hall.

Smith, F. (1971). Understanding Reading (1st edn). New York: Holt, Rinehart & Winston.

Smith, F. (1973). Psycholinguistics and Reading. New York: Holt, Rinehart & Winston.

Smith, F. (1979). Reading Without Nonsense. New York: Teachers College Press.

Smith, L. B. and Thelen, E. (Eds). (1993). A Dynamic Systems Approach to Development: Applications. Cambridge, MA: Bradford Book, MIT Press.

Smith, M. M. (1989). Reading without speech: A study of children with cerebral palsy. Irish Journal of Psychology, 10, 601–614.

Smith, M. M. (1992). Reading abilities of nonspeaking students: Two case studies. Augmentative and Alternative Communication, 8, 57–66.

Smith, M. (1996a, August). The bimodal situation of children learning language using AAC. Paper presented at the International Society for Augmentative and Alternative Communication Research Symposium, Vancouver, British Columbia, Canada.

Smith, M. (1996b) The medium or the message: A study of speaking children using communication boards. In S. von Tetzchner and M. H. Jensen (Eds), Augmentative and Alternative Communication: European Perspectives (pp. 119–136). London: Whurr.

Smith, M. M. (1997). The bimodal situation of children developing alternative modes of language. In E. Björck-Åkesson and P. Lindsay (Eds), Communication... Naturally: Theoretical and Methodological Issues in Augmentative and Alternative Communication. Proceedings of the Fourth ISAAC Research Symposium (pp. 12–18). Västerås, Sweden: Mälardalen University Press.

Smith, M. M. and Blischak, D. M. (1997). Literacy. In L. L. Lloyd, D. R. Fuller and H. H. Arvidson (Eds), Augmentative and Alternative Communication: A Handbook of Principles And Practices (pp. 414–444). Boston: Allyn and Bacon.

Smith, M. and Grove, N. (1996, August). Input/output asymmetries: Implications for language development in AAC. Paper presented at the Seventh Biennial Conference of the International Society for Augmentative and Alternative Communication, Vancouver, British Columbia, Canada.

Smith-Lewis, M. R. and Ford, A. (1987). A user's perspective on augmentative communication. Augmentative and Alternative Communication, 3, 12–17.

Snijders, J. T. H. and Snijders-Oomen, S. O. (1976). Non-verbal Intelligence Scale. Windsor, UK: NFER Nelson.

Snow, C. E. (1991). Diverse conversational contexts for the acquisition of various language skills. In J. Miller (Ed.), Research on Child Language Disorders: A Decade of Progress (pp. 105–124). Austin, TX: Pro-Ed.

Snow, C. (1995). Issues in the study of input: Functions, universality, individual and developmental differences and necessary causes. In P. Fletcher and B. MacWhinney (Eds), Handbook of Child Language (pp. 180–193). London: Blackwell.

Sontag, J. (1996). Toward a comprehensive theoretical framework for disability research: Bronfenbrenner revisited. Journal of Special Education, 30, 319–344.

Soto, G. (1997a). Multi-unit utterances and syntax in graphic symbol communication. In E. Björck-Åkesson and P. Lindsay (Eds), Communication... Naturally: Theoretical and Methodological Issues in Augmentative and Alternative Communication. Proceedings of the Fourth ISAAC Research Symposium (pp. 26–32). Västerås, Sweden: Mälardalen University Press.

Soto, G. (1997b). Special education teacher attitudes toward AAC: Preliminary survey. Augmentative and Alternative Communication, 13, 186–197.

Soto, G. (1998, August). Pressing levers or picking locks: An AAC Response. Paper presented at the Eighth Biennial Conference of the International Society for Augmentative and Alternative Communication, Dublin, Ireland.

Soto, G., Huer, M. B. and Taylor, O. (1997). Multicultural issues. In L. L. Lloyd, D. R. Fuller and H. H. Arvidson (Eds), Augmentative and Alternative Communication: A Handbook of Principles and Practices (pp. 406–413). Boston: Allyn and Bacon.

Soto, G. and Olmstead, W. (1993). A semiotic perspective on AAC. Augmentative and Alternative Communication, 9, 134–141.

Soto, G. and Toro-Zambrana, W. (1995). Investigation of Blissymbol use from a language research paradigm. Augmentative and Alternative Communication, 11, 118–130.

Sparck Jones, K. and Galliers, J. R. (1995). Evaluating Natural Language Processing Systems: An Analysis and Review. Berlin: Springer-Verlag.

Spelke, E. (1991). Physical knowledge in infancy: Reflections on Piaget's theory. In S. Carey and R. Gelman (Eds), The Epigenesis of Mind: Essays on Biology and Cognition (pp. 133–169). Hillsdale, NJ: Erlbaum.

Sperber, D. and Wilson, D. (1986). Relevance: Communication and Cognition. Oxford, UK: Blackwell.

Stalker, K. (1998). Some ethical and methodological issues in research with people with learning difficulties. Disability and Society, 13, 5–19.

Stanovich, K. E. (1980). Toward an interactive-compensatory model of individual differences in the development of reading fluency. Reading Research Quarterly, 1, 32–71.

Stanovich, K. E. (1986). Matthew effects in reading: Some consequences of individual differences in the acquisition of literacy. Reading Research Quarterly, 21, 360–407.

Stanovich, K. E. (1988). The right and wrong places to look for the cognitive locus of reading disability. Annals of Dyslexia, 38, 154–177.

Stanovich, K. E. (1992). Speculations on the causes and consequences of individual differences in early reading acquisition. In P. B. Gough, L. C. Ehri and R. Treiman (Eds), Reading Acquisition (pp. 307–342). Hillsdale, NJ: Erlbaum.

Stanovich, K. E. and West, R. F. (1989). Exposure to print and orthographic processing. Reading Research Quarterly, 24, 402–433.

Steciw, M. A. (1995, July). Hearing and vision considerations for meeting the needs of individuals with severe disabilities. Materials for AAC course at Purdue University, West Lafayette, IN.

Stephenson, J. and Linfoot, K. (1996). Pictures as communication symbols for students with severe intellectual disability. Augmentative and Alternative Communication, 12, 244–256.

Ström, N. (1997). Automatic continuous speech recognition with rapid speaker adaptation for human/machine interaction. Doctoral thesis, KTH, Department of Speech, Music and Hearing, Stockholm, Sweden.

Strömqvist, S. and Ahlsén, E. (Eds). (1998). Reading and Writing Strategies of Disabled Groups (Progress Report 1). Göteborg, Sweden: Göteborg University, Department of Linguistics.

Strömqvist, S. and Malmsten, L. (1998). ScriptLog Pro 1.04: User's Manual. Göteborg, Sweden: Göteborg University, Department of Linguistics.

Strömqvist, S. and Wengelin, Å. (1998). The temporal distribution of actions in on-line writing. In E. Esperét (Ed.), Writing and Learning to Write at the Dawn of the 21st Century. Proceedings from the 1998 European Writing Conference. Poitiers, France: Université de Poitiers.

Sutton, A. C. (1989). The social-verbal competence of AAC users. Augmentative and Alternative Communication, 5, 150–164.

Sutton, A. C. (1997). Language theory and intervention practice. In E. Björck-Åkesson and P. Lindsay (Eds), Communication... Naturally: Theoretical and Methodological Issues in Augmentative and Alternative Communication. Proceedings of the Fourth ISAAC Research Symposium (pp. 33–47). Västerås, Sweden: Mälardalen University Press.

Sutton, A. and Dench, C. (1998). Connected speech development in a child with limited language production experience. Journal of Speech-Language Pathology and Audiology, 22, 134–141.

Sutton, A. and Gallagher, T. (1993). Verb class distinctions and AAC language encoding limitations. Journal of Speech and Hearing Research, 36, 1216–1226.

Sutton, A. and Gallagher, T. (1995). Comprehension assessment of a child using an AAC system: A comparison of two techniques. American Journal of Speech-Language Pathology, 4, 60–67.

Sutton, A. and Morford, J. (1998). Constituent order in picture pointing sequences produced by speaking children using AAC. Applied Psycholinguistics, 19, 525–536.

Swain, J., Heyman, B. and Gillman, M. (1998). Public research, private concerns: Ethical issues in the use of open-ended interviews with people who have learning difficulties. Disability and Society, 13, 21–36.

Sweeney, L. A. (1988). Communication dependency profile: Manuscript and assessment tool. Manuscript in preparation.

Sweeney, L. A. (1989). Reducing learned dependency in potential and early augmentative communication users. In Proceedings of the Southeast Augmentative

Communication Conference (pp. 66–68). Birmingham, AL: Southeast Augmentative Communication Conference.

Sweeney, L. A. (1992, November). Profiling communicative dependency. Miniseminar presented at the Annual Convention of the American Speech-Language-Hearing Association, San Antonio, TX.

Sweeney, L. A. (1993). Helplessness, dependency, and explanatory style as variables of employment potential among augmented communicators. In Proceedings of the First Pittsburgh Employment Conference for Augmented Communicators, 1 (pp. 91–100). Pittsburgh, PA: Pittsburgh Employment Conference.

Sweeney, L. A. (1996, September). Fostering interactive communication: Developing partner skills that support the augmented communicator. Presented at Macomb Intermediate School District, Macomb, MI.

Sweeney, L. A. (1997). Toward identification of factors within and around the family that affect acceptance and use of AAC. In E. Björck-Åkesson and P. Lindsay (Eds), Communication... Naturally: Theoretical and Methodological Issues in Augmentative and Alternative Communication (pp. 217–230). Västerås, Sweden: Mälardalen University Press.

Sweeney, L. A. (1999). Family interactions with AAC: What about dad? Manuscript in preparation.

Sweeney, L. A. and Engwis, P. (1996, August). Perceived levels of initiation among individuals experiencing significant communication challenges. Presented at the Seventh Biennial Conference of the International Society for Augmentative and Alternative Communication, Vancouver, British Columbia, Canada.

Sweeney, L. A. and Van Tatenhove, G. (1998, November). Transitions through the life span for people who use AAC. Short course presented at the Annual Convention of the American Speech-Language-Hearing Association, San Antonio, TX.

Sweeney, L. A., Björck-Åkesson, E. and Granlund, M. (1998, August). Family issues in AAC: Establishing core learnings. Presented at the International Society for Augmentative and Alternative Communication Research Symposium, Dublin, Ireland.

Sweeney, L. A., Granlund, M., Björck-Åkesson, E., Basil, C., Soro-Camats, E., Jonker, V. M., Boendermaker-Meyer, M. and Heim, M. J. M. (1998, August). Family involvement in AAC: Common issues and international perspectives. Seminar presented at the Eighth Biennial Conference of the International Society for Augmentative and Alternative Communication, Dublin, Ireland.

Swiffin, A. L., Arnott, J. L. and Newell, A. F. (1987). The use of syntax in a predictive communication aid for the physically impaired. In Proceedings of the Tenth Annual Conference on Rehabilitation Technology (pp. 124–126). Washington, DC: RESNA.

Tannock, R., Girolometto, L. and Seigel, L. (1992). Language intervention with children who have developmental delay: Effects of an interactive approach. American Journal on Mental Retardation, 97, 145–160.

Taylor, S. J. and Bogdan, R. (1984). Introduction to Qualitative Research Methods: The Search for Meanings. New York: Wiley.

Tesch, R. (1990). Qualitative Research: Analysis Types and Software Tools. New York: Falmer Press.

Tharp, R. G. and Gallimore, R. (1989). Challenging Cultural Minds. London: Cambridge University Press.

Thomas, C. and Parry, A. (1996). Research on users' views about stroke services: Towards an empowerment research paradigm or more of the same? Physiotherapy, 82(1), 6–12.

Thompson, H. (1994). TEMAA: A testbed study of evaluation methodologies: Authoring aids. In Proceedings of the ELSNET Language Engineering Convention (pp. 147–148). Paris, France.

Todman, J. and Alm, N. (1997). Pragmatics and AAC approaches to conversational goals. In A. Copestake, S. Langer and S. Palazuelos-Cagigas (Eds). In Natural Language Processing for Communication Aids. Proceedings of the Workshop at the 35th Annual Meeting of the Association for Computational Linguistics and the 8th Conference of the European Chapter of the ACL (pp. 1–8). Madrid, Spain: Association for Computational Linguistics.

Todman, J., Alm, N. and Elder, L. (1994). Computer-aided conversation: A prototype system for non-speaking people with physical disabilities. Applied Psycholinguistics, 15, 45–73.

Todman, J., Elder, L. and Alm, N. (1995). An evaluation of the content of computer-aided conversations. Augmentative and Alternative Communication, 11, 229–234.

Todman, J. and Lewins, E. (1996). Conversational rate of a non-vocal person with motor neurone disease using the 'TALK' system. International Journal of Rehabilitation Research, 19, 285–287.

Todman, J., Lewins, E., File, P., Alm, N. and Elder, L. (1995). Use of a communication aid (TALK) by a non-speaking person with cerebral palsy. Communication Matters, 9, 18–21.

Todman, J., Rankin, D. and File, P. (in press). The use of stored text in computer-aided Conversation: a single-case experiment. Journal of Language and Social Psychology.

Trivette, C. M., Dunst, C. J. and Deal, A. G. (1997). Resource-based early intervention practices. In S. K. Thurman, J. R. Cornwell and S. R. Gottwald (Eds), The Contexts of Early Intervention: Systems and Settings. Baltimore: Paul H. Brookes.

Tunmer, W. E. and Hoover, W. A. (1993). Phonological recoding skill and beginning reading. Reading and Writing: An Interdisciplinary Journal, 5, 161–170.

Tunmer, W. E. and Nesdale, A. R. (1985). Phonemic segmentation skill and beginning reading. Journal of Educational Psychology, 77, 417–427.

Turnbull, A. P. and Turnbull, H. R., (1996). Participatory action research. In National Council on Disability (Ed.), Improving the Implementation of the Individuals with Disabilities Education Act: Making Schools Work for All of America's Children (pp. 685–710). Washington, DC: National Council on Disability.

Tyvand, S. and Demasco P. (1993). Syntax statistics in word prediction. In The Swedish Handicap Institute (Ed.), Proceedings of the ECART2 Conference (section 11.1). Stockholm: Kommentus.

Vaillant, P. (1998). Interpretation of iconic utterances based on contents representation: Semantic analysis in the PVI system. Journal of Natural Language Engineering, 4(1), 17–40.

van Balkom, H. (1998). Enhancing natural language compensation (NCL) through augmentative communication. Paper presented at the Eighth Biennial Conference of the International Society for Augmentative and Alternative Communication, Dublin, Ireland.

van Balkom, H. and Welle Donker-Gimbrére, M. (1996). A psycholinguistic approach to graphic language use. In S. von Tetzchner and M. H. Jensen (Eds), Augmentative and Alternative Communication: European Perspectives (pp. 153–170). London: Whurr.

Vanderheiden, G. C. and Lloyd, L. L. (1986). Communication systems and their components. In S. W. Blackstone (Ed.), Augmentative Communication: An Introduction (pp. 49–161). Rockville, MD: American Speech-Language-Hearing Association.

Vanderheiden, G. C. and Yoder, D. E. (1986). Overview. In S. W. Blackstone (Ed.), Augmentative Communication: An Introduction (pp. 1–28). Rockville, MD: American Speech-Language-Hearing Association.

Vanderheyden, P. B. (1995). An augmentative communication interface based on conversational schemata. In Proceedings of the IJCAI '95 Workshop on Developing AI Applications for Disabled People (pp. 203–212). Montreal, Québec, Canada.

Vandervelden, M. C. and Siegel, L. S. (1995). Phonological recoding and phoneme awareness in early literacy: A developmental approach. Reading Research Quarterly, 30, 854–875.

Vasta, R. (Ed.). (1992). Six Theories of Child Development. London: Jessica Kingsley.

Veneziano, E., Sinclair, H. and Berthoud, I. (1990). From one word to two words: Repetition patterns on the way to structured speech. Journal of Child Language, 17, 633–650.

von Bertalanffy, L. (1968). General Systems Theory. New York: Braziller.

von Tetzchner, S. (1985). Words and chips – Pragmatics and pidginization of computer-aided communication. Child Language Teaching and Therapy, 1, 295–305.

von Tetzchner, S. (1996, August). The contexts of early aided language acquisition. Presented at the Seventh Biennial Conference of the International Society for Augmentative and Alternative Communication, Vancouver, British Columbia, Canada.

von Tetzchner, S. (1997). The use of graphic language intervention among young children in Norway. European Journal of Disorders of Communication, 32, 217–234.

von Tetzchner, S., Dille, K., Jørgensen, K. K., Ormhaug, B. M., Oxholm, B. and Warme, R. (1998, August). From single signs to relational meanings. Presented at the Eighth Biennial Conference of the International Society for Augmentative and Alternative Communication, Dublin, Ireland.

von Tetzchner, S., Grove, N., Loncke, F., Barnett, S., Woll, B. and Clibbens, J. (1996). Preliminaries to a comprehensive model of augmentative and alternative communication. In S. von Tetzchner and M. H. Jensen (Eds), Augmentative and Alternative Communication: European Perspectives (pp. 19–36). London: Whurr.

von Tetzchner, S. and Jensen, M. H. (Eds). (1996a). Augmentative and Alternative Communication: European Perspectives. London: Whurr.

von Tetzchner, S. and Jensen, M. H. (1996b). Introduction. In S. von Tetzchner and M. H. Jensen (Eds), Augmentative and Alternative Communication: European Perspectives (pp. 1–18). London: Whurr.

von Tetzchner, S. and Martinsen, H. (1992). Introduction to Sign Teaching and the Use of Communication Aids. London: Whurr. (Norwegian edition, 1991, Gyldendal; North American edition, 1992, Taylor and Francis; Spanish edition, 1993, Aprendizaje-Visor)

von Tetzchner, S. and Martinsen, J. H. (1996). Words and strategies: Conversations with young children who use aided language. In S. von Tetzchner and M. H. Jensen (Eds), Augmentative and Alternative Communication: European Perspectives (pp. 65–88). London: Whurr.

Wakao, T., Ehara, T., Sawamura, E., Abe, Y. and Shirai, K. (1997). Application of NLP technology to production of close-caption TV programs in Japanese for the hearing impaired. In A. Copestake, S. Langer and S. Palazuelos-Cagigas (Eds), Natural Language Processing for Communication Aids. Proceedings of the Workshop at the 35th Annual Meeting of the Association for Computational Linguistics and the 8th Conference of the European Chapter of the ACL (pp. 55–58). Madrid, Spain: Association for Computational Linguistics.

Warrick, A. (1988). Sociocommunicative considerations within augmentative and alternative communication. Augmentative and Alternative Communication, 4, 45–51.

Wehmeyer, M. L. (1999). A functional model of self-determination: Describing development and implementing instruction. Manuscript in preparation, pp. 1 - 29.

Wehmeyer, M. L., Agran, M. and Hughes, C. (1998). Teaching Self-determination to Students with Disabilities: Basic Skills for Successful Transition. Baltimore: Paul H. Brookes.

Wehmeyer, M. and Schwartz, M. (1997). Self-determination and positive adult outcomes: A follow-up study of youth with mental retardation or learning disabilities. Exceptional Children, 63, 245–255.

Weir, R. H. (1962). Language in the Crib. The Hague, The Netherlands: Mouton.

Wengelin, Å. (1998a). Spelling in and out of context in Swedish adults with severe reading and writing difficulties. Unpublished manuscript, Göteborg University, Department of Linguistics, Göteborg, Sweden.

Wengelin, Å. (1998b, July). Writing management in Swedish adults with and without severe reading and writing difficulties. Paper presented at the Second European Conference of Writing, Speech and Context, University of Nottingham, Nottingham, UK.

Wengelin, Å. (1999). Spelling and grammar in dyslexic and deaf adults. In S. Strömqvist and E. Ahlsén (Eds), The Process of Writing – A Progress Report. Göteborg, Sweden: Göteborg University, Department of Linguistics.

Werner, H. (1948). The Comparative Psychology of Mental Development. New York: International Universities Press.

Wetherby, A. and Prizant, B. (1993). Communication and Symbolic Behavior Scales (CSBS). Chicago: Riverside.

Whitehurst, G. (1997). Language processes in context: Language learning in children reared in poverty. In R. Paul (Ed.), Exploring the Speech-Language Connection (pp. 233–266). Baltimore: Paul H. Brookes.

Whitney-Thomas, J. (1996). Participatory action research as an approach to enhancing quality of life for people with disabilities. In R. L. Schalock (Ed.), Quality of Life: Vol. II. Application to Persons with Disabilities. Washington, DC: American Association on Mental Retardation.

Willard-Holt, C. (1998). Academic and personality characteristics of gifted students with cerebral palsy: A multiple case study. Exceptional Children, 65, 37–50.

Williams, M. B. (1995). Talking about us. Alternatively Speaking, 4(2), 1–4.

Williams, M. B. (1996, August). How can you give a speech when you haven't said a word all your life? Words+ Lecture presented at Seventh Biennial Conference of the International Society for Augmentative and Alternative Communication, Vancouver, British Columbia, Canada.

Winton. (1990). Report of the New Mexico House Memorial 5 Task Force on Young Children and Families, 1.

Wittgenstein, L. (1953). Philosophical Investigations. Oxford, UK: Blackwell.

Wolf, M. M. (1978). Social validity: The case for subjective measurement, or how applied behavior analysis is finding its heart. Journal of Applied Behavior Analysis, 11, 203–214.

Wolfensberger, W. (1972). The Principle of Normalization in Human Services. Toronto, Ontario, Canada: National Institute on Mental Retardation.

Wolfensberger, W. and Glenn, L. (1973). Program Analysis of Service Systems: A Method for Quantitative Evaluation of Human Services. Toronto, Ontario, Canada: National Institute on Mental Retardation.

Yovetich, W. S. (1985). Cognitive processing of Blissymbols by normal adults. Unpublished doctoral dissertation, University of Western Ontario, London, Ontario, Canada.

Yovetich, W. S. and Paivio, A. (1980). Cognitive processing of Bliss-like symbols by normal populations: A report on four studies. In EASE 80 Communication and Handicap: The Conference for Special Education. Helsinki, Finland.

Yovetich, W. S. and Young, T. A. (1988). The effects of representativeness and concrete-
    ness on the 'guessability' of Blissymbols. Augmentative and Alternative
    Communication, 4, 35–39.

Zarb, G. (1992). On the road to Damascus: First steps towards changing the relations of
    disability research production. Disability, Handicap and Society, 7, 125–138.

Zuckerman, B. and Brazelton, T. B. (1994). Strategies for a family-supportive child
    health care system. In: S. L. Kagan and B. Weissbourd (Eds), Putting Families First:
    America's Family Support Movement and the Challenge of Change (pp. 73–92). San
    Francisco, CA: Jossey-Bass.

Index